HEART FAILURE

CONTEMPORARY CARDIOLOGY

CHRISTOPHER P. CANNON, MD
SERIES EDITOR

Heart Failure: A Clinician's Guide to Ambulatory Diagnosis and Treatment, edited by *Mariell L. Jessup, MD, FACC, FAHA, and Evan Loh, MD, FACC, FAHA, 2003*

Cardiac Repolarization: Bridging Basic and Clinical Science, edited by *Ihor Gussak, MD, PhD, Charles Antzelevitch, PhD, Stephen C. Hammill, MD,* co-edited by *Win-Kuong Shen, MD, and Preben Bjerregaard, MD, DMSc, 2003*

Cardiovascular Health Care Economics, edited by *William S. Weintraub, MD, 2003*

Nuclear Cardiology Basics: How to Set Up and Maintain a Laboratory, edited by *Frans J. Th. Wackers, MD, Wendy Bruni, CNMT, and Barry L. Zaret, MD, 2003*

Essentials of Bedside Cardiology: With a Complete Course in Heart Sounds and Murmurs on CD, Second Edition, by *Jules Constant, MD, FACC, 2003*

Minimally Invasive Cardiac Surgery, Second Edition, edited by *Mehmet C. Oz, MD and Daniel J. Goldstein, MD, 2003*

Platelet Glycoprotein IIb/IIIa Inhibitors in Cardiovascular Disease, Second Edition, edited by *A. Michael Lincoff, MD, 2003*

Management of Acute Coronary Syndromes, Second Edition, edited by *Christopher P. Cannon, MD, 2003*

Aging, Heart Disease, and Its Management, Facts and Controversies, edited by *Niloo M. Edwards, MD, Mathew S. Maurer, MD, and Rachel B. Wellner, MPH, 2003*

Peripheral Arterial Disease: Diagnosis and Treatment, edited by *Jay D. Coffman, MD and Robert T. Eberhardt, MD, 2003*

Primary Angioplasty in Acute Myocardial Infarction, edited by *James E. Tcheng, MD, 2002*

Cardiogenic Shock: Diagnosis and Treatment, edited by *David Hasdai, MD, Peter B. Berger, MD, Alexander Battler, MD, and David R. Holmes, Jr., MD, 2002*

Management of Cardiac Arrhythmias, edited by Leonard I. Ganz, MD, 2002

Diabetes and Cardiovascular Disease, edited by *Michael T. Johnstone and Aristidis Veves, MD, DSC, 2001*

Blood Pressure Monitoring in Cardiovascular Medicine and Therapeutics, edited by *William B. White, MD, 2001*

Vascular Disease and Injury: Preclinical Research, edited by *Daniel I. Simon, MD, and Campbell Rogers, MD 2001*

HEART FAILURE

A Clinician's Guide to Ambulatory Diagnosis and Treatment

Edited by

MARIELL L. JESSUP, MD, FACC, FAHA

Heart Failure/Transplant Program
University of Pennsylvania Health System,
Philadelphia, PA

EVAN LOH, MD, FACC, FAHA

University of Pennsylvania Health System,
Philadelphia, PA

Foreword
Robert O. Bonow, MD
President, American Heart Association

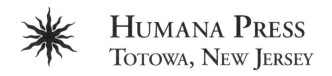

HUMANA PRESS
TOTOWA, NEW JERSEY

Production Editor: Robin B. Weisberg.
Cover Illustration: From Fig. 9 in Chapter 8, "Evaluation of Ventricular Function" by Craig H. Scott and Victor A. Ferrari.
Cover design by Patricia F. Cleary.

This publication is printed on acid-free paper. ∞
ANSI Z39.48-1984 (American National Standards Institute) Permanence of Paper for Printed Library Materials.

Printed in the United States of America. 10 9 8 7 6 5 4 3 2 1

Library of Congress Cataloging-in-Publication Data
Heart failure : a clinician's guide to ambulatroy diagnosis and treatment / edited by Mariell L. Jessup, Evan Loh.
    p. cm. -- (Contemporary cardiology)
  Includes bibliographical references and index.
  ISBN 1-58829-041-7 (alk. paper); 1-59259-347-X (e-ISBN)
   1. Heart failure. 2. Ambulatory medical care. I. Jessup, Mariell L. II. Loh, Evan.
   III. Contemporary cardiology (Totowa, N.J.: unnumbered)

RC685.C53H425 2003
616.1'29--dc21   2002191939

FOREWORD

During the past few decades, significant progress has been made in the prevention and treatment of cardiovascular disease in the United States. Despite these advances, national statistics indicate that the incidence and prevalence of chronic heart failure have been increasing in recent years. In fact, heart failure is the only category of cardiovascular disease in which the prevalence, incidence, and mortality have increased steadily in the past 25 years. These worrisome trends are paralleled by steady increases in the hospitalization rates and health care costs related to heart failure. The heart failure epidemic is fueled by several factors. Heart failure is age related, with a prevalence of 1% between the ages of 50 and 59. This rate increases to roughly 10% above the age of 75. With the aging of the population, a greater number of patients with chronic heart failure will undoubtedly occur. Additionally, improvement in the treatment of acute myocardial infarction translates into more patients surviving with left-ventricular dysfunction, which translates into more patients developing clinical heart failure over the course of subsequent decades. Finally, better management of heart failure itself, with the potential for improved survival through advances in medical therapy and implantable devices, could result in the paradoxical situation in which enhanced survival might be achieved at the expense of more patients alive with heart failure symptoms. The combination of an aging population and decline in mortality from other forms of cardiovascular diseases indicates that heart failure will continue to increase in public health importance. Hence, more and more patients will be diagnosed, treated, and followed in the primary outpatient setting.

Heart Failure: A Clinician's Guide to Ambulatory Diagnosis and Treatment, edited by Drs. Jessup and Loh, provides an in-depth, hands-on approach to the office-based evaluation and management of the patient with heart failure. Extensive coverage is provided regarding the presenting signs and symptoms of heart failure, as well as the tools with which to evaluate left-ventricular function, hemodynamics, and exercise performance. The chapters on treatment recommendations are up-to-date and evidence-based, consistent with current peer reviewed practice guidelines. Appropriate attention is placed on treatment options for the patient with advanced heart failure, including alternative therapies, emerging therapeutic alternatives, and surgical approaches and devices. A highly commendable feature of the book is the considerable

v

emphasis on patient education and disease management, and the many related references to web-based resources will be of great practical value. *Heart Failure: A Clinician's Guide to Ambulatory Diagnosis and Treatment* will prove an indispensable resource to physicians and nurses on the primary care team in the daily management of their patients with heart failure.

Robert O. Bonow, MD
Division of Cardiology
Northwestern University Feinberg School of Medicine,
Chicago, IL

PREFACE

Heart failure is a complex clinical syndrome manifested by dyspnea, fatigue, fluid retention, and decreased exercise tolerance. Heart failure may result from disorders of the pericardium, the myocardium, the endocardium, valvular structures, and the great vessels of the heart or from rhythm disturbances. Nearly 5 million Americans have heart failure today, an incidence approaching 10 per 1000 population after the age of 65 years. Heart failure is the reason for at least 20% of all hospital admissions in persons above age 65; hospitalizations for heart failure have increased by 159%. The prevalence of patients with heart failure has grown markedly as a result of the aging population and the number of patients who have survived heart attacks, heart valve surgery, and other cardiac procedures as a result of improvements in adjunctive medical therapies and surgical techniques. Thus, almost any practicing clinician will encounter a patient with the heart failure syndrome on a regular basis.

Heart Failure: A Clinician's Guide to Ambulatory Diagnosis and Treatment reviews all aspects of heart failure diagnosis and management, with a particular emphasis on office-based/ambulatory care. The volume discusses diagnostic and therapeutic options for clinicians in evaluating patients with dyspnea, fatigue, or edema. The recommendations contained herein are specific and directed at targeted symptoms. The many diagnostic-imaging modalities discussed focus on the practical utility of the tests. *Heart Failure: A Clinician's Guide to Ambulatory Diagnosis and Treatment* reviews the state-of-the-art pharmacologic, device, and surgical options for heart failure management, with care algorithms that are usually supervised by a nurse or nurse specialist.

Heart Failure: A Clinician's Guide to Ambulatory Diagnosis and Treatment is intended for generalists and internists, nurse practitioners, physician assistants, and general cardiologists who practice in the community setting. The epidemic of heart failure that faces our country necessitates a coordinated effort at prevention and optimal treatment of the disease. Unfortunately, all of the solutions to this enormous problem have yet to be elucidated, but additional efforts to educate and inform our busy clinicians will be important to keep up to date with the evolutions in heart failure care available today. We hope *Heart Failure: A Clinician's Guide to Ambulatory Diagnosis and Treatment* will serve as a platform for a systematic approach to the care of patients with heart failure for all clinicians.

We are very grateful for the excellent contributions from our authors, all of whom practice or trained at the University of Pennsylvania Health System. This work represents our approach to the plague of heart failure, a northeastern United States approach certainly, but a concerted and devoted one nevertheless.

Mariell L. Jessup, MD, FACC, FAHA
Evan Loh, MD, FACC, FAHA

CONTENTS

CONTRIBUTORS

MICHAEL A. ACKER, MD, *Division of Cardiothoracic Surgery, Department of Surgery, University of Pennsylvania Health System, Philadelphia, PA*

SUSAN C. BROZENA, MD, FACC, FAHA, *Heart Failure/Transplant Program, University of Pennsylvania Health System, Philadelphia, PA*

DAVID J. CALLANS, MD, *Electrophysiology Program of the Division of Cardiovascular Medicine, University of Pennsylvania Health System, Philadelphia, PA*

SHASHANK DESAI, MD, *Heart Failure/Transplant Program, University of Pennsylvania Health System, Philadelphia, PA*

VICTOR A. FERRARI, MD, *Noninvasive Imaging Program of the Division of Cardiovascular Medicine, University of Pennsylvania Health System, Philadelphia, PA*

RUCHIRA GLASER, MD, *Division of Cardiovascular Medicine, University of Pennsylvania Health System, Philadelphia, PA*

LEE R. GOLDBERG, MD, MPH, FACC, *Heart Failure/Transplant Program, University of Pennsylvania Health System, Philadelphia, PA*

IRVING M. HERLING, MD, *Division of Cardiovascular Medicine, University of Pennsylvania Health System, Philadelphia, PA*

HENRY H. HSIA, MD, FACC, *Division of Cardiovascular Medicine, University of Pennsylvania Health System, Philadelphia, PA*

MARIELL L. JESSUP, MD, FACC, FAHA, *Heart Failure/Transplant Program, University of Pennsylvania Health System, Philadelphia, PA*

JERRY JOHNSON, MD, *Division of Geriatric Medicine, University of Pennsylvania Health System, Philadelphia, PA*

ANDREW KAO, MD, FACC, *Heart Failure/Transplant Program, University of Pennsylvania Health System, Philadelphia, PA*

MARTIN G. KEANE, MD, *Division of Cardiovascular Medicine, University of Pennsylvania Health System, Philadelphia, PA*

BRUCE D. KLUGHERZ, MD, *Cardiac Catheterization Laboratory, Philadelphia Veterans Affairs Hospital, University of Pennsylvania Health System, Philadelphia, PA*

DUSAN Z. KOCOVIC, MD, *Division of Cardiovascular Medicine, University of Pennsylvania Health System, Philadelphia, PA*

DANIEL M. KOLANSKY, MD, *Division of Cardiovascular Medicine, University of Pennsylvania Health System, Philadelphia, PA*

EVAN LOH, MD, FACC, FAHA, *University of Pennsylvania Health System, Philadelphia, PA*

DAVID M. MCCARTHY, MD, *Division of Cardiovascular Medicine, University of Pennsylvania Health System, Philadelphia, PA*

KATHLEEN M. MCCAULEY, PhD, RN, CS, FAAN, *School of Nursing, University of Pennsylvania Health System, Philadelphia, PA*

SRIHARI S. NAIDU, MD, *Division of Cardiovascular Medicine, University of Pennsylvania Health System, Philadelphia, PA*

VICKAS V. PATEL, MD, PhD, *Division of Cardiovascular Medicine, University of Pennsylvania Health System, Philadelphia, PA*

DANIELA PINI, MD, *Heart Failure/Transplant Program, University of Pennsylvania Health System, Philadelphia, PA*

ERIC D. POPJES, MD, *Penn State Milton S. Hershey Medical Center, Hershey, PA*

ROBERT W. RHO, MD, *Division of Cardiovascular Medicine, University of Pennsylvania Health System, Philadelphia, PA*

CRAIG H. SCOTT, MD, *Noninvasive Imaging Program of the Division of Cardiovascular Medicine, University of Pennsylvania Health System, Philadelphia, PA*

ROBERT L. WILENSKY, MD, *Division of Cardiovascular Medicine, University of Pennsylvania Health System, Philadelphia, PA*

DAVID ZELTSMAN, *Division of Cardiothoracic Surgery, University of Medicine and Dentistry of New Jersey, Robert Wood Johnson Medical School, New Brunswick, NJ*

ROSS ZIMMER, MD, *Division of Cardiovascular Medicine, University of Pennsylvania Health System Philadelphia, PA*

1 Heart Failure

The Economic Burden of a Deadly Disease

Daniela Pini, MD

CONTENTS

INTRODUCTION

Descriptions of heart failure exist from as early as ancient Egypt, Greece, Rome, and India. The description of the circulatory system by William Harvey in 1628 represented an important step in the understanding of the nature of the condition. Roentgen's discovery of X-rays and Einthoven's development of electrocardiography in the 1890s led to further improvements in the investigation of heart failure. The advent of echocardiography, cardiac catheterization, and nuclear medicine has since improved the diagnosis and investigation of patients with heart failure.

For many centuries, bloodletting was used as a treatment of heart failure. In 1785, William Withering first reported the benefits of digi-

From: *Contemporary Cardiology: Heart Failure:*
A Clinician's Guide to Ambulatory Diagnosis and Treatment
Edited by: M. L. Jessup and E. Loh © Humana Press Inc., Totowa, NJ

talis. In the 19th and early 20th centuries, Southey's tubes were used to treat fluid retention associated with heart failure. The tubes were inserted into edematous peripheries, allowing some drainage of fluid. It was not until the 20th century that diuretics were developed. However, the early mercurial agents were associated with substantial toxicity. The much safer thiazide diuretics were introduced in the 1950s. Vasodilators began to be widely used when angiotensin-converting enzyme (ACE) inhibitors were developed in the 1970s. In 1987, the CONSENSUS-I study *(1)* documented the unequivocal survival benefits of enalapril in patients with severe heart failure. In 1996, the US carvedilol heart failure study *(2)*, the first large randomized controlled trial involving a β-blocking agent, showed a substantial reduction in mortality in patients with moderate heart failure treated with carvedilol.

Heart failure is now recognized as a major and escalating public health problem in industrialized countries with aging populations. Heart failure is the end stage of all diseases of the heart and is a major cause of morbidity and mortality. It is estimated to account for about 5% of admissions to hospital medical wards, with more than 100,000 annual admissions in the United Kingdom and more than 2.5 million annual admissions in the United States *(3,4)*. The number of admissions for heart failure in the United Kingdom now exceeds the number for myocardial infarction *(5)*. In the United States, heart failure is the most common principal diagnosis among hospitalized adults aged 65 years and older *(6)*. As in the United Kingdom, there are more discharges for heart failure than for myocardial infarction in this age group *(7)*. It has been estimated that the risk for persons aged ≥ 70 years requiring hospitalization for heart failure within 8 years might be as high as 15% in the United States *(3)*. Reports from several countries suggest that approximately 1 to 2% of the total health care budget is expended on the management of heart failure *(8)*.

Despite advances in drug therapy, the prognosis of patients with heart failure remains poor. Heart failure mortality data are comparable to data for the worst forms of malignant disease, although they are not generally taken to be so.

PREVALENCE OF HEART FAILURE

Population-based studies in heart failure are difficult to compare because of the lack of universal agreement on a definition of heart failure, which is primarily a clinical diagnosis. The data vary widely with varying methods of ascertainment, but they do provide a perspective on the size of the problem.

Table 1
Prevalence of Heart Failure

Study	Location	Year of publication	Overall prevalence rate	Prevalence rate in older population
Physician records/prescriptions				
RCGP (11)	UK national data	1958	3/1000	—
Gibson et al. (12)	Rural cohort, US	1966	9–10/1000	65/1000 (>65 years)
RCGP (76)	UK national data	1986	11/1000	—
Parameshwar et al. (13)	London, UK	1992	4/1000	28/1000 (> 65 years)
Rodeheffer et al. (17)	Rochester, US	1993	3/1000	-
Mair et al. (14)	Liverpool, UK	1994	15/1000	80/1000 (> 65 years)
RCGP (77)	UK national data	1995	9/1000	74/1000 (65–74 years)
Clarke et al. (15)	Notcinghamshire, UK	1995	8–16/1000	40–60/1000 (> 70 years)
Lip et al. (16)	Birmingham, UK	1997	24/1000	—
Clinical criteria				
Droller and Pemberton (78)	Sheffield, UK	1953	—	30–50/1000 (> 62 years)
Garrison et al. (20)	Georgia, US	1966	21/1000	35/1000 (65–74 years)
Framingham (18,19)	Framingham, US	1971,1993	7/1000	24/1000 (≥45 years)
Landahl et al. (79)	Sweden	1984	—	80–170/1000 (70–75 years)
Eriksson et al. (21)[a]	Gothenburg, Sweden	1989	—	130/1000 (69 years)
NHANES-I (20)	US national data	1992	20/1000	—
Glasgow (24)[b]	Glasgow, UK	1997	15/1000	—
Rotterdam (27)[b]	Rotterdam, Holland	1997	15/1000	—
Helsinki (28)[b]	Helsinki, Finland	1997	—	22/1000 (75–86 years)

[a]Men only.
[b]Echocardiographic studies.
Adapted with permission from ref. 32.

3

Table 1 summarizes the prevalence of heart failure as estimated from population studies based on physician records and prescriptions, population studies based on clinical criteria, and population studies based on echocardiographic surveys. It has been shown that approximately 30–50% of patients with heart failure have a normal or nearly normal ejection fraction *(9)*. In these patients, heart failure is usually a result of left-ventricular diastolic dysfunction. The epidemiology of diastolic heart failure has been incompletely described. Diastolic heart failure affects women disproportionately *(9)* and blacks may be more susceptible than non-blacks *(10)*.

Population Studies Based on Physician Records and Prescriptions

The earliest large prevalence survey was undertaken in England and Wales between May 1955 and April 1956 *(11)*. The survey was conducted among 171 general practitioners. The number of patients consulting for congestive heart failure (CHF) and left-ventricular failure was 2.2 and 0.8 per 1000 of population, respectively.

In 1962–1963, Gibson et al. *(12)* measured the prevalence of CHF in the white population in two US rural communities. The study estimated a 6-month population prevalence of 8.8 per 1000 in one community and 10.2 per 1000 in the other. Those figures increased to 64.9 and 64.7 in persons over age 65.

Parameshwar et al. *(13)* examined the clinical records of diuretic-treated patients in three general practices in Northwest London in 1992 to identify possible cases of CHF. From 30,204 patients, a clinical diagnosis of CHF was made in 117 cases (47 male and 71 female), giving an overall prevalence of 3.9 cases per 1000. However, in those aged under 65 years, the prevalence was 0.6 per 1000, whereas in those over 65 years it was 28 per 1000.

In 1994, in a similar study conducted in Liverpool, Mair et al. *(14)* identified 266 cases of CHF from 17,400 patients belonging to two general practices (a prevalence rate of 15 per 1000). The prevalence increased to 80 per 1000 in those aged 65 years or more.

Clarke et al. *(15)* analyzed prescriptions for loop diuretics for all residents of the English county of Nottinghamshire. In 1995, they reported that between 13,107 and 26,214 patients had been prescribed furosemide in this region. Case note review of a random sample of these patients showed that 56% were being treated for heart failure. This equated to an overall prevalence of 8–16 per 1000. Once again, the prevalence of CHF increased with advancing age, rising to 40–60 per 1000 in patients over 70 years of age.

In 1997, Lip et al. *(16)* reported the results of a study carried out in a general practice population of 25,819 in Birmingham. They found that the prevalence of CHF was 24 per 1000 in patients aged over 40 years.

In January 1982, Rodeheffer et al. *(17)* identified the prevalence of CHF in all persons aged 0-74 living in Rochester, MN. The overall prevalence was 2.7 per 1000 and increased with age, rising to 2.8 per 1000 in men aged 70–74 years.

Population Studies Based on Clinical Criteria

The Framingham Heart Study *(18,19)* was initiated for the purpose of defining precursive factors and the natural history of cardiovascular diseases. In 1948, 5209 residents of Framingham, MA, aged 28–62 years, were enrolled in the study. Members of the original cohort were subsequently evaluated at 2-year intervals with medical histories, physical examinations, and laboratory tests. In 1971, children of the original study participants and spouses of these children, aged 6–70 years, were entered in the Framingham Offspring Study. Serial evaluations were performed on the 5135 members of the Framingham Offspring study 8 and 12 years after enrollment. Among 9405 participants (47% male) followed up from September 1948 to June 1988, CHF developed in 652 participants. There were 17 additional cases of CHF diagnosed at the first Framingham Heart Study examination (prevalence 3 per 1000); all these individuals were less than 63 years of age. The prevalence of CHF increased dramatically with age. Among men, the prevalence of CHF climbed from 8 cases per 1000 in those 50–59 years of age to 66 cases per 1000 in those aged 80–89 years. In women the prevalence of CHF increased from 8 cases per 1000 in those aged 50–59 years to 79 cases per 1000 in those 80–89 years of age. During the 1980s, the age-adjusted prevalence of CHF was 7.4 per 1000 in men and 7.7 per 1000 in women. Among persons aged ≥ 45 years, the age-adjusted prevalence of CHF was 24 per 1000 in men and 25 per 1000 in women.

In Evans County, GA, in 1960–1962, CHF was found in 17 per 1000 of persons aged 45–64 and 35 per 1000 of those aged 65–74 years *(20)*. The overall prevalence in persons aged 45–74 years was 21 per 1000.

Eriksson et al. *(21)* evaluated for the presence of CHF a cohort of 855 men born in Gothenburg, Sweden, in 1913, at the age of 50, 54, 60, and 67 years. A prevalence was found of 21 per 1000 at 50 years, 24 at 54 years, and 43 per 1000 at 60 years and 130 per 1000 at 67 years.

The National Health and Nutrition and Examination Survey (NHANES-I) *(22)* reported the prevalence of CHF in the United States. This study screened 14,407 persons of both sexes, aged 25–74 years, between 1971 and 1975 and reported a prevalence of 20 cases per 1000. However, detailed evaluations were carried out in only 6913 subjects.

Prevalence of Left-Ventricular Systolic Dysfunction on BasedEchocardiographic Surveys

Wheeldon and colleagues (23) documented that many patients with a clinical diagnosis of CHF do not have left-ventricular systolic dysfunction or, indeed, any significant cardiac abnormality. Population-based echocardiographic studies were subsequently carried out to estimate the prevalence of left-ventricular systolic dysfunction.

The Glasgow study (24) drew its 1640 subjects from the 2000 people (age 25–74 years) who had attended the third Glasgow MONICA coronary-risk-factor survey in 1992 (25,26). Left-ventricular systolic dysfunction was defined as a left-ventricular ejection fraction ≤ 30%. The overall prevalence of left-ventricular systolic dysfunction was 2.9%; the prevalence of symptomatic left-ventricular dysfunction was 1.5%. The prevalence was greater in men and increased with age to 6.4% in men aged 65–74 years.

The Rotterdam study (27) examined individuals aged 55–74 years, but the findings were similar to those of the Glasgow study. Left-ventricular systolic dysfunction was defined as a fractional shortening ≤ 25%. The overall prevalence of left ventricular systolic dysfunction was 3.7%; 40% of cases were symptomatic.

The Helsinki aging study (28) examined 501 subjects (367 females) aged 75–86 years. CHF was diagnosed based on clinical criteria in 8.2% of the participants. However, echocardiography showed left ventricular systolic dysfunction (defined as a fractional shortening ≤ 25% and left ventricular dilatation) in only 28% of the patients diagnosed with CHF. The prevalence of left-ventricular systolic dysfunction in asymptomatic subjects was 9%. The overall prevalence of left-ventricular systolic dysfunction was therefore 10.8%.

INCIDENCE OF HEART FAILURE

Incidence data (Table 2) are much more limited than prevalence data. In the Framingham study (19) the incidence of CHF increased dramatically with age. During the 1980s, the age-adjusted annual incidence of congestive heart failure was 2.3 cases per 1000 in men. In women, the corresponding age-adjusted annual incidence was 1.4 cases per 1000. Among individuals aged ≥ 45, the age-adjusted annual incidence of CHF was 7.2 cases per 1000 in men and 4.7 cases per 1000 in women.

Table 2
Incidence of Heart Failure

Study	Location	Year of publication	Overall incidence rate	Incidence rate in older population
Framingham (19)	Framingham, US	1993	2/1000	27/1000 (80–89 years)[a]
Eriksson et al. (21)	Gothenburg, Sweden	1989	—	10/1000 (61–67 years)[a]
Remes et al. (29)	Finland	1992	1–4/1000	8/1000 (≥ 75 years)[a]
Rodeheffer et al. (17)	Rochester, US	1993	1/1000	1–6/1000 (65–67 years)[a]
Cowie et al. (30)[b]	London, UK	1990	1.3/1000	7.4 (75–84 years)

[a]Men.
[b]Echocardiographic study.
Adapted with permission from ref. 32.

Similar rates were reported by Eriksson and coworkers *(21)* and Remes and coworkers *(29)*. Markedly lower rates were reported by Rodeheffer and coworkers *(17)*. During 1981, they reported the incidence of heart failure in the population of the city of Rochester in persons aged 0–74 years. The annual incidence was 1.1 per 1000. Incidence increased with age: 0.76, 1.6 and 0.94 per 1000 of men aged 45–49, 65–69, and 70–74 years, respectively.

The most recent incidence study by Cowie and coworkers studied a population of 151,000 in Hillingdon District, London *(30)*. The authors adopted the criteria recommended by the European Society of Cardiology to determine the presence of CHF *(31)*. According to the guidelines of the European Society of Cardiology, objective evidence of cardiac dysfunction, preferably demonstrated by echocardiography, has to be present, in addition to symptoms and signs attributable to heart failure, to establish the presence of the syndrome. The crude incidence rate in the population aged over 25 years was 1.3 cases per 1000. The incidence rate increased steadily from 0.02 per 1000 in those aged 25–34 years to 11.6 in those aged 85 years or over and was higher in males than females (age-standardized incidence ratio 1.75).

The incidence and prevalence of CHF are likely to increase in the future because of both an aging population and therapeutic advances in the management of acute myocardial infarction, leading to improved survival in patients with impaired cardiac function. An analysis of demographic trends in The Netherlands has predicted that the prevalence of CHF as a result of coronary artery disease will rise by 70% by the year 2010 (using 1985 as the base year) *(32)*. Similar increases have been predicted for Australia *(33)*. In Northern Europe, it is estimated that there will be about 15,000 prevalent symptomatic cases with left-ventricular systolic function per million of the (adult) population, possibly a further 15,000 per million who are asymptomatic and 15,000 per million who have features of heart failure without major systolic dysfunction *(8)*.

ETIOLOGY OF HEART FAILURE

In western countries, coronary artery disease, either alone or in combination with hypertension, seems to be the most common cause of heart failure *(19,24,30,34)*. In the Framingham Heart Study *(19)*, 70% of men and 78% of women with heart failure had an antecedent diagnosis of hypertension. Forty percent of men and women with CHF had a prior history of both hypertension and coronary artery disease. Coronary artery disease was found in 59% of men and 48% of women with new CHF. However, from 1948 to 1988, the age-adjusted prevalence of coronary artery disease with new CHF increased by 46% per calendar decade. The prevalence of coronary artery disease, as the identified cause of new cases of CHF, increased from 22% in the 1950s to nearly 70% in the 1970s. During this period, the relative contribution of hypertension and valvular heart disease decreased dramatically *(35)*. However, valvular heart disease remains an important cause of heart failure in many regions of the world *(36)*. Diabetes mellitus is also an important risk factor for heart failure *(37)*.

The chief risk factors of diastolic heart failure are advancing age, hypertension, diabetes, left-ventricular hypertrophy, and coronary artery disease *(38)*.

MORBIDITY OF HEART FAILURE

Quality of Life

Two large studies from the United States have shown that self-reported quality of life is impaired more by heart failure than by any other common chronic medical disorder *(39,40)*.

Outpatient/Ambulatory Care

In the United States, it has been estimated that 85% of patients with CHF are treated primarily in the ambulatory setting *(7)*. From 1980 through 1993, the number of physician office visits for CHF increased by 71% from 1.7 million to 2.9 million annually *(41)*. Heart failure ranks second only to hypertension as a cardiovascular reason for an office visit *(7)*. In addition, more than 65,000 patients with heart failure receive home health care each year *(41)*.

Hospitalization

On a global scale, hospitalization for CHF appears to be a growing problem. Heart failure accounts for al least 5% of admissions to general medical and geriatric wards in British hospitals, and admission rates for CHF in various European countries (Sweden, The Netherlands and Scotland) and in the United States have doubled in the past 10–15 years *(4)*. In the United States, in 1995, there were more than 2.6 million hospitalizations among adults with CHF as one of the diagnosis *(3)*. Almost four of five hospitalizations occurred among adults aged ≥ 65 years; thus, the federal government was the expected source of payment for almost 80% of these hospital claims. Indeed, CHF is the leading indication for hospitalization in older adults in industrialized countries *(6,42,43)*. Hospitalization for CHF is not only common, but also prolonged. In the United States, the average length of stay has been estimated to be between 6 and 11 days *(44,45)*. In the United Kingdom, the mean length of stay for a CHF-related hospitalization is 11.4 days on acute medical wards and 28.5 days on acute geriatric wards *(46)*.

Hospital readmissions and general practice consultations often occur soon after the diagnosis of CHF. In elderly patients with CHF, readmission rates range from 29% to 47% within 3 to 6 months of the initial hospital discharge *(4)*. Among a sample of patients hospitalized with CHF in 1987 in the United States, one-half of 90-day readmissions were potentially preventable *(47)*. Factors that contribute to preventable readmissions include patient nonadherence with medications or diet, inadequate discharge planning or follow-up, a failed social support system, and failure to seek medical attention promptly when symptoms recurred *(47)*. Factors also associated with readmission within 6 months in patients 65 years or older are prior admission within 1 year, prior heart failure, diabetes, and creatinine level > 2.5 mg/dL at discharge *(48)*.

MORTALITY OF HEART FAILURE

Heart failure is a lethal condition. In the original and subsequent Framingham cohort *(19)*, the overall 1-year survival rates in men and women were 57% and 64%, respectively. The overall 5-year survival rates in men and women were 25% and 38%, respectively. In comparison 5-year survival for all cancers among men and women in the United States during the same period was approximately 50%. Hospital series, which include more severe cases, show a 1-year mortality of 30–50% *(49–51)*. By contrast, annual mortality for patients with chronic stable CHF is approximately 10% *(36)*. The annual mortality from diastolic heart failure is uncertain, with estimates varying widely from 9 to 28% *(52,53)*. In the general population, the mortality rate among patients with diastolic heart failure is four times that among persons without heart failure, but it is half that among patients with systolic heart failure *(52)*.

Mortality rates increase with age. In a study conducted in New Zealand, only 5% of deaths occurred in patients younger than 45 years and approximately 30% in patients younger than 75 years *(50)*. Heart failure appears to be more lethal in men than in women *(54)*. Black patients with both asymptomatic and symptomatic mild-to-moderate left-ventricular systolic dysfunction seem to have higher overall mortality than similarly treated white patients *(55)*.

The underlying cause of CHF is independently associated with survival. The presence of ischemic heart disease appears to influence prognosis adversely *(56)*. Felker et al. *(57)* recently reported the outcomes of 1230 patients with CHF, grouped into the following categories according to the underlying disease: idiopathic cardiomyopathy, peripartum cardiomyopathy, cardiomyopathy owing to myocarditis, ischemic heart disease, infiltrative myocardial disease (amyloidosis, sarcoidosis, and hemocromatosis), hypertension, HIV infection, connective tissue disease, substance abuse, and therapy with doxorubicin and other causes. The patients with peripartum cardiomyopathy had the best prognosis, being the only group to have a significantly better rate of survival than the patients with idiopathic cardiomyopathy. As compared to the patients with idiopathic cardiomyopathy, the patients with ischemic heart disease and connective tissue disease had significantly worse survival. No significant difference in survival was found between the patients with idiopathic cardiomyopathy and those with cardiomyopathy owing to myocarditis, hypertension, substance abuse, or other causes. Patients with cardiomyopathy owing to amyloidosis, hemocromatosis, HIV infection, and doxoubicin therapy had an especially poor prognosis.

COSTS OF HEART FAILURE

Heart failure is a considerable economic burden. Reports from several countries suggest that about 1–2% of the total health care budget is expended on the management of CHF (58–61). Because of its high prevalence and associated high medical resource consumption, heart failure is now the single most costly cardiovascular illness in the United States, with total costs for 1998 estimated at $20.2 billion (6).

The costs of hospitalization are a major component of the costs of treating CHF and are relatively constant between health care systems as a proportion, representing 67–75% of the total cost of treating a patient (7,8,43,59–61). An important determinant of the costs of hospital care is the average length of hospital stay, which is often prolonged in patients with CHF (44–46). Health care utilization increases with the severity of CHF and so does the health care cost. Progression to more severe CHF results in frequent presentation at emergency departments, and consequently, a high number of hospital admissions. The relation between the cost of heart failure treatment and the severity of disease is nonlinear and the cost arises almost exponentially as the New York Heart Association (NYHA) class of heart failure goes up (62). Health care costs for patients with NYHA class IV CHF are 8–30 times greater than for patients with NYHA class II disease (5). The cost of ambulatory care for CHF accounts for approx 15% of the total health care cost for CHF (7,42,59,61,63). Drug treatment accounts for approximately 10% of the total health care cost for CHF (42,59,61). The cost of surgery, which includes heart transplantation or similar procedures, coronary artery bypass grafting and percutaneous transluminal coronary angioplasty, represents only about 1% of the total expenditure for CHF *(8,42,59,61)*.

If it is indisputable that CHF is a considerable economic burden, it is also one of the few conditions in which, under some circumstances, lives may be saved by significantly reducing costs. Treatment can alleviate symptoms and improve prognosis. Treatments that reduce the risk of thrombotic events can have a dramatic impact on hospitalization. In fact, patients with CHF are prone to events such as myocardial infarction and stroke, which may account for up to 25% of bed-days occupancy related to CHF *(64)*. Optimal drug therapy can delay the progression to severe heart failure and reduce, over a finite period, the rate of hospitalization *(2,65)*. However, treatments that also delay death have the potential to increase costs, as surviving patients still need to be treated, and these patients will often deteriorate in the long term. Although rates of hospitalization may be reduced by effective treatment, any treatment that improves survival exposes the patients to a longer period during which they are at risk of requiring hospitalization. In addition, if drugs reduce the risk of hospitalization and improve longevity, they can become the dominant cost. However, the current available reports indicate that digoxin, ACE inhibitors, and β-blockers all appear to be cos-effective *(43,61,66–75)*. Estimates range from substantial cost savings to a few thousand dollars per life-year gained. Indeed, the major factor limiting the reduction in costs associated with effective treatment for CHF (with the exception of digoxin, that does not affect survival) is the costs incurred as a consequence of improved longevity *(8)*.

REFERENCES

1. The CONSENSUS Trial Study Group. Effects of enalapril on mortality in severe congestive heart failure. Results of the Cooperative North Scandinavian Enalapril Survival Study (CONSENSUS). N Engl J Med 1987;316:1429–1435.
2. Packer M, Bristow MR, Cohn JN, et al. The effect of carvedilol on morbidity and mortality in patients with chronic heart failure. N Engl J Med 1996;334:1349–1355.
3. Haldeman GA, Croft JB, Giles WH, Rashidee A. Hospitalization of patients with heart failure: National Hospital Discharge Survey, 1985 to 1995. Am Heart J 1999;137:352–360.
4. Davis RC, Hobbs FDR, Lip GYH. History and epidemiology. (Clinical Review: ABC of heart failure). Br Med J 2000;320:39–42.
5. McMurray JJV, Petrie MC, Murdoch DR, et al. Clinical epidemiology of heart failure: public and private health burden. Eur Heart J 1998;19:P9–16.
6. American Heart Association. 1998 heart and stroke statistical update, Dallas, Texas, 1998.
7. O'Connell JB, Bristow MR. Economic impact of heart failure in the United States: time for a different approach. J Heart Lung Transplant 1994;13:S107–112.
8. Cleland JGF. Health economic consequences of the pharmacological treatment of heart failure. Eur Heart J 1998;19:P32–39.

9. Vasan RS, Benjamin EJ, Levy D. Prevalence, clinical features and prognosis of diastolic heart failure: an epidemiologic perspective. J Am College Cardiol 1995;26:1565–1574.

10. Topol EJ, Traill TA, Fortuin NJ. Hypertensive hypertrophic cardiomyopathy of the elderly. N Engl J Med 1985;312:277–283.

11. Logan WPD, Cushion AA. Morbidity statistics from general practice. Studies on medical and population subjects (No. 14). Vol. 1. London: HMSO, 1958.

12. Gibson TC, White KL, Klainer LM. The prevalence of congestive heart failure in two rural communities. J Chronic Dis 1996;19:141–152.

13. Parameshwar J, Shackell MM, Richardson A, Poole-Wilson PA, Sutton GC. Prevalence of heart failure in three general practices in north west London. Br J Gen Pract 1992;42:287–289.

14. Mair FS, Crowley TS, Bundred PE. Prevalence, aetiology and management of heart failure in general practice. Br J Gen Pract 1996;46:77–79.

15. Clarke KW, Gray D, Hampton JR. How common is heart failure? Evidence from PACT (Prescribing Analysis and Cost) data in Nottingham. J Public Health Med 1995;17:549–564.

16. Lip GYH, Sawar S, Ahmed I, et al. A survey of heart failure in general practice. Eur J Gen Pract 1997;3:85–89.

17. Rodeheffer RJ, Jacobsen SJ, Gersh BJ, et al. The incidence and prevalence fo congestive heart failure in Rochester, Minnesota. Mayo Clinic Proceedings 1993;68:1143–1150.

18. McKee PA, Castelli WP, McNamara PM, Kannel WB. The natural history of congestive heart failure: the Framingham study. N Engl J Med 1971;285:1441–1446.

19. Ho KK, Pinsky JL, Kannel WB, Levy D. The epidemiology of heart failure: the Framingham Study. J Am College Cardiol 1993;22:6A–13A.

20. Garrison GE, McDonough JR, Hames CG, Stulb SC. Prevalence of chronic congestive heart failure in the population of Evans County, Georgia. Am J Epidemiol 1966;83:338–344.

21. Eriksson H, Svardsudd K, Larsson B, et al. Risk factors for heart failure in the general population: the study of men born in 1913. Eur Heart J 1989;10:647–656.

22. Schocken DD, Arrieta MI, Leaverton PE, Ross EA. Prevalence and mortality rate of congestive heart failure in the United States. J Am Coll Cardiol 1992;20:301–306.

23. Wheeldon NM, MacDonald TM, Flucker CJ, McKendrick AD, McDevitt DG, Struthers AD. Echocardiography in chronic heart failure in the community. Q J Med 1993;86:17–23.

24. McDonagh TA, Morrison CE, Lawrence A, et al. Symptomatic and asymptomatic left-ventricular systolic dysfunction in an urban population. Lancet 1997;350:829–833.

25. Smith WC, Shewry MC, Tunstall-Pedoe H, Crombie IK, Tavendale R. Cardiovascular disease in Edinburgh and north Glasgow—a tale of two cities. J Clin Epidemiol 1990;43:637–643.

26. Tunstall-Pedoe H, Kuulasmaa K, Amouyel P, Arveiler D, Rajakangas AM, Pajak A. Myocardial infarction and coronary deaths in the World Health Organization MONICA Project. Registration procedures, event rates, and case fatality rates in 38 populations from 21 countries in four continents. Circulation 1994;90:583–612.

27. Mosterd A, de Bruijne MC, Hoes AW, Deckers JW, Hofman A, Grobbee DE. Usefulness of echocardiography in detecting left ventricular dysfunction in population-based studies (The Rotterdam Study). Am J Cardiol 1997;79:103,104.

28. Kupari M, Lindroos M, Iivanainen AM, Heikkila J, Tilvis R. Congestive heart failure in old age: prevalence, mechanisms and 4-year prognosis in the Helsinki Ageing Study. J Intern Med 1997;241:387–394.

29. Remes J, Reunanen A, Aromaa A, Pyorala K. Incidence of heart failure in eastern Finland: a population-based surveillance study. Eur Heart J 1992;13:588–593.

30. Cowie MR, Wood DA, Coats AJ, et al. Incidence and aetiology of heart failure; a population-based study. Eur Heart J 1999;20:421–428.

31. The Task Force on Heart Failure of the European Society of Cardiology. Guidelines for the diagnosis of heart failure. Eur Heart J 1995;16:741–751.

32. Bonneux L, Barendregt JJ, Meeter K, Bonsel GJ, van der Maas PJ. Estimating clinical morbidity due to ischemic heart disease and congestive heart failure: the future rise of heart failure. Am J Public Health 1994;84:20–28.

33. Kelly DT. Paul Dudley White International Lecture. Our future society. A global challenge. Circulation 1997;95:2459–2464.

34. McMurray JJ, Stewart S. Epidemiology, aetiology and prognosis of heart failure. Heart 2000;83:596–602.

35. Kannel WB, Ho K, Thom T. Changing epidemiological features of cardiac failure. Br Heart J 1994;72:S3–S9.

36. Sharpe N, Doughty R. Epidemiology of heart failure and ventricular dysfunction. Lancet 1998;352:S3–S7.

37. Levy D, Larson MG, Vasan RS, Kannel WB, Ho KK. The progression from hypertension to congestive heart failure. JAMA 1996;275:1557–1562.

38. Vasan RS, Benjamin EJ. Diastolic heart failure - no time to relax. N Engl J Med 2001;344:56–59.

39. Stewart AL, Greenfield S, Hays RD, et al. Functional status and well-being of patients with chronic conditions. Results from the Medical Outcomes Study. JAMA 1989;262:907–913.

40. Fryback DG, Dasbach EJ, Klein R, et al. The Beaver Dam Health Outcomes Study: initial catalog of health-state quality factors. Med Decis Making 1993;13:89–102.

41. National Heart Lung and Blood Institute. Congestive heart failure in the United States: a new epidemic, Bethesda, MD. US Department of Health and Human Services, 1996.

42. Ryden-Bergsten T, Andersson F. The health care costs of heart failure in Sweden. J Intern Med 1999;246:275–284.

43. Scott WG, Scott HM. Heart failure. A decision analytic analysis of New Zealand data using the published results of the SOLVD Treatment Trial. Studies of Left Ventricular Dysfunction. Pharmacoeconomics 1996;9:156,157.

44. Weingarten SR, Riedinger MS, Shinbane J, et al. Triage practice guideline for patients hospitalized with congestive heart failure: improving the effectiveness of the coronary care unit. Am J Med 1993;94:483–490.

45. Polanczyk CA, Rohde LE, Dec GW, DiSalvo T. Ten-year trends in hospital care for congestive heart failure: improved outcomes and increased use of resources. Arch Intern Med 2000;160:325–332.

46. McMurray J, McDonagh T, Morrison CE, Dargie HJ. Trends in hospitalization for heart failure in Scotland 1980-1990. Eur Heart J 1993;14:1158–1162.

47. Vinson JM, Rich MW, Sperry JC, Shah AS, McNamara T. Early readmission of elderly patients with congestive heart failure. J Am Geriatr Soc 1990;38:1290–125.

48. Krumholz HM, Chen YT, Wang Y, Vaccarino V, Radford MJ, Horwitz RI. Predictors of readmission among elderly survivors of admission with heart failure. Am Heart J 2000;139:72–77.

49. Franciosa JA, Wilen M, Ziesche S, Cohn JN. Survival in men with severe chronic left ventricular failure due to either coronary heart disease or idiopathic dilated cardiomyopathy. Am J Cardiol 1983;51:831–836.

50. Wilson JR, Schwartz JS, Sutton MS, et al. Prognosis in severe heart failure: relation to hemodynamic measurements and ventricular ectopic activity. J Am Coll Cardiol 1983;2:403–410.

51. Brophy JM, Deslauriers G, Rouleau JL. Long-term prognosis of patients presenting to the emergency room with decompensated congestive heart failure. Can J Cardiol 1994;10:543–547.

52. Vasan RS, Larson MG, Benjamin EJ, Evans JC, Reiss CK, Levy D. Congestive heart failure in subjects with normal versus reduced left ventricular ejection fraction: prevalence and mortality in a population-based cohort. J Am Coll Cardiol 1999;33:1948–1955.

53. Pernenkil R, Vinson JM, Shah AS, Beckham V, Wittenberg C, Rich MW. Course and prognosis in patients > or = 70 years of age with congestive heart failure and normal versus abnormal left ventricular ejection fraction. Am J Cardiol 1997;79:216–219.

54. Ho KK, Anderson KM, Kannel WB, Grossman W, Levy D. Survival after the onset of congestive heart failure in Framingham Heart Study subjects. Circulation 1993;88:107–115.

55. Dries DL, Exner DV, Gersh BJ, Cooper HA, Carson PE, Domanski MJ. Racial differences in the outcome of left ventricular dysfunction. N Engl J Med 1999;340:609–616.

56. Adams KF, Jr., Dunlap SH, Sueta CA, et al. Relation between gender, etiology and survival in patients with symptomatic heart failure. J Am Coll Cardiol 1996;28:1781–1788.

57. Felker GM, Thompson RE, Hare JM, et al. Underlying causes and long-term survival in patients with initially unexplained cardiomyopathy. N Engl J Med 2000;342:1077–1084.

58. Yancy CW, Firth BG. Congestive heart failure. Dis Mon 1988;34;465–536.

59. McMurray J, Hart W, Rhodes G. An evaluation of the cost of chronic heart failure to the National Health Service in the UK. Br J Med Econom 1993;6:99–110.

60. Launois R, Launois B, Reboul-Marty J, Battais J, Lefebvre P. The cost of chronic illness severity: the heart failure case. J Med Econom 1990;8:395–412.

61. van Hout BA, Wielink G, Bonsel GJ, Rutten FF. Effects of ACE inhibitors on heart failure in The Netherlands: a pharmacoeconomic model. Pharmacoeconomics 1993;3:387–397.

62. Malek M. Health economics of heart failure. Heart 1999;82:IV11–IV13.

63. Konstam D, Dracup K, Baker D, et al. Heart failure: evaluation and care of patients with left ventricular systolic dysfunction. Clinical Practice Guideline No. 11. AHCPR Publication No. 94-0612. Rockville, MD: Agency for Health Care Policy and Research, Public Health Service, US Department of Health and Human Services, June, 1994.

64. Brown AM, Cleland JG. Influence of concomitant disease on patterns of hospitalization in patients with heart failure discharged from Scottish hospitals in 1995. Eur Heart J 1998;19:1063–1069.

65. The SOLVD Investigators. Effect of enalapril on survival in patients with reduced left ventricular ejection fractions and congestive heart failure. N Engl J Med 1991;325:293–302.

66. Ward RE, Gheorghiade M, Young JB, Uretsky B. Economic outcomes of withdrawal of digoxin therapy in adult patients with stable congestive heart failure. J Am Coll Cardiol 1995;26:93–101.

67. The Digitalis Investigation Group. The Effect of Digoxin on Mortality and Morbidity in Patients with Heart Failure. N Engl J Med 1997;336:525–533.
68. Hart W, Rhodes G, McMurray J. The cost effectiveness of enalapril in the treatment of chronic heart failure. Br J Med Econom 1993;6:91–98.
69. Paul SD, Kuntz KM, Eagle KA, Weinstein MC. Costs and effectiveness of angiotensin converting enzyme inhibition in patients with congestive heart failure. Arch Intern Med 1994;154:1143–119.
70. Cook JR, Glick HA, Gerth W, Kinosian B, Kostis JB. The cost and cardioprotective effects of enalapril in hypertensive patients with left ventricular dysfunction. Am J Hypertens 1998;11:1433–1441.
71. Butler JR, Fletcher PJ. A cost-effectiveness analysis of enalapril maleate in the management of congestive heart failure in Australia. Aust N Z J Med 1996;26:89–95.
72. Kleber FX, Niemoller L, Doering W. Impact of converting enzyme inhibition on progression of chronic heart failure: results of the Munich Mild Heart Failure Trial. Br Heart J 1992;67:289–296.
73. Malek M, Cunningham-Davis J, Malek L, et al. A cost minimisation analysis of cardiac failure treatment in the UK using CIBIS trial data. Cardiac Insufficiency Bisoprolol Study. Int J Clin Pract 1999;53:19–23.
74. Delea TE, Vera-Llonch M, Richner RE, Fowler MB, Oster G. Cost effectiveness of carvedilol for heart failure. Am J Cardiol 1999;83:890–896.
75. Levy P, Lechat P, Leizorovicz A, Levy E. A cost-minimization of heart failure therapy with bisoprolol in the French setting: an analysis from CIBIS trial data. Cardiac Insufficiency Bisoprolol Study. Cardiovasc Drugs Ther 1998;12:301–305.
76. Royal College of General Practitioners. Office of Population Census and Survey and Department of Health and Social Security. Morbidity statistics from general practice: third national study, 1981–1982. London: HMSO, 1988.
77. Royal College of General Practitioners. Office of Population Census and Survey and Department of Health and Social Security. Morbidity statistics from general practice: fourth national study, 1991–1992. London: HMSO, 1995.
78. Droller H, Pemberton J. Cardiovascular disease in a random sample of elderly people. Br Heart J 1953;15:199–204.
79. Landahl S, Svanborg A, Astrand K. Heart volume and the prevalence of certain common cardiovascular disorders at 70 and 75 years of age. Eur Heart J 1984;5:326–331.

2 Taking a History in a Patient with Heart Failure

Irving M. Herling, MD

CONTENTS

INTRODUCTION

Identification of the etiology of heart failure early in the course of the disease will allow the physician to institute pharmacologic therapies. These therapies may not only effectively ameliorate the symptoms of heart failure, but may also favorably alter the natural history of this disease process by addressing the neurohormonal influences that perpetuate injury in the failing heart. Furthermore, the identification of the pathophysiologic processes that have resulted in myocardial injury or dysfunction may allow the institution of therapies specifically directed at alleviating or reconciling those disorders. The identification of myocardial ischemia (e.g., contributing to myocardial hibernation) may direct the physician to provide therapies directed at improving myocar-

From: *Contemporary Cardiology: Heart Failure:*
A Clinician's Guide to Ambulatory Diagnosis and Treatment
Edited by: M. L. Jessup and E. Loh © Humana Press Inc., Totowa, NJ

dial blood flow and thereby improve cardiac function. Similarly, the identification of valvular lesions producing either pressure or volume overload may be reconciled by valve replacement or repair. A history of excessive alcohol consumption, a common cause of myocardial dysfunction, and subsequent avoidance of alcohol use, often results in improved cardiac function.

In addition to the identification of the pathophysiologic processes initiating myocardial injury, the exacerbation of heart failure in patients with known cardiac dysfunction can often be avoided or reconciled if the physician is astute in taking the history that identifies alterations in dietary sodium intake, or the concurrent use of drugs negatively impacting on fluid retention or cardiac function.

PRESENTING SYMPTOMS
OF THE HEART FAILURE PATIENT

Frequently, patients present complaints of fatigue, effort-related dyspnea, orthopnea, paroxysmal nocturnal dyspnea, edema, and occasionally, palpitations or embolic events as a result of intramyocardial thrombi. These symptoms often trigger noninvasive cardiovascular testing, which effectively identifies the presence of both diastolic and systolic ventricular dysfunction.

However, on other occasions, myocardial dysfunction is identified incidentally during echocardiographic testing in patients with heart murmurs or nondescript symptoms. Once such dysfunction is found, the physician must seek to identify the etiology of myocardial injury.

WHEN TO SUSPECT ISCHEMIC HEART DISEASE
IN THE PATIENT WITH HEART FAILURE

Ischemic heart disease is currently the most common etiology of congestive heart failure (CHF) in the United States. Patients often provide a history of prior myocardial infarction or classical angina pectoris. Noninvasive testing provides a tool to assess the severity of myocardial ischemia and quantitate to the extent of the myocardial scar. However, patients frequently do not report classical angina pectoris, but instead complain of dyspnea that represents their ischemic equivalent. The presence of cardiac risk factors contributing to the development of coronary disease, such as tobacco abuse, diabetes mellitus, dyslipidemia, hypertension, a family history of premature coronary disease, male gender, as well as increasing age, make it more likely that the patient's symptomatology may well be a result of coronary atherosclerosis. However, some patients are entirely asymptomatic despite the presence of substantial coronary disease *(1)*. In particular, diabetics seem to be more likely to have "silent ischemia" and therefore may not complain of angina. Some of these patients may have sustained silent myocardial infarctions or have significant myocardial hibernation from severe ischemia in the absence of classical anginal symptomatology. The occurrence of silent or symptomatic myocardial infarction will often initiate or exacerbate heart failure. New Q waves on the electrocardiogram or exercise imaging studies will often confirm the diagnosis.

Valvular Heart Disease

Valvular heart disease may also produce heart failure or asymptomatic ventricular dysfunction. Aortic and mitral regurgitation may over time produce left-ventricular volume overload, resulting in systolic ventricular dysfunction. The presence of a heart murmur has often been recorded during prior examinations. Other patients with stenotic lesions of the aortic or mitral valves, or patients with congenital pulmonic stenosis, or tricuspid valvular disease, may also develop symptomatic heart failure. Echocardiography testing defines the magnitude of the valvular lesion, as well as its impact on ventricular function.

Occasionally, a patient with trivial pre-existent valvular disease may develop bacterial endocarditis that may produce an acute or subacute alteration in valvular incompetence and new volume overload, resulting in CHF *(2)*. A febrile illness after dental work, urologic manipulation, or skin- or soft-tissue infection may raise suspicion for the presence of either acute or subacute bacterial endocarditis. When the infection is subacute, clinical deterioration is of more gradual onset and is often associated with malaise, anorexia, weight loss, myalgias, and systemic emboli. Acute endocarditis, especially with *Staphylococcus aureus*, may present a septic syndrome with acute CHF. At times, the presenting complaint may result from an embolic event to the brain or extremities.

Congenital Heart Disease

Most patients with significant congenital heart disease have already undergone cardiologic evaluation. These lesions may produce CHF in adulthood. Occasionally, patients with patent ductus arteriosus or atrial septal defect may be undiagnosed until they develop heart failure later in life. Noninvasive imaging and cardiac catheterization will define these lesions.

Hypertension

Long-standing hypertension, especially when poorly controlled, not only contributes to the presence of coronary atherosclerosis, but also may produce myocardial dysfunction as a result of long-standing pressure overload. A history of poorly controlled or severe hypertension is often obtained.

Diabetes Mellitus

Although most patients with diabetes mellitus will develop myocardial dysfunction from concomitant coronary disease, myocardial dysfunction from diabetes, particularly in the setting of hypertension, is well recognized *(3)*. This diagnosis is made by excluding the presence of coronary disease or other known etiologies of myocardial dysfunction in the diabetic, hypertensive patient.

Myocardial Toxins

Excessive alcohol intake is a frequent cause of myocardial dysfunction in our society *(4)*. An accurate history assessing the magnitude and duration of alcohol consumption must be obtained in any patient with heart failure. Patients will often underreport the amount of alcohol they consume. A more accurate history may be forthcoming from a spouse or other family member. Quantitation of alcohol intake is very relevant because abstinence from alcohol in these patients may produce substantial improvement in myocardial function. Concomitant, excessive alcohol use in the setting of other etiologies of ventricular dysfunction will potentiate the severity of heart failure. Furthermore, alcohol may trigger supraventricular and ventricular arrhythmias in these patients.

Cocaine abuse, a common problem in urban societies, is a common cause of myocardial injury, resulting in cardiomyopathy along with coronary vasospasm and acute myocardial infarction. A history regarding illicit drug use must be obtained in any patient with heart failure. In addition to the direct toxicity associated with the use of illicit drugs, these patients are often at risk for developing HIV, which may result in clinical AIDS and cardiomyopathy associated with severe AIDS involvement.

Chemotherapeutic agents used to treat neoplastic disease may likewise produce myocardial injury. The anthracycline derivatives are the most frequent agents associated with myocardial toxicity. Although oncologists attempt to limit the exposure of their patients to these agents in order to prevent cardiotoxicity, idiosyncratic injury occurs at times, particularly when associated with other myocardial disease or concomitant radiation therapy in which the heart is included in the radiation field *(5)*. Radiation itself may produce myocardial injury and initiate premature atherosclerotic and valvular disease.

Nutritional deficiencies that lead to severe anemia, such as beri beri or other chronic anemic states, may produce high-output CHF. Reconciliation of the anemia and/or nutritional deficiency may reverse myocardial dysfunction.

TACHYCARDIA-INDUCED MYOCARDIAL DYSFUNCTION

It is also well recognized that chronic tachycardia, as a result of incessant tachyarrhythmias or poorly controlled atrial fibrillation, can produce reversible myocardial dysfunction (6). It is now recognized that patients with atrial fibrillation often require the addition of β-blockers or calcium channel blockers to modulate their ventricular response. Treadmill testing or ambulatory electrocardiographic monitoring will often provide the physician with evidence of excessive heart rates. In these patients, the heart rate may exceed 110–140 beats per minute for much of the day, or if the heart rate increases to 120–140 beats per minute within the first 2 minutes of exercise, tachycardia-related cardiomyopathy should be considered.

Sleep Apnea

Some patients with right-sided CHF may suffer from obstructive sleep apnea. In these patients, chronic pulmonary hypertension and hypoxemia produce right-ventricular dysfunction along with systemic hypertension. Such patients are often obese and snore heavily, reporting daytime somnolence, early morning headache, or developing nocturnal tachyarrhythmias that bring them to the care of the cardiologist. Treatment for sleep apnea may ameliorate heart failure in these patients.

Other Causes of Ventricular Dysfunction

In some patients who develop myocardial dysfunction and CHF, no apparent etiology can be identified. Occasionally, patients may report a viral syndrome in the weeks to months before the onset of their symptomatology, suggesting a postviral myocardiopathy. Some patients may have a fulminant course of acute myocarditis resulting in severe and rapid clinical deterioration. Myocardial biopsy may be required to identify these individuals.

Some patients may suffer from congenital cardiomyopathy. There is often a family history of sudden cardiac death or early myocardial dysfunction. Hemochromatosis, hypertrophic cardiomyopathy, and the muscular dystrophies are heritable disorders that lead to significant cardiac involvement. Family histories of cardiac death or heart failure can often be obtained.

Unexplained heart failure in women postpartum was described in the 1930s and has become a well-recognized form of cardiomyopathy.

Peripartum cardiomyopathy should be suspected in patients who develop signs or symptoms of CHF in the third trimester of pregnancy or postpartum. The prognosis in these patients is excellent in comparison to other patients with cardiomyopathy, with one-third recovering to normal function and one-third stabilizing for prolonged periods of time *(7)*. Because the disease often recurs with subsequent pregnancies, the recognition of this syndrome is essential to prevent the patient from being exposed to additional myocardial injury.

CHRONIC HEART FAILURE ASSESSMENT

Fluid Retention: Why Is it Occurring?

In addition to identifying potential etiology of the myocardial dysfunction, the patient history will often assist in identifying factors contributing to a deterioration in the patient's clinical status.

The most frequent cause of fluid overload and a worsening of congestive symptoms is excessive dietary intake of salt. Detailed questioning should be undertaken in regard to a change in diet, such as eating meals outside of the patient's home or the consumption of salt-laden substances. Educated patients may augment their diuretic dosing to prevent such dietary alterations from producing decompensation.

Another common cause of clinical deterioration is the failure to comply with the prescribed medical regimen. The most common medications that are not taken as prescribed are the loop diuretics. Patients often complain that the brisk diuresis that accompanies the administration of these drugs fequently limits their ability to leave their homes and impacts their ability to attend social activities. They usually will not volunteer this information, but will admit to their omission of their prescribed doses with direct questioning. The physician will often find that compliance will improve when diuretics are prescribed at times when the patient has easy access to toilet facilities.

DRUGS IMPACTING ON HEART FAILURE

Many patients with CHF suffer from arthritic infirmities and may be prescribed nonsteroidal anti-inflammatory drugs by other physicians or may obtain them over the counter. These drugs may produce salt retention and blunt the effect of angiotensin-converting enzyme (ACE) inhibitors. The physician must inquire about the use of these drugs in patients with heart failure who decompensate and seek alternative drugs or augment their current regimens. In general, however, these drugs should be avoided in patients with severe heart failure.

Other pharmacologic agents used in the management of cardiovascular disorders may impact adversely on patients with heart failure. Drugs such as the nondihydropyridine calcium channel blockers (e.g., verapamil, diltiazem) used to treat angina, hypertension, or supraventricular dysrhythmias and certain antiarrhythmic drugs such as flecainide or disopyramide, may significantly impair left-ventricular fuction. β-blockers, although now indicated for the long-term treatment of heart failure patients, may produce transient deterioration in ventricular function and promote fluid retention. An occasional patient may decompensate when prescribed eyedrops for glaucoma that contain β-blockers because these may be systemically absorbed through the lacrimal ducts. Alternative therapy for glaucoma should be provided.

MYOCARDIAL ISCHEMIA

Myocardial ischemia or infarction may be superimposed on preexistent heart failure, which may cause acute or subacute decompensation. A history of accelerating angina or prolonged ischemic discomfort may be elicited in these patients, although some may not report classical ischemic symptomatology.

DYSRHYTHMIAS

Palpitations occur commonly in heart failure patients. Ventricular ectopy is nearly ubiquitous in patients with substantial left-ventricular dysfunction, but when extremely frequent or occurring in runs, may reduce cardiac output substantially.

The development of atrial fibrillation in patients with compensated heart failure may produce rapid deterioration as a consequence of the loss of atrial contribution to ventricular filling, as well as rapid heart rates that in and of themselves may cause further deterioration of ventricular function. In the patient with ischemic disease, atrial fibrillation with rapid rates may also produce significant ischemic dysfunction.

Bradyarrhythmias may also produce a reduction in cardiac output that may trigger decompensation. Symptoms of light headedness or worsening fatigue may be reported. Ambulatory echocardiographic monitoring is useful in defining these dysrhythmias.

OTHER FACTORS

Anemia is poorly tolerated by heart failure patients because it requires an increase in cardiac output and promotes fluid retention. Patients with severely impaired left-ventricular function often receive oral anticoagulants that may promote bleeding. The physician must inquire as to the occurrence of melena or hematochezia.

A decline in renal function and progressive renal insufficiency may also result in fluid overload and diminished diuretic efficacy. Furthermore, the metabolism of drugs excreted via the kidneys will be altered potentially resulting in an accumulation of these drugs, such as β-blockers and digoxin. Accumulation of these drugs may produce bradycardia or heart block along with life-threatening digitalis toxicity.

Hypo- or hyperthyroidism may contribute to CHF decompensation. Amiodarone, a commonly prescribed antiarrhythmic drug in heart failure patients, may produce hyper- or hypothyroidism. Thyroid function studies should be followed closely in patients taking this drug.

Therefore, the history provides insights as to the etiology of the patient's heart failure syndrome, as well as identifying factors contributing to subsequent deterioration in function and quality of life. When possible, the identification of these factors and their reconciliation will substantially assist in the management of these patients.

REFERENCES

1. Kellerman JJ, Braunwald E, eds. Silent Myocardial Ischemia: A Critical Appraisal. Basel, Karger: 1990.
2. Agostino RS, Miller DC, Stinson EB, et al. Valve replacement in patients with native valve endocarditis: what really determines operative outcome? Ann Thorac Surg 1985;40(5):429–438.
3. Hamby RI, Zoneraich S, Sherman S. Diabetic Cardiomyopathy. JAMA 1974;229:1749–1754.
4. Burch GE, Giles TD. Alcoholic cardiomyopathy: concept of the disease and its treatment. Am J Med 1971;50:141–145.
5. Minow RA, Benjamin RS, Lee ET, Gottlieb JA. Adriamycin cardiomyopathy-risk factors. Cancer 1977;39:1397–1402.
6. Packer DL, Bardy GH, Worley SJ, et al. Tachycardia-induced cardiomyopathy: a reversible form of left ventricular dysfunction. Am J Cardiol 1986;57:563–570.
7. DeMakis JG, Rhamitoola SH, Sutton GC, et al. Natural course of peripartum cardiomyopathy. Circulation 1971;44:1053–1061.

3 Evaluation of Dyspnea

David M. McCarthy, MD

CONTENTS

INTRODUCTION
TYPES OF DYSPNEA
APPROACH TO THE PATIENT WITH DYSPNEA
CONCLUSION
REFERENCES

INTRODUCTION

Dyspnea is derived from Greek (*dys*—hard or bad; *pnoe*—breathing) and means difficult or laborious breathing *(1)*. It is a symptom, as opposed to a sign, and is therefore subjective, dependent on both the degree of disturbance and the patient's perception of the intensity of the problem: "an unpleasant sensation of difficulty in breathing" *(2)*. Dyspnea "alerts individuals when they are in danger of receiving inadequate ventilation" *(3)* and is different from tachypnea. If pain can be described as "a complex subjective sensation reflecting real or potential tissue damage and the affective response to it" *(4)*, then dyspnea is not far behind in the ranks of subjective and frequently encountered symptoms.

Dyspnea can be experienced by normal subjects (e.g., while exercising) and patients with many conditions, but most frequently, by those patients with cardiac or pulmonary disease *(5)*. Indeed, dyspnea on exertion is the most common symptom in patients with heart failure *(6)*. However, because it is also seen in a variety of other conditions, the clinician must identify the source of dyspnea before prescribing treatment, which may be quite different based on the etiology (e.g., diuretics for heart failure, inhalers and/or antibiotics for chronic obstructive pulmonary disease [COPD]).

From: *Contemporary Cardiology: Heart Failure:*
A Clinician's Guide to Ambulatory Diagnosis and Treatment
Edited by: M. L. Jessup and E. Loh © Humana Press Inc., Totowa, NJ

This task is made even more difficult by the frequent co-existence of cardiac and pulmonary disease in the same patient.

The purpose of this chapter is to outline an approach to the patient with dyspnea, with particular attention to the heart failure patient, so that the cause of dyspnea can be accurately determined and appropriate therapy can be prescribed.

TYPES OF DYSPNEA

In order to accurately characterize dyspnea, the nature of the condition must be understood. A recent consensus statement of the American Thoracic Society addressed this in detail, pointing out that there are multiple types of dyspnea and proposed that the term *dyspnea* be "used to characterize a subjective experience of breathing discomfort that consists of qualitatively distinct sensations that vary in intensity" *(7)*. This is a broad definition, and the multiple mechanisms of dyspnea (particularly in pulmonary disease) are beyond the scope of this discussion. However, it is necessary to understand the types of dyspnea that heart failure patients experience along with the pathophysiologic mechanism(s).

Generally, the first presentation is dyspnea with exertion, and as previously noted, this is a normal response to strenuous exercise. A brief discussion of the physiology of exercise is important in order to understand why patients experience dyspnea in this setting *(8)*.

When physical work (exercise) is undertaken, the skeletal muscles must produce energy through oxidative metabolism. Because there is little oxygen stored in the muscle, muscle blood flow must increase to supply the oxygen consumed in this process. This is accomplished by increasing the cardiac output, initially by augmenting the stroke volume, and subsequently by progressively increasing the heart rate. As the exercising muscles consume oxygen, they generate carbon dioxide, which is eliminated in the lungs through increased ventilation. This normal cardiopulmonary response to exercise maintains normal acid-base balance in the blood during moderate exercise, but as the muscles utilize oxygen to a greater degree than can be supported by oxygen delivery (i.e., cardiac output), the aerobic metabolism is supplemented by anaerobic pathways within the muscle cell, with the conversion of pyruvate to lactate and the generation of lactic acid in the blood. The point at which this develops is termed the *anaerobic threshold*. The lactic acid generated is immediately buffered by bicarbonate ion with the release of further carbon dioxide into the bloodstream. This results in further increases in ventilation, both by the need to eliminate the

additional CO_2 and because the lowered serum bicarbonate level stimulates the respiratory control mechanism in the carotid bodies.

Thus, exercise involves a complex interaction of metabolic pathways
and physiologic responses to maintain homeostasis. Organic causes of
dyspnea relate to inadequacy of oxygen delivery, CO_2 elimination, or
both (8). It is therefore understandable why patients with cardiac or
pulmonary conditions experience dyspnea, because the delivery of
oxygen requires both adequate ventilation and adequate cardiac output,
as does the elimination of CO_2. In heart failure, not only is the cardiac
output response blunted, but the increased pulmonary venous pressure
causes pulmonary congestion and interferes with the exchange of oxygen and carbon dioxide in the alveoli. In pulmonary disease, there can
be abnormalities in ventilation, gas exchange, or both.

Exertional dyspnea is clinically important when it occurs at an
unexpectedly (or unacceptably) low workload for a given patient (9).
Because exercise performance can be limited by a variety of conditions
other than cardiopulmonary disease, including anemia, obesity, peripheral vascular disease, physical deconditioning, and psychological causes
(8), it is important to eliminate these noncardiopulmonary causes before
trying to identify a cardiopulmonary source. It must also be considered
whether the patient's dyspnea is actually an anginal equivalent. This is
usually exertional but is a result of myocardial ischemia, which the patient
perceives as breathlessness rather than chest pain or discomfort. There
may be associated pulmonary congestion (from ischemic papillary muscle
dysfunction or left ventricular failure on the basis of acute ischemia and
transient left-ventricular dysfunction). Again, the treatment of this type of
dyspnea would be directed at preventing or relieving myocardial ischemia.

We often try to quantify the degree of exertional dyspnea by identifying activities that provoke the symptom; we will record "one flight
DOE" in the patient record, as if that were an objective measure.
Although the patient may indeed experience dyspnea when climbing
one flight of stairs, as the earlier discussion indicates, this may relate
both to the speed at which the stairs are climbed and the patient's perception of the degree of breathlessness. It is, therefore, a decidedly
unobjective measurement, but may still be useful quantitatively because
the serial assessment in a given patient can be helpful in following the
course of the disease or the response to therapy. On the other hand, the
New York Heart Association (NYHA) functional classification is a
useful means of classifying patients based on what type of physical
activity is limited by dyspnea (or other symptoms).

In addition to exertional dyspnea, there are other forms of dyspnea or
breathing difficulties that are associated with cardiac disease. *Orthop-*

nea is dyspnea that occurs in the recumbent position and generally indicates severe heart failure. The mechanism is the increased venous return from edematous legs when the patient assumes the recumbent position. Patients learn to avoid this by using extra pillows (hence, the origin of another *nonquantitative* term "two-pillow orthopnea"). Of course, a patient may use extra pillows for comfort reasons (e.g., cervical spine disease) without having orthopnea; it is important not only to ask how many pillows a patient sleeps with, but also why. Some cardiac patients have such severe orthopnea that they sleep sitting up in a chair or recliner.

There are unusual forms of positional dyspnea that can indicate cardiac or pulmonary disease. *Trepopnea* is shortness of breath that occurs in one lateral decubitus position but not the other. Originally thought to be a result of distortion of the great vessels in one lateral position, it is actually felt to be from ventilatory-perfusion mismatching that can occur in either cardiac or pulmonary conditions *(10)*. Another unusual condition is *platypnea*, which is hypoxia and dyspnea occurring in the upright position (the opposite of orthopnea); it is sometimes referred to as *platypnea orthodeoxia*. This is seen in patients with atrial septal defect or patent foramen ovale in the setting of pulmonary disease, especially following pneumonectomy. It is a result of right-to-left shunting in the upright position and is relieved by closure of the interatrial defect.

Paroxysmal nocturnal dyspnea is a type of acute dyspnea that occurs in patients with chronic heart failure. The description by Fuster *(11)* is classic:

> *One to two hours after going to bed, the patient suddenly awakens with a smothering sensation; he or she must sit up or even go to the window for air. Occasionally the episode is accompanied by cough or wheezing as a result of pulmonary congestion which narrows the bronchiolar tubes. The smothering sensation and asphyxia, which are at times accompanied by palpitations, vertigo, or constrictive retrosternal pain, often last for 10 to 30 minutes. Then, the symptoms subside and the patient returns to bed and usually sleeps peacefully for the rest of the night.*

The wheezing component is called *cardiac asthma* and can also occur with exertional dyspnea or orthopnea. The physical findings are similar to bronchial asthma, and the clinician must use the history as a clue to which mechanism is operative (and therefore which form of treatment—bronchodilator vs diuretic—to prescribe). A related symptom is *cough*, which is commonly associated with lung disease but can be a manifestation of heart disease (not to mention a side effect of angiotensin-converting enzyme [ACE] inhibitor therapy for heart failure). When cough is associated with heart failure, it is frequently nonproductive and occurs in situations that otherwise might produce dyspnea, such as exertion or recumbency *(12)*. In addition, dyspnea precedes cough in congestive heart failure (CHF) patients with orthopnea, whereas it results from coughing in patients with COPD *(13)*.

Other breathing disturbances can occur during sleep. *Cheyne-Stokes* periodic breathing is a rare manifestation of advanced heart failure, often with concomitant neurologic disease, although it can also be seen in isolated neurologic disease (e.g., stroke or head trauma). The original description is very revealing:

> *For several days his breathing was irregular; it would entirely cease for a quarter of a minute, then it would become perceptible, though very low, then by degrees it became heaving and quick, and then it would gradually cease again. This revolution in the state of his breathing occupied about a minute....* (14)

The mechanism of this phenomenon relates to prolonged left heart-to-brain circulation time, which results in disturbance of the normal feedback mechanism controlling respiration *(11)*. Because the patient is sleeping there is usually no symptomatic perception of this; thus, it is really not a type of dyspnea but rather an abnormal breathing pattern observed by others.

Another breathing disorder during sleep that can be seen in patients with heart disease is *obstructive sleep apnea*, where there are periods of apnea that terminate with brief arousal. As this frequently occurs in the setting of loud snoring, family members are generally those who report this condition. It is a contributing factor to arrhythmias and hypertension and should be thought of in this context. The patient may report arousals from sleep but not necessarily identify these with dyspnea. Unlike Cheyne-Stokes breathing, which has a predictable periodicity, the apneic periods in obstructive sleep apnea are often more prolonged and terminate abruptly with arousal.

The most severe form of dyspnea is *acute pulmonary edema*, which is usually a result of acute left-ventricular failure in the setting of an abrupt change in cardiac status. Examples would include acute myocardial infarction, acute mitral or aortic regurgitation, hypertensive crisis, and acute tachyarrhythmias. The patient may have a prior history of heart disease, but often this is the first manifestation. There is an accumulation of extravascular fluid in the alveoli or pulmonary interstitium with severe hypoxia and dyspnea: the patient may feel as if he or she is drowning in his or her own secretions *(12)*. This is a life-threatening emergency that requires immediate therapy to relieve symptoms and correct hypoxia. However, one must always bear in mind that there are conditions of *noncardiogenic* pulmonary edema *(15)* for which the treatment is quite different.

APPROACH TO THE PATIENT WITH DYSPNEA

The first step in evaluating dyspnea is taking a careful clinical history, with attention to the clues enumerated previously about the type of dyspnea and the situations in which it becomes manifest. The patient's description of what is experienced and when is unique in that only the patient knows what he or she is feeling. As mentioned earlier, dyspnea is a very subjective phenomenon, and there have been attempts to characterize the patient descriptors according to the type of disease process (i.e., heart failure, various types of lung disease, deconditioning, etc.). In one such study *(16)*, the various types of pulmonary disease each had unique clusters of descriptors when patients were asked to complete a questionnaire. However, the clinical utility of such an approach in an individual patient is limited, because there is considerable overlap in the patient responses.

There are obvious historical clues that come to mind, however. For example, a patient with a history of childhood asthma is less likely to have cardiac asthma than a patient who develops new onset wheezing later in life. Similarly, a heavy smoker who wakes up coughing, but after sitting up to clear is phlegm can immediately go back to sleep, is probably not experiencing paroxysmal nocturnal dyspnea. Another cause of nocturnal cough is esophageal reflux with aspiration, which has nothing to do with either cardiac or pulmonary disease. A patient with severe emphysema may become orthopneic, but the basis is likely to be the inability to use the abdominal muscles as accessory to the diaphragm when lying down.

Dyspnea at rest is more likely to be associated with pulmonary disease than with heart failure, with the exception of acute pulmonary edema. On the other hand, exertional provocation of dyspnea is very nonspecific, because it may occur in the setting of lung disease, heart failure, ischemic heart disease, or deconditioning. Sometimes the patient's description of his breathing discomfort is a clue to the etiology (e.g., tightness in the chest suggests either angina or bronchospasm). Rapid shallow breathing, either at rest or with exercise, is more common in lung disease. Heavy breathing or sighing is often a sign of deconditioning.

No matter how good we think we are at taking a careful history, our ability to correctly identify the cause of dyspnea based on history alone is not very good; in fact, in one study the initial diagnostic impression based on history alone was correct in only two-thirds of the patients *(5)*. We obviously need to be more accurate in ascribing the cause of dyspnea in order to prescribe the correct treatment.

We can improve our diagnostic accuracy by performing a thorough *physical examination*, with particular attention to the heart and lungs. But as we have seen, findings on exam are not specific (e.g., wheezing can be associated with both cardiac and pulmonary conditions). Also, the findings may vary depending on whether the patient is dyspneic during the examination, or is being assessed for a history of dyspnea. Nevertheless, there are exam findings that frequently point us in the right direction.

There are certain obvious clues to look for: distended neck veins, pulmonary rales, cardiac murmurs, and peripheral edema. Other sentinel findings include tachypnea, pursed lips, cyanosis, clubbing, chest deformities (e.g., the "barrel chest" of COPD; severe kyphoscoliosis, which can be associated with restrictive lung disease), and prominent use of accessory muscles of respiration. We can also see if the patient has the appearance of a "blue bloater" or a "pink puffer," both of which indicate chronic lung disease (obstructive and emphysematous, respectively).

However, it is easy to be fooled because patients may have physical findings pointing to both cardiac and pulmonary disease. A good example is the finding of *rales*, which can be associated with pulmonary congestion or interstitial lung disease. Of course, the absence of rales does not rule out CHF as a cause of dyspnea, as patients with chronic CHF may have compensatory factors that prevent the accumulation of fluid within the alveoli *(12)*.

Another example of an overlapping examination finding is *pulsus paradoxus*, which cardiologists usually associate with pericardial disease. What is seen is a significant drop in systolic BP during inspiration; normally there is a fall of up to 10 mm Hg, from impaired LV filling during inspiration, and in a patient with pericardial disease, a fall of more than 20 mm Hg indicates possible tamponade or constriction. However, some of the largest blood pressure variations during respiration are seen in patients with severe COPD, as a result of the marked change in intrathoracic pressure in these patients during inspiration. Thus, the physical examination findings must be considered in light of the clinical situation: if one is evaluating a patient with *chronic* dyspnea who has severe pulsus paradoxus, the patient probably has pulmonary disease, because cardiac tamponade is not usually associated with chronic dyspnea (although patients may have orthopnea).

With the availability of echocardiography, cardiac examination has lost some of its allure. Indeed, the most frequent reason given for requesting an echo is "murmur." Cardiologists are trained to discern the type of lesion based on the character of the murmur: its timing, location, intensity, radiation, and response to various maneuvers. Because many cardiac conditions associated with murmurs can cause dyspnea, the finding of a murmur tends to focus attention more on the heart and away from the lungs as the source of dyspnea.

Ancillary Testing

There are several studies that can be performed in order to better define the cause of dyspnea. Among the simplest in the office is the *electrocardiogram*, which can reveal unsuspected infarction pattern or arrhythmia. There might also be a "pulmonary disease pattern" (vertical axis, right-atrial enlargement, poor R wave progression, and low voltage) *(17)*. Another office test that can be helpful is the *hematocrit*, which can point to anemia as either a cause of dyspnea or a contributing factor in a cardiac or pulmonary patient.

The *chest X-ray* is frequently performed to assess dyspnea, and there are certainly findings that are specific to cardiac or pulmonary disease. Obvious indicators pointing to cardiac or pulmonary disease include cardiomegaly, flattened diaphragms, pulmonary blebs, pneumothorax, pulmonary infiltrate, pleural effusion, or acute pulmonary edema. Once again, however, the patient with both cardiac and pulmonary disease may pose a diagnostic dilemma (e.g., a patient with severe emphysema may not demonstrate classic X-ray findings of pulmonary edema). Despite these limitations, the chest X-ray is useful in the initial evaluation of a patient with dyspnea.

Pulmonary Function Testing

In the evaluation of dyspnea, a relatively inexpensive and noninvasive but specialized procedure is *pulmonary function testing* (PFT). This would include spirometry, measurement of lung volumes, and assessment of diffusing capacity. These procedures are generally performed on patients with known or suspected lung disease and do not assess cardiac function. However, because patients with heart failure can have abnormalities in pulmonary function, PFTs are sometimes useful in deciding whether a patient has intrinsic lung disease or abnormal gas exchange as a result of CHF.

In chronic CHF, there can be obstructive and restrictive defects on spirometry from interstitial edema and bronchial wall congestion. With treatment of CHF, these PFT abnormalities may improve but do not always completely normalize. Heart failure patients can also have abnormalities of carbon monoxide diffusing capacity (DL_{CO}), but this test is not routinely ordered or especially useful in assessing CHF. Similarly, pre- and postbronchodilator spirometry is best applied to patients with COPD rather than CHF. Finally, heart failure patients can have respiratory muscle fatigue as a cause of exertional dyspnea, presumably a result of poor respiratory muscle blood flow and resultant metabolic abnormalities. In general, however, PFT abnormalities are imprecise in patients with heart failure, although serial assessment can be used to demonstrate response to therapy or assess degree of disability in selected patients (18).

Cardiopulmonary Exercise Testing

Because heart failure patients frequently complain of exertional symptoms (fatigue, dyspnea, or both), exercise testing can be very helpful. In the patient with exertional dyspnea, exercise measurement of gas exchange can sometimes determine whether performance is limited by cardiac or pulmonary disease. In fact, the American College of Cardiology/American Heart Association (ACC/AHA) practice guidelines for exercise testing list this procedure as a class I indication for differentiating cardiac vs pulmonary limitations as a cause of exertional dyspnea (19).

The details of the *cardiopulmonary exercise test* (CPET) procedure are described elsewhere in this volume. We have already seen the discrepancy, which can be found on physical examination when a patient is not symptomatic at the time of the exam. During CPET, the patient is exercised to the point of symptoms, and the analysis of gas exchange data relates specifically to those symptoms. Of course, because the patient is unable to talk during exercise (from the mouthpiece), the exact nature and severity of the symptoms must be determined at the conclusion of the test. However, the patient can indicate the severity of symptoms by pointing to the appropriate rating on the Borg scale (20). If the limiting symptom is dyspnea, the cause could be cardiac, pulmonary, a combination of the two, or deconditioning.

Because all patients are limited by symptoms, they all have reduced exercise capacity in comparison with normals. Pulmonary patients, however, are often limited by their inability to increase ventilation as a result of lung disease. The *dyspnea index*, which is the ratio of maximum minute ventilation during exercise (VE) to the maximum voluntary ventilation at rest (MVV) can be used to separate cardiac from pulmonary causes of dyspnea (21). The COPD patient will approach his MVV during exercise (i.e., the VE/MVV approximates 1.0), whereas a heart failure patient may have adequate ventilatory reserve (VE/MVV 0.7) but is limited by inability to further increase cardiac output. Thus, the heart failure patient will have reached his or her anaerobic threshold before stopping, whereas the pulmonary patient may have to stop exercise before that level, as his or her inability to increase ventilation develops at submaximal (aerobic) levels of exercise. The deconditioned subject neither reaches the aerobic threshold nor is limited by ventilatory factors; his or her exercise is submaximal on the basis of poor muscle tone.

Even among pulmonary disease patients there can be a variable response to CPET. Some COPD patients reach the anaerobic threshold but do so at a heart rate below that predicted, reflecting the fact that their ventilatory limitation causes them to stop exercise before they actually stress the cardiovascular system. On the other hand, in restrictive lung disease, there is a low anaerobic threshold because of hypoxemia caused by inability to increase pulmonary blood flow (rather than impaired ventilation); such patients will reach predicted maximal heart rate at a very low exercise workload *(22)*. A similar pattern is seen in patients with pulmonary hypertension.

CONCLUSION

In summary, the evaluation of dyspnea is a complex issue that the clinician is frequently called upon to perform. It calls for a systematic approach, which always includes a careful history and physical examination. Ancillary testing can be employed, and specialized procedures such as pulmonary function testing and exercise testing with gas exchange analysis are often helpful. An accurate diagnosis combined with properly directed treatment can afford great benefit to a symptomatic patient.

REFERENCES

1. The Oxford English Dictionary. 2nd ed. Oxford: Clarendon Press, 1989.
2. Beers MH, Berkow R, eds. The Merck Manual of Diagnosis and Therapy. 17th ed. Merch Research Laboratories; Whitehouse Station, NJ: 1999, p. 514.
3. Stulbarg MS, Adams L. Dyspnea. In: Murray JF, Nadel JA, eds. Textbook of respiratory medicine. Saunders; Philadelphia: 1994, p. 541.
4. Beers MH, Berkow R, eds. The Merck Manual of Diagnosis and Therapy. 17th ed. Merck Research Laboratories Whitehouse Station, NJ: 1999, p. 1363.
5. Pratter MR, Curley FJ, Dubois J, et al. Cause and evaluation of chronic dyspnea in a pulmonary disease clinic. Arch Intern Med 1989;149:2277–2282.
6. Harlan WR, Oberman A, Grimm R, et al. Chronic congestive heart failure in coronary artery disease: clinical criteria. Ann Intern Med 1977;86:133–138.
7. Meek PM, Schwartzstein RM, Adams L., et al. Dyspnea: mechanisms, assessment, and management: a consensus statement of the American Thoracic Society. Am J Respir Crit Care Med 1999;159:321–340.
8. Wasserman K. Dyspnea on exertion: is it the heart or the lungs? JAMA 1982;248: 2039–2043.
9. Adams L, Chronos N, Lane R, et al. The measurement of breathlessness induced in normal subjects: individual differences. Clin Sci 1986;70:131–140.
10. Fuster V, Dines DE, Rodarte JR, et al. Relationships between disease of the heart and disease of the lungs. In: Giuliani ER, et al., eds. Cardiology: fundamentals and practice. Mosby-Year Book Inc., St. Louis, MO: 1991; pp. 2037–2050.

11. Fuster V. The clinical history. In: Giuliani ER, et al., eds. Cardiology: fundamentals and practice. Mosby-Year Book, Inc., St. Louis, MO: 1991; pp. 189–203.
12. Young JB, Farmer JA. The diagnostic evaluation of patients with heart failure. In Hosenpud JD, Greenberg BH, eds. Congestive heart failure: pathophysiology, diagnosis, and comprehensive approach to management. Springer-Verlag, New York: 1994, pp. 597–621.
13. Braunwald E. The history. In: Braunwald E, ed. Heart disease: a textbook of cardiovascular medicine. 5th ed. W.B. Saunders, Philadelphia, PA: 1997; pp.1 14.
14. Cheyne J. A case of apoplexy in which the fleshy part of the heart was converted into fat. In: Major RH, ed. Classic descriptions of disease. 3rd ed. Charles C. Thomas, Springfield, IL: 1945, pp. 550–552.
15. Ingraham RH Jr, Braunwald E. Dyspnea and pulmonary edema. In Wilson JD, et al., eds. Harrison's principles of internal medicine. 12th ed. McGraw-Hill, New York: 1991, pp. 223,224.
16. Mahler DA, Harver A, Lentine T, et al. Descriptors of breathlessness in cardiorespiratory diseases. Am J Respir Crit Care Med 1996:154:1357–1363.
17. Sgarbossa E, Wagner G. Electrocardiography. In Topol EJ, ed. Textbook of cardiovascular medicine. Lippincott-Raven, Philadelphia, PA: 1998, p. 1582.
18. Waxman AB. Pulmonary function test abnormalities in pulmonary vascular disease and chronic heart failure. Clin Chest Med 2001;22:751–758.
19. Gibbons RJ, Balady GJ, Beasley JW, et al. ACC/AHA guidelines for exercise testing: a report of the American College of Cardiology/American Heart Association task force on practice guidelines. J Amer Coll Cardiol 1997;30:260–315.
20. Borg G. Subjective effort and physical activities. Scand J Rehab Med 1978;6:108–113.
21. Myers J, Madhavan R. Exercise testing with gas exchange analysis. Cardiology Clinics 2001;19:433–445.
22. Wasserman K. Diagnosing cardiovascular and lung pathophysiology from exercise gas exchange. Chest 1997;112:1091–1101.

4 Heart Failure and Fatigue

Eric D. Popjes, MD

INTRODUCTION

Fatigue is one of the hallmark symptoms of heart failure and is present in a majority of patients. It leads to great limitation in physical activity and has a negative impact on quality of life. It occurs regardless of the etiology of the heart failure, is usually insidious in onset, and is an important part of the classification of symptom severity. Despite these facts, it is a symptom that can be difficult to quantify and difficult to distinguish from dyspnea, the other hallmark symptom of heart failure. It is a subjective complaint that has no single objective test to measure it. In addition, it can be multifactorial in origin. It is not adequately explained by a reduced cardiac output alone, and other factors such as peripheral muscle and vasculature abnormalities, neuroendocrine

From: *Contemporary Cardiology: Heart Failure:*
A Clinician's Guide to Ambulatory Diagnosis and Treatment
Edited by: M. L. Jessup and E. Loh © Humana Press Inc., Totowa, NJ

changes, depression, side effects of therapy, sleep disturbances, and other concomitant diseases all need to be considered as etiologic factors.

REDUCED CARDIAC OUTPUT

Regardless of the etiology, heart failure is defined as the inability to provide adequate oxygen supply in order to meet the body's demands. This applies to both the resting and active states and results in significant vasoconstriction and the shunting of blood toward vital organs and away from peripheral structures. Given this information, it makes sense to say that fatigue in heart failure is secondary to a lack of adequate skeletal muscle perfusion, oxygen delivery, and subsequent anaerobic metabolism. However, reduced cardiac output alone is insufficient to explain fatigue in all patients.

Dyspnea, or a feeling of breathlessness, is perhaps the most common complaint of heart failure patients. It is classically explained using the backward heart failure theory. A failing heart results in an elevation of intracardiac pressures, which then results in elevated pulmonary vein and intra-alveolar pressures. The end results are increased alveolar stiffness, reduced area for gas exchange, and resistance to airflow, all of which contribute to the perception of breathlessness.

The problem with distinguishing between dyspnea and fatigue, or backward and forward heart failure, is that there is much overlap. Frequently, there is no clinically significant difference between patients with dyspnea, fatigue, or both, yet their perceptions are clearly different. Monitoring hemodynamics with exertion may show similar results between patients, but the patients themselves describe very different symptoms (1,2). In addition, different forms of exercise can result in different symptoms despite similar workloads and hemodynamics (3). Slow gradual protocols result in more fatigue, whereas fast ramping protocols may result in dyspnea as the major complaint.

The inadequacy of explaining fatigue solely on the basis of a low cardiac output has also been demonstrated in other studies. Venous oxygen content of veins draining exercising muscle is little changed in some cases despite fatigue. Also, normalizing cardiac output with medical therapy such as inotropes is still inadequate to relieve symptoms in some (4). These facts suggest that some of the symptoms are a result of abnormalities in oxygen use rather than its delivery.

Low cardiac output and forward flow have significant effects on the rest of the body that may also explain fatigue. Hypotension will result in central nervous effects. Decreased renal perfusion results in elevation of the blood urea nitrogen level and stimulation of the release of antidiuretic hormone. Uremia and hyponatremia (a harbinger of poor outcome [5]) can ensue, either of which can cause fatigue and lethargy. Long-standing renal insufficiency results in low erythropoetin levels and anemia. Anemia may also be secondary to chronic disease in those with long-standing heart failure. Gastrointestinal congestion from right-ventricular failure can lead to fatigue by causing anorexia, poor nutrition or liver dysfunction and its subsequent effects. Hypoxia, secondary to pulmonary congestion, is rare in heart failure except in severe or acute cases but may cause fatigue at rest or with minimal exertion.

PERIPHERAL MUSCLE ABNORMALITIES

In many respects, the peripheral muscles of patients with heart failure are abnormal. Atrophy, malnutrition, decreased perfusion, disuse, and neurohormonal and immunologic effects all contribute to abnormal muscle function, which result in muscle fatigue and poor exercise tolerance. These effects occur in both skeletal and respiratory muscle and can be partially attenuated by consistent exercise and training.

Muscle atrophy can be obvious in patients with cachexia but is less obvious in many others. However, magnetic resonance imaging (MRI) and creatinine/height index have demonstrated lower muscle mass in patients with heart failure in comparison to those without heart failure (6). In addition, biopsy specimens have also shown atrophy of individual fibers (7). The degree of atrophy is associated with VO_2, suggesting that this is a component of the mechanism underlying exercise intolerance Data on peripheral muscle strength in heart failure is not consistent, but there appears to be a trend toward increased weakness. On the other hand, testing of muscle endurance has shown early fatigue with repetitive contractions and maintenance of contraction (7).

Histologically, there are many abnormalities seen in the muscle of heart failure patients. There appears to be an increase in the percentage of type II fibers, mostly a result of decrease in the type I fibers that are associated with endurance (8,9). Evaluation of mitochondria reveals a decrease in their density, a decrease in surface area of the cristae, and staining for cytochrome oxidase (10). These findings suggest a decrease in oxidative metabolism and less reliance on aerobic metabolism. There is also a decrease in intracellular lipid and glycogen content, signifying fewer energy stores (8,11).

Evaluation of phosphate metabolism and muscle pH with the use of MRI also suggests a move toward an increase in anaerobic or glycolytic metabolism (12,13). With exercise, there is a more pronounced increase in the inorganic phosphate to phosphocreatine ratio, which correlates with adenosine diphosphate (ADP) concentration. An increase in ADP means less adenosine triphosphate (ATP) and less oxidative metabolism. Postexertion recovery of phosphocreatine in heart failure patients is also delayed. Muscle pH decreases progressively with and at all levels of exercise, as opposed to control patients, who have no decrease until peak exercise. Lactate production and release occurs more rapidly in heart failure patients as well *(14–16)*. These metabolic changes do not immediately normalize after restoration of normal blood flow and take time to reverse.

Nervous system activation of the muscle seems to be intact and not contributing to muscle fatigue. Central motor drive and signaling and the neuromuscular junction both appear to have normal function, indicating that the problem lies within the muscle alone. Importantly, however, afferent nerve fibers that originate in the muscles themselves may sense the abnormalities that occur and send signals back to the central nervous system, leading to perceptions of fatigue and dyspnea (frequently called the ergoreflex).

Abnormal action potentials within the muscles may also contribute to fatigue and weakness. There appears to be perturbations of sodium and potassium balance that favors depolarization and, hence, smaller action potentials. With continued exercise, muscle weakness may occur secondary to abnormal calcium handling (release and reuptake) as well *(17)*.

Consistent exercise and training play a vital role in the treatment of heart failure. Multiple studies from clinical, biochemical, and cellular aspects have shown marked improvements in muscle abnormalities, exercise tolerance, and fatigue in patients with heart failure who undergo training. These investigations occurred with concurrent medical therapy and were done with at least 3 weeks of training. They have also shown that these improvements quickly revert with restriction of activity and occur independent of central hemodynamics *(18,19)*.

Clinically, heart rate decreases, perceptions of fatigue and dyspnea lessen, and exercise tolerance improves. Physiologic improvements include improved O_2 uptake and consumption and decreased lactate production *(19)*. There is a delay in reaching the anaerobic threshold, an increase in oxidative capacity and cytochrome oxidase activity, and increased ATP synthesis and phosphocreatine recovery *(18,20)*. Histologically, there is an increase in type I and II fibers, decreased fiber atrophy, and increased muscle mass *(21)*. On the vascular level, blood flow to trained muscles is increased.

The abnormalities that are seen in the peripheral muscles of heart failure patients are also seen in muscles of respiration. There is atrophy, increased lactate production, and muscle hypoxia. Diaphragmatic work increases and maximal voluntary and sustainable ventilation is decreased (22). The mechanisms responsible are thought to be the same as elsewhere. Significantly, the benefits of exercise seen in peripheral muscles are manifest in the muscles of respiration as well.

VASCULAR ABNORMALITIES

As mentioned previously, part of the body's response to a reduced cardiac output is to increase vasoconstriction in order to maintain flow and pressure to vital organs. The normal response to exercise is to increase cardiac output and vasodilatation, but in the setting of heart failure, both of these responses are blunted. Because the peripheral muscles are structures that blood flow is shunted away from, the fatigue induced by exertion in heart failure may be, in part, owing to inadequate flow of blood (and therefore oxygen and nutrients) to skeletal muscles.

The vasoconstriction that occurs in heart failure is thought to be caused by two basic mechanisms—endothelial dysfunction and neurohormonal activation. The former is apparently closely associated with a reduced stimulation of nitric oxide release from endothelial cells and elevated levels of tumor necrosis factor-alpha (TNF-α) (23). TNF-α appears to increase endothelial permeability, cause changes in cell structure, and decrease expression of constitutive nitric oxide synthetase (24). To some degree, endothelial dysfunction can improve with exercise training (25). Neurohormonal activation in heart failure includes activation of the sympathetic nervous and renin-angiotensin systems and stimulation of vasopressin release.

The use of vasodilators to improve muscle flow has met with marginal success. The maximal effects do not occur acutely but after chronic use (26). The full benefits of vasodilatation occur over time, perhaps because of structural abnormalities of the vessels that can not be overcome in the acute setting. In addition, restoration of flow to normal levels does not necessarily result in an increase in exercise tolerance or a decrease in muscle fatigue, indicating that vasoconstriction by itself is not sufficient to explain these symptoms.

NEUROENDOCRINE CHANGES

As mentioned, heart failure is a condition in which there is significant neurohormonal activation. Catecholamines are elevated and intricately involved in vasoconstriction and left-ventricular remodeling. Activation of the renin-angiotensin system leads to sodium and water retention and vasoconstriction. Vasopressin causes vasoconstriction but also leads to free water retention and, potentially, hyponatremia. All of these effects can cause fatigue via electrolyte abnormalities, further reduction in cardiac output, reduced skeletal muscle blood flow, renal insufficiency, or other mechanisms.

Recently, TNF-α levels have been found to be significantly elevated in heart failure. Levels appear to correlate with prognosis and the severity of hemodynamic disarray and increase directly with New York Heart Association (NYHA) class *(27)*. TNF-α itself can induce heart failure when infused into experimental animals (directly via effects on calcium and indirectly through changes in nitric oxide production), stimulate apoptosis and activation of the renin-angiotensin system, and cause endothelial dysfunction *(28–32)*. One hypothesis that has been proposed is its potential role in idiopathic/viral-induced cardiomyopathy. TNF-α production and release are stimulated by viral replication. If it is truly toxic to cardiac myocytes, it may play a critical immunologic role in the pathogenesis and progression of certain viral-related cardiomyopathies. The exact cause and effect role that TNF-α plays is not clearly defined and further investigation is needed in this field.

One striking characteristic of some heart failure patients is marked and progressive cachexia, profound muscle wasting, and decreases in lean tissue, fat, and bone mass *(33,34)*. They are weaker, more anemic and anorexic, quicker to fatigue, and have a worse prognosis than patients without cachexia independent of age, left ventricular ejection fraction (LVEF), peak VO_2, sodium levels, and NYHA class *(35)*. Mortality at 18 months in cachectic heart failure patients is 50% *(36)*. Interestingly, TNF-α levels are elevated mainly in patients with cachexia *(37,38)*. It is believed to have significant direct catabolic effects and other indirect effects via cortisol, which itself is catabolic and is also increased in heart failure patients with cachexia *(39)*. In experimental animals, implantation of TNF-α-producing tumors into skeletal muscle results in wasting of that muscle, whereas implantation in the brain causes anorexia *(40)*. The apoptosis-inducing effect of TNF-α may also play a role in cachexia. However, TNF-α and cortisol may not be the only cachexia-inducing culprits. Epinephrine and norepinephrine levels are generally higher in cachectic heart failure patients and can cause a shift toward the catabolic state *(41)*. The renin-angiotensin system is also activated, but the significance of this in the etiology of cachexia is not known.

The presence of cachexia and neurohormonal and cytokine activation stress the importance of several critical aspects of the treatment of the heart failure patient. Nutritional aspects, such as the help of dietitians and consideration of drug side effects that effect nutrition (nausea and vomiting with many drugs, effects on the sense of taste by angiotensin-converting enzyme [ACE] inhibitors) need to considered throughout. Routine exercise, perhaps with the help of physical therapists, can reduce atrophy and neurohormone levels and improve peripheral blood flow. Newer drug therapies are under investigation to block cytokines and their apparent effects (TNF-α receptor blockers), and other drugs (growth hormone, anabolic steroids) that counter the catabolic state that exists in many heart failure patients may be of theoretical benefit in some patients.

DEPRESSION

The Diagnostic and Statistical Manual defines major depression by the presence of a depressed mood or sadness and or a lack of interest or pleasure in life events accompanied by varying degrees of appetite changes, sleep disturbances, weight gain or loss, guilt, hopelessness, suicidal ideation, and fatigue (42). The complaints must be at least 2 weeks in duration and must not be organic in origin or secondary to bereavement or grief.

In general, fatigue is present in a majority of patients with depression and depression has been estimated to be present in 13 to 35% of patients with heart failure (43–45). It tends to be more prevalent in heart failure patients than in those with other cardiac diseases (46), such as chronic angina, and is more commonly diagnosed in women with heart failure (although in the population at large, women are also diagnosed with depression more frequently) (47). Potential explanations for the higher prevalence in women may be that men tend to tolerate their symptoms better or minimize them more.

There is no doubt that depression plays a major role in terms of overall well-being and life satisfaction. Heart failure is a demanding physical and emotional stress to both the patient and family and can greatly impact quality of life. In the study by Dracup et al. (46), 134 heart failure patients reported that depression was the greatest factor affecting their quality of life, more so than dyspnea, edema, or physical limitation, although each are all closely associated with depression. Importantly, there was significant improvement in the patients in this group who underwent transplantation, and those who refused transplant were more severely depressed.

The presence of depression in the heart failure patient seems to affect the perception of limitation. Data indicates that those who are depressed subjectively perceive themselves as more limited than those without depression, although objective evidence (stress testing with VO_2 or invasive hemodynamic monitoring) indicates little difference in exercise tolerance between the two groups. In addition, there appears to be an association between NYHA classification (of which fatigue is a major component) and depression, indicating that both the patient and clinician's assessments can be influenced by the presence of depression in the patient *(44)*.

In many instances, it has been shown that heart failure patients with depression have a higher mortality than those without depression *(44,48)*. The reasons for this association are not known, but theories abound. Some have speculated that it is secondary to an underlying neurohormonal abnormality that causes the central nervous system effects of depression (serotonin, dopamine) and perpetuates cardiac failure *(49)*. Others have suggested that depressed patients are simply less compliant with their medical regimen, which leads to less benefit and shortened survival. Still others have suggested that those who are depressed often have other lifestyle risks, such as cigarette and alcohol use, poor nutrition, or a lack of exercise that increases mortality.

The key to treatment of depression in heart failure patients (or any patient for that matter) is to ask the patients about it. Ask about their mood, interests, sleep, appetite, degree of fatigue, and energy level. Asking and talking about it is often revealing for the doctor and patient alike and may make patients feel better knowing that all the aspects of their care are covered and considered. In addition to asking, one should listen to patient concerns and worries and to those of family members. Providing support individually or through heart failure support groups can do more than any antidepressant ever will. Finally, do not minimize complaints. They may be subtle clues to major problems.

Throughout all these aspects of care, the use of an antidepressant should be considered. In general, the serotonin reuptake inhibitors are well tolerated by most heart failure patients. Side effects from antidepressants are few but can vary from drug to drug (i.e., insomnia, somnolence, and impotence). Wellbutrin is also relatively safe in heart failure patients and, given its negative effects on cigarette cravings, may be particularly useful in patients who are smokers. Tricyclic antidepressants are generally avoided or used when others fail because of their potential side effects (tachycardia, QRS and QT prolongation on ECG, cardiac depressant effects).

SLEEP DISTURBANCES

Whether they are aware of it or not, many patients with heart failure have difficulty with or abnormalities of sleep. If patients do not give a history of this, their spouses or other family members often will. Nights are often spent in a restless state with frequent arousals or limited time in the deep stages of sleep. This inevitably leads to daytime drowsiness and fatigue.

Patients with heart failure resulting in pulmonary congestion with the supine position suffer from orthopnea and paroxysmal nocturnal dyspnea. This necessitates sitting propped up in bed on pillows or sleeping in a chair, positions that usually lack comfort for adequate rest. More aggressive medical treatment, especially with daytime diuretics, and the purchase of an adjustable bed may provide some relief in these circumstances.

Another significant nightime complaint of heart failure patients is nocturia. During the day when the patient is in upright and active, there is constriction of the renal vasculature, thereby limiting urine production. When the patient assumes the resting, supine position at night, there is a decrease in vasoconstriction and an increase in renal blood flow and urine production. Compounding this physiology is the use of diuretics. Most heart failure patients take duiretics. Many need twice-a-day dosing of a loop diuretic, the second dose of which may have lingering effects into the night. Others are taking once-daily diuretics (metolazone, hydrochlorothiazide), whose effects can last throughout the night. The end result is several trips to the bathroom during the night and interrupted sleep.

Perhaps one of the interesting aspects of heart failure is its association with Cheyne-Stokes respiration and central sleep apnea (CSR-CSA). Research in the last 10 years has shown that up to 40–50% of heart failure patients suffer from CSR-CSA, regardless of the etiology of the heart failure (50,51). CSR-CSA has been shown to occur with systolic and diastolic dysfunction and is an independent risk factor for increased mortality and atrial and ventricular arrhythmias (50,52,53). CSR-CSA is defined in terms of the number of episodes of apnea or hypopnea that occur per hour of sleep (the apnea-hypopnea index [AHI]) and is manifested by frequent episodes of arousal, hypoxia, hypercapnia, and hypertension. Most investigators use an AHI of 10–20 per hour to distinguish patients with CSR-CSA.

The sleep of patients with CSR-CSA is greatly disrupted and certainly not restful. They spend more time in the early, less deep stages of sleep (stages 1 and 2) and less time in stages 3 and 4 and REM sleep (54). Consequently, by the time these patients awake in the morning, the amount of time spent in restful and quality sleep was limited, and their subsequent waking hours are marked by fatigue and drowsiness.

The mechanism of the association between heart failure and CSR-CSA appears to be quite complex and is probably self-perpetuating via the initiation of a vicious cycle of events. A common link between the two is sympathetic activation and an elevation in catecholamine levels (55,56). Heart failure stimulates the sympathetic system via low cardiac output and hypotension, whereas CSR-CSA revs up the system via repetitive arousals and desaturations. The end result of each is an increase in afterload, reduction in cardiac output, hypoxia, myocardial ischemia, and a worsening of each causative process.

In addition, it is possible that heart failure patients are hypersensitive to changes in CO_2 that occur during sleep (57,58). The medullary chemoreceptors in the brainstem are the central point of feedback loops that regulate respiration. Normally, small changes in CO_2 stimulate changes in respiration and ventilation to bring levels back to baseline. During sleep, average CO_2 levels tend to rise slightly to a higher baseline. In heart failure patients, this small fluctuation seems to stimulate a hyperventilatory response that results in marked decreases in CO_2, which in turn causes apnea. CO_2 levels then begin to rise again, and the process repeats itself.

Treatment of CSR-CSA is both direct and indirect. Various therapies have been studied in order to improve breathing and respiration. Respiratory stimulants, such as theophylline and diamox, can result in a reduction of the AHI and duration of desaturations but data on symptoms is not present (59,60). Nasal O_2 at night also reduces the AHI, and has also been shown to decrease sensitivity to CO_2 and daytime sleepiness and improve exercise tolerance (61–63). It is also a therapy that is well tolerated by most patients.

Mechanical support of breathing with the use of continuous and bilevel positive airway pressure (CPAP and BiPAP) and newer devices are the most studied of all the direct therapies. These devices work by providing forced breaths during episodes of apnea and support during periods of ventilation. The downfalls of some of these machines are that they can work against breathing at times and are poorly tolerated by some. Despite this, there is good evidence for their usage. O_2 saturation increases, CO_2 levels are elevated above apneic levels, and the AHI can be greatly reduced (52). Heart rate and afterload decrease and inspiratory muscle strength has been shown to improve (64). Substantial increases in LVEF, reductions in the degree of mitral regurgitation, and improved hemodynamics have all been shown after the use of CPAP, and there are also decreases in catecholamine and natriuretic peptide levels (55,65). Most importantly, however, the use of these devices has made patients feel better as a result of decreased fatigue, daytime drowsiness, and dyspnea (64).

The indirect treatment of CSR-CSA involves the treatment of the underlying heart failure. The use of ACE inhibitors has been shown to decrease the AHI and to improve some symptoms (66), but data for diuretics and digoxin is lacking or unconvincing. Of particular interest is the recent advance in recognizing the utility of β-blockers in the treatment of heart failure. Given their effects on the sympathetic nervous system, it will be interesting to see if their use will have significant effects on CSR-CSA. Most of the trials that have shown improvements in CSR-CSA with treatment (CPAP, BiPAP, O_2, ACE inhibitors) did not involve a great percentage of patients on β-blockers. Perhaps their use will be of greater benefit than other currently available therapies.

Finally, surgical treatment has shown to improve CSR-CSA. In studies of patients who have undergone cardiac transplantation, there is improvement or resolution of their breathing disorder and great improvement in symptoms (67). Other surgical procedures to correct or improve the underlying heart failure, such as coronary artery bypass or valve replacement, may also be of great benefit.

TREATMENT SIDE EFFECTS

The list of medications taken by a heart failure patient at any one particular time is usually long. Most are on anywhere from two to seven medications for heart failure alone, then other medications to treat their other medical problems. If one medication does not give them side effects, another one likely will, and then they may be prescribed another medication to treat these side effects. In addition, there are potential interactions of all of these drugs together—it is no wonder the patient gets tired of swallowing pills, and the doctor has trouble keeping track of all the potential interactions and effects.

Many of the drugs used to treat heart failure can cause fatigue by one mechanism or another. Fatigue may be caused by hypotension, bradycardia, central nervous depression, worsened cardiac output, hypovolemia, electrolyte disturbances, or depressed mood from taking so many pills and enduring their side effects.

Vasodilators, such has ACE inhibitors, angiotensin receptor blockers (ARBs), and hydralazine, can have profound effects in heart failure patients even in small doses. ACE inhibitors may need to be discontinued in up to 4–5% of patients because of hypotension and subsequent fatigue and dizziness (68). They may also induce significant renal insufficiency, which can lead to uremia, fatigue, and lethargy. For these reasons, doses should be started small and increased slowly and renal function and electrolytes should be closely monitored. ARBs have similar effects but are also reported to cause somnolence, confusion, depression, and fatigue as direct side effects. Hydralazine is known to cause a lupus-like syndrome, depression, profound hypotension, and anemia—all of which can result in significant fatigue.

β-Blockers are notorious for causing fatigue in many patients to whom they are prescribed, especially early after induction. The mechanisms of this fatigue are usually numerous. Some patients experience significant bradycardia or other cardiac conduction abnormalities that can result in hypotension and a reduction in cardiac output. In patients with heart failure, initiation of β-blocker therapy can result in a clinically important effect on myocardial contractility and, therefore, directly worsen forward flow and symptoms. Direct central nervous effects of β-blockers, which can occur in 1–2% of patients, include depression, lassitude, and sleep disturbances *(68)*. Using a β-blocker that tends to be more water-soluble (tenormin) as opposed to lipid-soluble (metoprolol) may lesson some of these effects. Whereas the chronic use of these drugs in heart failure patients has been shown to be of great benefit in mortality and morbidity of heart function, their acute effects may be difficult to overcome and may require patience, time, persistence, and adjustment of other medications.

Diuretics play a critical role in the treatment of most heart failure patients, greatly improving dyspnea and peripheral edema, but they can affect changes that can result in fatigue. Loop diuretics can cause profound dehydration, hypovolemia, hypotension, renal insufficiency, and electrolyte disturbances (hypokalemia, hypomagnesemia, hypernatremia) and each one of these can, in turn, cause significant fatigue. Other effects include muscle aches and weakness, lethargy, and drowsiness. Although aldactone and metolazone are not potent diuretics, when they are combined with loop diuretics, they can greatly increase urine production and potentiate all of the above effects. Aldactone is also known to cause drowsiness, confusion, and lethargy probably through a central depressant effect. Finally, with all diuretics, nocturia can lead to limited sleep at night and excessive daytime drowsiness and fatigue. Minor changes in the timing of diuretic doses can result in a great reduction in nocturia and improvement in nightime sleep.

Most people tolerate digoxin very well. As long as electrolytes are closely monitored and the dose of the drug is adjusted for renal insufficiency, side effects are rare and toxicity exceptional. However, in any heart failure patient presenting with fatigue, lassitude, nausea, bradycardia, or visual complaints, an EKG and serum digoxin level should be considered in order to evaluate the possibility of toxicity. Like other heart failure medications, digoxin can cause certain central nervous effects, such as apathy and psychosis.

CONCOMITANT DISEASE

Simply stated, fatigue is a complex symptom. It is a nonspecific complaint that can result from numerous disease processes. Abnormali-

Table 1
Differential Diagnosis of Fatigue

Heart failure
Depression
Sleep disturbances
Medication side effects
Anemia
Renal insufficiency
Liver dysfunction
Thyroid disease
Pulmonary disease
Diabetes
Infection
Collagen vascular disorder
Alcoholism
Malnutrition
Poor physical conditioning
Chronic fatigue syndrome

ties in nearly every organ system can result in fatigue, making the differential diagnosis extensive. The presence of heart failure only makes the problem more complicated because many patients with heart failure also have concomitant diseases, related or unrelated to their heart failure, that should not be forgotten. The typical patient with heart failure is not infrequently anemic, deconditioned, diabetic, and depressed, and has obstructive lung disease and/or renal insufficiency. This patient may also be at higher risk for certain cancers because of age or may be prone to infection because of age or chronic disease. Considering all of these problems and others, and distinguishing the role of each in the etiology of the patient's symptoms is often a clinical nightmare. Table 1 is a partial list of the causes of fatigue, many of which can be caused by or are a cause of heart failure.

Despite a potentially complicated situation, the approach to the patient remains the same in most cases. A detailed history and review of systems (or symptoms) and a complete physical examination, including a mental status exam, will provide much of the information needed to narrow down or make the diagnosis or will direct the need for further laboratory testing.

REFERENCES

1. Lipkin DP, Poole-Wilson PA. Symptoms limiting exercise in chronic heart failure. Br Med J (Clin Res Ed) 1986;292:1030,1031.

2. Clark AL, Sparrow JL, Coats AJ. Muscle fatigue and dyspnoea in chronic heart failure: two sides of the same coin? Eur Heart J 1995;16:49–52.

3. Lipkin DP, Canepa-Anson R, Stephens MR, et al. Factors determining symptoms in heart failure: comparison of fast and slow exercise tests. Br Heart J 1986;55:439–445.

4. Mancini DM, Schwartz M, Ferraro N, et al. Effect of dobutamine on skeletal muscle metabolism in patients with congestive heart failure. Am J Cardiol 1990;65:1121–1126.

5. Panciroli C, Galloni G, Oddone A, et al. Prognostic value of hyponatremia in patients with severe chronic heart failure. Angiology 1990;41:631–638.

6. Mancini DM, Walter G, Reichek N, et al. Contribution of skeletal muscle atrophy to exercise intolerance and altered muscle metabolism in heart failure. Circulation 1992;85:1364–1373.

7. Minotti JR, Pillay P, Oka R, et al. Skeletal muscle size: relationship to muscle function in heart failure. J Appl Physiol 1993;75:373–381.

8. Lipkin DP, Jones DA, Round JM, et al. Abnormalities of skeletal muscle in patients with chronic heart failure. Int J Cardiol 1988;18:187–195.

9. Mancini DM, Coyle E, Loggan A, et al. Contribution of intrinsic skeletal muscle changes to 31P NMR skeletal muscle metabolic abnormalities in patients with chronic heart failure. Circulation 1989;80:1338–1346.

10. Drexler H, Riede U, Munzel T, et al. Alterations of skeletal muscle in chronic heart failure. Circulation 1992;85:1751–1759.

11. Sullivan MJ, Green HJ, Cobb FR. Skeletal muscle biochemistry and histology in ambulatory patients with long-term heart failure. Circulation 1990;81:518–527.

12. Massie BM, Conway M, Yonge R, et al. 31P nuclear magnetic resonance evidence of abnormal skeletal muscle metabolism in patients with congestive heart failure. Am J Cardiol 1987;60:309–315.

13. Wilson JR, Fink L, Maris J, et al. Evaluation of energy metabolism in skeletal muscle of patients with heart failure with gated phosphorus-31 nuclear magnetic resonance. Circulation 1985;71:57–62.

14. Wilson JR, Martin JL, Schwartz D, et al. Exercise intolerance in patients with chronic heart failure: role of impaired nutritive flow to skeletal muscle. Circulation 1984;69:1079–1087.

15. Weber KT, Janicki JS. Lactate production during maximal and submaximal exercise in patients with chronic heart failure. J Am Coll Cardiol 1985;6:717–724.

16. Sullivan MJ, Higginbotham MB, Cobb FR. Increased exercise ventilation in patients with chronic heart failure: intact ventilatory control despite hemodynamic and pulmonary abnormalities. Circulation 1988;77:552–559.

17. Lunde PK, Verburg E, Vollestad NK, et al. Skeletal muscle fatigue in normal subjects and heart failure patients. Is there a common mechanism? Acta Physiol Scand 1998;162:215–228.

18. Minotti JR, Johnson EC, Hudson TL, et al. Skeletal muscle response to exercise training in congestive heart failure. J Clin Invest 1990;86:751–758.

19. Meyer K, Schwaibold M, Westbrook S, et al. Effects of short-term exercise training and activity restriction on functional capacity in patients with severe chronic congestive heart failure. Am J Cardiol 1996;78:1017–1022.

20. Hambrecht R, Niebauer J, Fiehn E, et al. Physical training in patients with stable chronic heart failure: effects on cardiorespiratory fitness and ultrastructural abnormalities of leg muscles. J Am Coll Cardiol 1995;25:1239–1249.

21. Belardinelli R, Georgiou D, Scocco V, et al. Low intensity exercise training in patients with chronic heart failure. J Am Coll Cardiol 1995;26:975–982.

22. Mancini DM, Henson D, La Manca J, et al. Respiratory muscle function and dyspnea in patients with chronic congestive heart failure. Circulation 1992;86:909–918.

23. Tracey KJ, Cerami A. Tumor necrosis factor, other cytokines and disease. Annu Rev Cell Biol 1993; 9:317–343.

24. Linke A, Schoene N, Gielen S, et al. Endothelial dysfunction in patients with chronic heart failure: systemic effects of lower-limb exercise training. J Am Coll Cardiol 2001;37:392–397.
25. Hambrecht R, Fiehn E, Weigl C, et al. Regular physical exercise corrects endothelial dysfunction and improves exercise capacity in patients with chronic heart failure. Circulation 1998;98:2709–2715.
26. Jeserich M, Pape L, Just H, et al. Effect of long-term angiotensin-converting enzyme inhibition on vascular function in patients with chronic congestive heart failure. Am J Cardiol 1995;76:1079–1082.
27. Kapadia SR, Yakoob K, Nader S, et al. Elevated circulating levels of serum tumor necrosis factor-alpha in patients with hemodynamically significant pressure and volume overload. J Am Coll Cardiol 2000;36:208–212.
28. Habib FM, Springall DR, Davies GJ, et al. Tumour necrosis factor and inducible nitric oxide synthase in dilated cardiomyopathy. Lancet 1996;347:1151–1155.
29. Satoh M, Nakamura M, Tamura G, et al. Inducible nitric oxide synthase and tumor necrosis factor alpha in myocardium in human dilated cardiomyopathy. J Am Coll Cardiol 1997;29:716–724.
30. Kubota T, Miyagishima M, Frye CS, et al. Overexpression of tumor necrosis factor-alpha activates both anti- and pro-apoptotic pathways in the myocardium. J Mol Cell Cardiol 2001;33:1331–1344.
31. Agnoletti L, Curello S, Bachetti T, et al. Serum from patients with severe heart failure downregulates eNOS and is proapoptotic: role of tumor necrosis factor-alpha. Circulation 1999;100:1983–1991.
32. Dalla Libera L, Sabbadini R, Renken C, et al. Apoptosis in the skeletal muscle of rats with heart failure is associated with increased serum levels of TNF-alpha and sphingosine. J Mol Cell Cardiol 2001;33:1871–1878.
33. Anker SD, Ponikowski PP, Clark AL, et al. Cytokines and neurohormones relating to body composition alterations in the wasting syndrome of chronic heart failure. Eur Heart J 1999;20:683–693.
34. Anker SD, Clark AL, Texeira MM, et al. Loss of bone mineral in patients with cachexia due to chronic heart failure. Am J Cardiol 1999;83:612–615, A10.
35. Anker SD, Swan JW, Volterrani M, et al. The influence of muscle mass, strength, fatigability and blood flow on exercise capacity in cachectic and non-cachectic patients with chronic heart failure. Eur Heart J 1997;18:259–269.
36. Anker SD, Coats AJ. Cachexia in heart failure is bad for you. Eur Heart J 1998;19:191–193.
37. Levine B, Kalman J, Mayer L, et al. Elevated circulating levels of tumor necrosis factor in severe chronic heart failure. N Engl J Med 1990;323:236–241.
38. McMurray J, Abdullah I, Dargie HJ, et al. Increased concentrations of tumour necrosis factor in "cachectic" patients with severe chronic heart failure. Br Heart J 1991;66:356–358.
39. Anker SD, Clark AL, Kemp M, et al. Tumor necrosis factor and steroid metabolism in chronic heart failure: possible relation to muscle wasting. J Am Coll Cardiol 1997;30:997–1001.
40. Tracey KJ, Morgello S, Koplin B, et al. Metabolic effects of cachectin/tumor necrosis factor are modified by site of production. Cachectin/tumor necrosis factor-secreting tumor in skeletal muscle induces chronic cachexia, while implantation in brain induces predominantly acute anorexia. J Clin Invest 1990;86:2014–2024.
41. Anker SD, Chua TP, Ponikowski P, et al. Hormonal changes and catabolic/anabolic imbalance in chronic heart failure and their importance for cardiac cachexia. Circulation 1997;96:526–534.

42. Diagnostic and Statistical Manual for Mental Disorders: DSM-IV. American Psychiatric Association, Washington, DC: 1994, p. 358.
43. Koenig HG. Depression in hospitalized older patients with congestive heart failure. Gen Hosp Psychiatry 1998;20:29–43.
44. Murberg TA, Bru E, Srebak S, et al. Depressed mood and subjective health symptoms as predictors of mortality in patients with congestive heart failure: a two-years follow- up study. Int J Psychiatry Med 1999;29:311–326.
45. Freedland KE, Carney R, Rich MW, et al. Depression in elderly patients with congestive heart failure. J Geriatric Psychiatry 1991;24:59–71.
46. Dracup K, Walden JA, Stevenson LW, et al. Quality of life in patients with advanced heart failure. J Heart Lung Transplant 1992;11:273–279.
47. Murberg TA, Bru E, Aarsland T, et al. Functional status and depression among men and women with congestive heart failure. Int J Psychiatry Med 1998;28:273–291.
48. Vaccarino V, Kasi SV, Abramson J, et al. Depressive symptoms and risk of functional decline and death in patients with heart failure. J Am Coll Cardiol 2001;38:199–205.
49. Guiry E, Conroy RM, Hickey N, et al. Psychological response to an acute coronary event and its effect on subsequent rehabilitation and lifestyle change. Clin Cardiol 1987;10:256–260.
50. Javaheri S, Parker TJ, Liming JD, et al. Sleep apnea in 81 ambulatory male patients with stable heart failure. Types and their prevalences, consequences, and presentations. Circulation 1998;97:2154–2159.
51. Javaheri S, Parker TJ, Wexler L, et al. Occult sleep-disordered breathing in stable congestive heart failure. Ann Intern Med 1995;122:487–492.
52. Chan J, Sanderson J, Chan W, et al. Prevalence of sleep-disordered breathing in diastolic heart failure. Chest 1997;111:1488–1493.
53. Burgess KR. Central sleep apnoea and heart failure (part II). Respirology 1998;3:1–11.
54. Hanly P, Zuberi-Khokhar N. Daytime sleepiness in patients with congestive heart failure and Cheyne- Stokes respiration. Chest 1995;107: 952–958.
55. Naughton MT, Benard DC, Liu PP, et al. Effects of nasal CPAP on sympathetic activity in patients with heart failure and central sleep apnea. Am J Respir Crit Care Med 1995;152:473–479.
56. Bradley TD, Floras JS. Pathophysiologic and therapeutic implications of sleep apnea in congestive heart failure. J Card Fail 1996;2:223–240.
57. Javaheri S. A mechanism of central sleep apnea in patients with heart failure. N Engl J Med 1999;341:949–954.
58. Wilcox I, McNamara SG, Dodd MJ, et al. Ventilatory control in patients with sleep apnoea and left ventricular dysfunction: comparison of obstructive and central sleep apnoea. Eur Respir J 1998;11:7–13.
59. Javaheri S, Parker TJ, Wexler L, et al. Effect of theophylline on sleep-disordered breathing in heart failure. N Engl J Med 1996;335:562–567.
60. DeBacker WA, Verbraecken J, Willemen M, et al. Central apnea index decreases after prolonged treatment with acetazolamide. Am J Respir Crit Care Med 1995;151:87–91.
61. Franklin KA, Eriksson P, Sahlin C, et al. Reversal of central sleep apnea with oxygen. Chest 1997;111:163–169.
62. Javaheri S, Ahmed M, Parker TJ, et al. Effects of nasal O2 on sleep-related disordered breathing in ambulatory patients with stable heart failure. Sleep 1999;22:1101–1106.
63. Andreas S, Clemens C, Sandholzer H, et al. Improvement of exercise capacity with treatment of Cheyne-Stokes respiration in patients with congestive heart failure. J Am Coll Cardiol 1996;27:1486–1490.

64. Granton JT, Naughton MT, Benard DC, et al. CPAP improves inspiratory muscle strength in patients with heart failure and central sleep apnea. Am J Respir Crit Care Med 1996;153:277–282.
65. Tkacova R, Rankin F, Fitzgerald FS, et al. Effect of continuous positive airway pressure on mitral regurgitant fraction and atrial natriuretic peptide in patients with heart failure. J Am Coll Cardiol 1997;30:739–745.
66. Walsh JT, Andrews R, Starling R, et al. Effects of captopril and oxygen on sleep apnoea in patients with mild to moderate congestive cardiac failure. Br Heart J 1995;73:237–241.
67. Skobel E, Kaminski R, Breuer C, et al. (Remission of nocturnal pathological respiratory patterns after orthotopic heart transplantation. A case report and overview of current status of therapy). Med Klin 2000;95:706–711.
68. Physicians' Desk Reference. 55th ed. Medical Economics Company, 2001.

5 Evaluation of Edema

Srihari S. Naidu, MD *and Ross Zimmer,* MD

INTRODUCTION

Edema is often the first clinical indication of significant heart failure. It is estimated that 5 L of water retention must occur prior to the development of overt edema *(1)*. Once detected by the patient or clinician, a thorough history and physical examination can lead to the tentative diagnosis of heart failure and can form the basis for further diagnostic testing to elucidate the underlying type of cardiac dysfunction.

In the patient with known heart failure, the development of new or worsening edema may indicate a decompensated state. Decompensation may be a result of medical or dietary noncompliance, an intercurrent new cardiac or renal insult, or progressive cardiac dysfunction despite medical therapy. The presence of new or worsening edema therefore warrants a complete re-evaluation of the patient and his or her medical regimen in order to reduce morbidity and improve survival.

Whereas the diagnosis of edema is simple, assigning a cardiac etiology often proves more difficult, as a variety of noncardiac etiologies can result in the development of edema. This chapter reviews the co-existent findings in the physical examination that indicate a cardiac cause of

From: *Contemporary Cardiology: Heart Failure:*
A Clinician's Guide to Ambulatory Diagnosis and Treatment
Edited by: M. L. Jessup and E. Loh © Humana Press Inc., Totowa, NJ

edema. Subsequent invasive and noninvasive testing then confirms or refutes a specific form of cardiac dysfunction, and the resolution of edema with tailored therapy can serve as indirect proof that the edema was, in fact, cardiac in origin.

For years, edema was believed to be a simple derangement in volume distribution, easily reversed by the judicious use of potent diuretic agents. However, it is now clear that the pathogenesis of edema is a complex process involving multiple neurohormonal pathways of abnormal salt and water handling by the kidneys. These complex pathways culminate in both salt and water retention, resulting in an expanded extravascular space. A complete understanding of these pathways, as well as the Starling forces responsible for extravasation of fluid into the interstitial space, results in a sophisticated approach to the treatment of edema in heart failure. Such an approach utilizes not only diuretics, but also agents that more fully block the abnormal renal homeostatic response to heart failure. Through this comprehensive approach to the management of edema, symptoms are alleviated and a positive effect on mortality is obtained.

ETIOLOGY OF EDEMA IN HEART FAILURE

Extracellular space is composed of two primary compartments: the intravascular space and the interstitial space. Typically, interstitial space contributes 75% of this extracellular space *(2)*. When total body volume increases because of an expansion of the interstitial space, edema formation is the result. Such edema may be localized to dependent areas or generalized to include the peritoneal, pleural, pericardial or diffuse subcutaneous spaces. This latter condition is known as anasarca and may occur in a variety of disease processes including severe congestive heart failure (CHF) *(3)*.

The rules governing edema formation at the microvascular level are based on the Starling forces, which are: (1) arteriolar hydrostatic pressure, (2) arteriolar oncotic pressure, (3) venular hydrostatic pressure, and (4) venular oncotic pressure. Oncotic pressure (primarily from intravascular albumin concentration) remains relatively constant from the arteriolar to the venular side of the capillary bed, being slightly higher in the venule as a result of fluid loss. In contrast, hydrostatic pressure is significantly higher in the arteriole than in the venule. Therefore, under normal circumstances, fluid leaves the intravascular space at the arteriolar level primarily because of hydrostatic driving force and returns to the intravascular space at the venular level primarily as a result of oncotic driving force. Although most extravasated fluid is reabsorbed at the venular level, the remainder is brought back to the systemic circulation via the lymphatic system. In the normal patient, the overall result is a steady-state fluid balance between the intravascular and interstitial spaces without edema formation (4).

It is clear that three derangements result in edema formation. These are (1) an increase in intravascular hydrostatic pressure, (2) a decrease in plasma oncotic pressure, and (3) an impairment of lymphatic drainage. To this may be added a fourth derangement, (4) the renal retention of salt and water. In retaining salt and water, there is an increase in the intravascular hydrostatic pressure, favoring extravasation of fluid to the interstitium. In addition, by retaining water in excess of salt, there is a drop in the intravascular oncotic pressure, reducing the driving force to reabsorb extravasated fluid. In CHF, all four of these derangements occur and contribute to edema formation (2).

Renal Retention of Salt and Water

Despite the fact that most patients with CHF have normal or increased plasma volume (5), the primary driving force toward renal salt and water retention appears to be the detection of a decrease in the effective arterial blood volume (EABV). An as yet poorly defined parameter, the EABV is loosely defined as blood volume in relation to vascular capacity (6). The reduced cardiac output of CHF results in a decreased EABV, sensed by baroreceptors in the left ventricle, the aortic arch, the carotid sinus, and the renal afferent arterioles (7). A sequence of neurohormonal activation then occurs that includes the sympathetic nervous system, the renin-angiotensin-aldosterone (RAA) system, and the nonosmotic release of vasopressin (antidiuretic hormone [ADH]), resulting in salt and water retention by the kidneys. Counter-balancing these systems, release of atrial and brain natriuretic peptides (ANP and BNP), occurs from the atria and ventricles, respectively. These peptides serve to augment renal excretion of salt and water in an attempt to counteract the other systems (8).

Catecholamine release in response to sympathetic nervous system activation results in renal vasoconstriction and reduced renal blood flow, decreasing the ability of the kidneys to excrete salt and water. In addition, intrarenal hemodynamic and oncotic changes that occur because of this vasoconstriction result in increased proximal tubular reabsorption of salt and water. Finally, catecholamines lead to further salt and water retention by directly activating both the RAA and ADH systems (4).

In heart failure, the juxtaglomerular apparatus (JGA) secretes renin by three mechanisms. First, baroreceptors in the renal afferent arterioles directly stimulate renin release. Second, reduced sodium delivery to the distal tubules as a result of the reduction in glomerular filtration rate (GFR) is sensed by the macula densa, which signals the JGA to secrete renin. Finally, sympathetic nervous system activation directly stimulates renin release via β-receptors in the JGA *(4)*.

Renin cleaves the circulating protein angiotensinogen to release angiotensin I, which is converted to angiotensin II by angiotensin-converting enzyme (ACE). Angiotensin II, in a manner similar to the catecholamines, produces renal vasoconstriction as well as proximal tubular salt and water reabsorption. Additionally, angiotensin II stimulates the release of aldosterone from the adrenal cortex. Aldosterone contributes to salt and water retention by enhancing sodium reabsorption in the distal and collecting tubules *(4)*. Finally, angiotensin II also appears to directly stimulate the nonosmotic release of ADH *(9)*.

Although the primary stimulus for ADH release from the hypothalamus is an increase in serum osmolality, it is clear that ADH may be released via nonosmotic mechanisms. Although not definitively understood, it is believed that baroreceptors detecting a decrease in EABV stimulate ADH release via the sympathetic nervous system *(8)*. In addition, it is known that angiotensin II directly stimulates the nonosmotic release of ADH *(9)*. By way of these two nonosmotic mechanisms of release, ADH levels rise and remain elevated despite the low osmolar state typical of CHF. In addition to being a potent vasoconstrictor, ADH has its primary effect in the collecting tubules, where it acts to maximally concentrate the urine by enhancing water reabsorption *(4,8)*.

Counter-balancing these three systems, ANP and BNP are produced and secreted by the myocardium in response to increased intracardiac pressure and myocardial stretch *(3)*. These peptides enhance glomerular filtration, block salt and water reabsorption in the proximal tubules, inhibit the release of renin and aldosterone, and inhibit the vasoconstrictor actions of angiotensin II, ADH, and the catecholamines. In this manner, the natriuretic peptides work to oppose salt and water retention in heart failure. However, for unclear reasons, the effect of these peptides is blunted and overcome in patients with heart failure, despite high circulating blood levels *(4)*.

Increased Hydrostatic Pressure

In heart failure, an increase in the venous intravascular hydrostatic pressure initially occurs. This increase is because of the impairment of cardiac output that results in elevated pulmonary, right-ventricular, right-atrial and, finally, central venous pressures. The increase in central venous pressure is relayed to the venules, inhibiting reabsorption of fluid from the interstitial space. In this manner, a portion of fluid that extravasates at the arteriolar level is unable to be returned to the intravascular space, and edema forms *(10)*.

More importantly, however, intravascular hydrostatic pressure increases significantly as a result of salt and water retention by the kidneys. By first expanding the intravascular volume, hydrostatic pressure increases from the limited compliance of the vasculature. The result is increased extravasation of fluid into the interstitium at the arteriolar level, and impaired reabsorption at the venular level *(2)*.

Decreased Plasma Oncotic Pressure

The etiology of decreased plasma oncotic pressure is multifactorial. The primary factor is renal retention of water in excess of salt, mediated by the excessive release of ADH. Additionally, ADH stimulates thirst and the ingestion of free water. Both of these effects of ADH serve to decrease plasma osmolality and oncotic pressure *(9)*.

An additional cause of decreased plasma oncotic pressure is the reduction in serum albumin concentration that occurs mainly in the late stages of heart failure. This occurs as a result of both malnutrition and liver dysfunction. Malnutrition is from cardiac cachexia, anorexia, negative protein balance, and intestinal malabsorption from bowel edema. Malnutrition thus impairs the ability of the patient to acquire protein necessary for the synthesis of albumin. Liver dysfunction results from chronic passive congestion and organ ischemia, directly impairing the synthesis of albumin. As albumin is the major protein in plasma contributing to oncotic pressure, a reduction in albumin from malnutrition and liver damage favors edema formation *(2)*.

Impaired Lymphatic Drainage

Impaired lymphatic drainage occurs as a direct result of elevated central venous hydrostatic pressure. This elevated pressure, which results from the reduced cardiac output and the retention of salt and water by the kidneys (*see* above), is transmitted directly to the thoracic duct as it empties into the venous system at the junction of the left-internal jugular and left-subclavian veins *(11)*. The result is an impairment in the return of lymphatic drainage from the periphery to the intravascular space. Whereas it is clear that this mechanism contributes to edema in heart failure, the exact magnitude of this contribution in an individual patient is variable *(4)*.

EXAMINATION OF EDEMA IN HEART FAILURE

There are two components to the adequate assessment of peripheral edema on physical examination. First, edema characteristic of CHF

Table 1
Common Causes of Edema

Congestive heart failure
Liver disease
  • Cirrhosis
  • Portal hypertension
Renal disease
  • Nephrotic syndrome
  • Chronic renal insufficiency
  • Glomerulonephritis
Severe malnutrition of malabsorption
Drugs
  • Calcium channel blockers
  • Estrogen
  • Steroids
  • Minoxidil
  • ACE inhibitors
Other causes
  • Venous/lymphatic obstruction
  • Varicose veins
  • Idiopathic edema/angioedema
  • Cellulitis
  • Myxedema

must be diagnosed. Second, the remainder of the physical examination must provide confirmatory evidence for a diagnosis of volume overload and cardiac dysfunction. The clinician must remain vigilant that a multitude of noncardiac etiologies can result in the formation of peripheral edema (see Table 1). In addition, one must remember that there are many forms of cardiac dysfunction that can lead to edema formation. Whereas myocardial systolic dysfunction with reduced ejection fraction is the etiology most sought when characteristic peripheral edema is found, valvular stenosis or regurgitation, isolated right heart failure, pericardial disease or diastolic dysfunction may be the underlying cardiac etiology of edema. Thus, a thorough physical examination focusing on the cardiac, lung, and vascular systems is necessary to fully characterize peripheral edema in terms of both magnitude and etiology.

In CHF, edema is typically in dependant regions. Thus, in ambulatory patients, edema is localized to the distal lower extremities in a symmetrical manner, rising higher up the legs as the edematous state worsens. In patients who are bedridden or in the supine position for a majority of the time, edema is localized to the sacral and presacral areas (9). Characteristically, the patient with edema complains of leg pain,

Table 2
Grading of Peripheral Edema *(12)*

1 (+): Mild edema
2 (+): Moderate edema
3 (+): Severe edema, legs clearly puffy
4 (+): Severe edema, legs clearly swollen

decreased exercise tolerance from "heavy" legs, or an inability to fit into shoes. Additionally, edema of heart failure often worsens as the day progresses, while the patient is upright, with little to no edema remaining by morning after a night of recumbency.

When edema is present in the legs, there is often obscuration of the veins, tendons, and bony prominences. Pitting edema is characteristic of CHF, and should be tested on the dorsum of each foot, over the shins, and behind each medial malleolus. The magnitude of pitting edema is recorded on a four-point scale *(see* Table 2) *(12)*. When a result of elevated hydrostatic pressure, as in CHF, the edema must be symmetric unless unilateral venous or lymphatic disease is concomitantly present. While examining the edematous legs, the clinician must exclude other common etiologies of edema, such as deep venous thrombosis, cellulitis, chronic venous insufficiency, and varicose veins. Less common etiologies such as advanced liver or renal disease must likewise be excluded.

Deep venous thrombosis often leads to asymmetric edema that is pitting in nature. There may be unilateral calf tenderness, a palpable cord, or calf pain on active foot dorsiflexion (Homan's sign). Cellulitis is typically nonpitting and unilateral. There is often pain, erythema and warmth, findings consistent with inflammation. Chronic venous insufficiency is suggested by brownish discoloration of the skin and by ulcers immediately above the ankle. Varicose veins are visibly dilated and tortuous. Asking the patient to stand may bring out obvious varicosities. Lymphedema, a relatively rare cause of edema, is typically nonpitting. From the accumulation of protein in the interstitial space, the skin is often thickened and fibrotic *(12)*.

Other causes of symmetric edema include liver disease, renal disease, and syndromes that result in hypoalbuminemia (malabsorption syndromes, severe malnutrition). Often, the patient will present with total body edema or anasarca because of low plasma oncotic pressure. Splenomegaly and other signs of portal hypertension indicate significant liver disease. Edema because of nephrotic syndrome is typically present around the eyelids and on the face. Further blood testing is required to make these diagnoses. Thyroid function tests should be performed if signs or symptoms of myxedema are present.

Finally, a number of medications have been shown to produce edema (*see* Table 1). A careful review of both prescription and nonprescription medications is needed. The dihidropyridine class of calcium channel blockers is particularly implicated as a common cause of peripheral edema. Additionally, ACE inhibitors are known to rarely cause angioedema.

Once the diagnosis of edema characteristic of CHF is made, the remainder of the physical examination focuses on finding confirmatory evidence for a cardiac etiology of volume overload. Although the astute clinician should inspect, auscultate, and palpate carefully for a variety of findings, including elevated jugular venous pressure, pericardial rub, systolic and diastolic murmurs, gallops, pulmonary rales, and decreased breath sounds, the main findings consistent with the hypervolemic state of CHF are elevation of the jugular venous pressure and the presence of an S3 gallop.

The evaluation of jugular venous pressure remains one of the most difficult examination techniques. However, it remains the most important clinical indicator of volume status and accurately represents right-atrial pressure. The right-internal jugular vein pressure is typically estimated. The external jugular vein may be utilized but has been shown to be less reliable. The sternal angle is the standard reference point, remaining roughly 5 cm above the right atrium regardless of patient position.

Typically, the patient is made supine with the head elevated 15 to 30° and turned slightly toward the contralateral side. By noting the highest location at which oscillations are seen, the level of venous pressure is identified. There are commonly two quick elevations, signifying *a* and *v* waves in the standard atrial pressure tracing. Once the level is identified, the *vertical* distance to the sternal angle is determined in centimeters. To this must be added 5 cm, representing the distance from the sternal angle to the right atrium, resulting in an estimation of jugular venous pressure in centimeters of water. A number greater than 8 or 9 is considered abnormally elevated, indicating intravascular volume overload. Importantly, in states of extreme volume overload, the patient may need to be more upright in order to make the jugular pulsations visible. In contrast, in states of volume depletion, the patient may need to be more supine. Regardless of the angulation, however, estimation of jugular venous pressure by this method remains accurate *(12)*.

The diagnosis of an S3 gallop is further confirmatory evidence of significant volume overload and a cardiac etiology of edema. The S3 may be either right- or left-sided and occurs early in diastole, coinciding with early, rapid ventricular filling. It is dull, low-pitched, and later than an opening snap, heard with the bell of the stethoscope held lightly against the chest. Whereas normal in young adulthood and in the third trimester of pregnancy, an S3 in an individual older than 40 years of age is almost always pathologic. The left-sided S3 is heard at the apex with the patient in the left-lateral position. A right-sided S3 is heard along the lower left-sternal border with the patient in the supine position. As opposed to a left-sided S3, a right-sided S3 changes with respiration, being notably louder on inspiration as venous return to the right side of the heart is augmented. Changes in pulmonary venous return with respiration are not of significant magnitude to impact on the intensity of a left-sided S3 (12).

In the patient with characteristic edema, elevated jugular venous pressure, and an S3, the diagnosis of CHF is likely. Further testing, such as echocardiography, is then necessary to elucidate the nature of cardiac dysfunction. In the patient with known heart failure and cardiac dysfunction, the presence of these three physical findings is indicative of a degree of decompensation. In addition to modifying the dietary or medical regimen, an effort must be made to determine the etiology of the decompensation. This may require further testing, such as echocardiography, left-heart catheterization, or the evaluation of cardiac enzymes.

TREATMENT OF EDEMA IN HEART FAILURE

It has become increasingly clear that optimal treatment of the edematous state of heart failure requires targeting the neurohormonal pathways responsible for its pathogenesis. The validity of this approach has been proven in multiple studies, showing improved morbidity and mortality with the use of ACE inhibitors and β-blockers, agents that block two of the primary neurohormonal systems involved in heart failure. It is for this reason that ACE inhibitors in particular have replaced diuretics as first-line therapy for CHF. Optimal management of edema in heart failure requires specific patient education, coupled with pharmacologic therapy to include ACE inhibitors, β-blockers, digoxin, and diuretics.

Patient Education

The patient with cardiac edema needs adequate education regarding the nature of their disease. In particular, the chronic and progressive nature of CHF must be conveyed. If possible, a family meeting is optimal in order to both convey the significance of the disease process and reduce the burden on the patient. Once the patient is educated about the disease, issues of medical compliance need to be addressed. Patients need to be aware that they will likely be on multiple medications for the remainder of life. Additionally, the importance of not missing doses needs to be stressed. As failure to comply with a prescribed medical regimen or diet accounts for up to 64% of all decompensations, extreme vigilance in patient education at the time of diagnosis should improve morbidity and mortality for the individual patient *(13)*.

Dietary changes are necessary to minimize edema. In particular, restriction of salt is recommended for all patients with heart failure and edema. Typically, the patient is advised to avoid the use of salt at the table and to avoid foods rich in salt content (such as canned foods, nuts, and sandwich meat). In extreme edematous states, salt restriction may be severe, as low as 2 g per day. In these extreme states, water restriction is often necessary, to levels of 1 to 2 L per day.

Leg elevation is beneficial in reducing edema. In severe cases, periods of bed rest may be required. These maneuvers increase reabsorption of fluid from the intersitium back into the intravascular space and, either via direct pressure natriuresis or augmentation of natriuretic peptide levels (ANP, BNP), results in improved diuresis. Compression stockings also serve this purpose and are very well tolerated.

Finally, the patient should be instructed to check his or her weight daily, preferably at the same time of day and with the same scale. As weight increases before symptoms of heart failure occur, the use of a log to document daily weights will allow the patient to communicate significant weight gain to the doctor prior to decompensation and hospitalization. Adjustments to the dose of diuretics or other medications at this early sign of heart failure will prevent the development of edema and obviate the need for hospitalization.

Angiotensin-Converting Enzyme Inhibitors

Because of the underlying neurohormonal pathophysiology, ACE inhibitors have replaced diuretics as first-line therapy for systolic dysfunction and CHF *(14)*. The Cooperative North Scandinavian Enalapril Survival Study (CONSENSUS) trial showed improved survival with the use of enalapril in patients with Class IV heart failure. The majority of the mortality benefit was a reduction in death due to progressive heart failure *(15)*. In addition to reducing mortality in both symptomatic and asymptomatic patients, the Study of Left-Ventricular Dysfunction (SOLVD) trial showed a reduction in hospitalizations from heart failure with the use of enalapril *(16)*. In these trials, the dose of enalapril was started low (2.5–5 mg per day) and titrated up to 10 or 20 mg twice a day. Other studies utilizing ramipril, lisinopril and captopril have shown similar results *(17-19)*. In contrast, however, angiotensin receptor blockers (ARBs) have not shown benefit over ACE inhibitors *(20)*. As such, ARBs are typically reserved for patients intolerant of ACE inhibitors.

Diuretics

With the exception of the unique diuretic spironolactone, diuretics have not been evaluated in large-scale placebo-controlled trials of mortality in heart failure. Therefore, there is no evidence that loop or thiazide diuretics reduce mortality in CHF. However, common experience has shown that optimal use of diuretics significantly improves morbidity in heart failure, including fatigue, exercise tolerance, and frequency of hospitalizations.

Whereas patients with mild heart failure and edema may respond to a thiazide diuretic alone, most patients with heart failure require a loop diuretic, such as furosemide and bumetanide *(3)*. These two loop diuretics have shown similar efficacy in patients with heart failure *(21)*. Patients with proven sulfa allergy require ethacrynic acid, as both furosemide and bumetanide contain sulfa moieties. In cases where high doses of loop diuretics are needed, the addition of a thiazide may produce significant diuresis and allow a reduction in the dose of the loop diuretic. This is important as ototoxicity will result with the continued use of loop diuretics at such high doses.

The extent of diuresis necessary is often difficult to gauge. Excessive diuresis can result in a fall in cardiac output, especially in patients with significant concomitant or primary diastolic dysfunction. Reduced cardiac output would further drive the neurohormonal pathways involved in the retention of salt and water. In general, diuresis should proceed until edema, elevated jugular venous pressure, and the S3 are absent, or until a significant complication occurs. The most frequent complication noted is a deterioration of renal function, heralded by a rising blood urea nitrogen (BUN) or creatinine concentration. However, it bears noting that a rising BUN or creatinine is often more indicative of the rate of diuresis, and renal function may improve if the dose or rate of diuresis is decreased. A mild deterioration in renal function is often tolerated in order to improve the functional status and symptoms of the patient *(22)*.

Unique to the diuretic class, spironolactone has shown mortality benefit in patients with severe Class IV heart failure *(23)*. Accordingly, patients with severe heart failure symptoms should be on 25 mg of spironolactone per day. Whereas the effect on mortality was significant, the absolute effect on diuresis is often modest.

With the use of diuretics, careful attention to potassium level is mandatory, as loop and thiazide diuretics cause potassium-wasting and hypokalemia. In contrast, spironolactone causes potassium retention. Unfortunately, the combination of medications utilized in heart failure (ACE inhibitors, diuretics, spironolactone) has variable effects on potassium in the individual patient, making frequent assessment of electrolyte levels mandatory. This is especially true when modifying or adding these agents to a regimen.

Digitalis

Digitalis remains a somewhat controversial agent in the management of heart failure. By increasing cardiac output, digitalis has potential in downregulating the neurohormonal activation of heart failure. Despite this, studies have failed to show a mortality benefit with the use of digitalis (24).

However, digitalis has been shown to improve the morbidity of heart failure in patients with systolic dysfunction. Specifically, studies in which digitalis therapy was withdrawn resulted in worsening heart failure symptoms, decreased functional capacity, and poorer quality-of-life scores (25,26). In a major prospective trial of digitalis, therapy resulted in fewer heart failure hospitalizations (24).

Based on these studies, digitalis therapy is recommended for patients with systolic dysfunction and symptomatic heart failure in order to decrease the frequency of hospitalizations and improve the quality of life. The dose of 0.25 mg per day is typically used. Lower or every-other-day dosing may be required in patients with renal insufficiency, and blood levels will need to be monitored at least initially. Toxicity results in neurologic, visual, gastrointestinal, and arrhythmic disturbances. Digitalis may cause tachycardia as a result of increased automaticity or bradycardia because of atrioventricular block. Hypokalemia exacerbates digitalis toxicity and must be monitored routinely while on therapy. Severe digitalis toxicity may require treatment with digitalis-specific antibody fragments.

β-Blockers

In directly blocking the sympathetic nervous system neurohormonal pathway, β-blockers have shown efficacy in reducing morbidity and mortality in heart failure. Both the nonspecific adrenergic blocker carvedilol and the β1-specific blocker metoprolol have improved survival, reduced hospitalizations, and improved symptoms of heart failure (27,28). In these trials, metoprolol was titrated to a target dose of 150–200 mg per day and carvedilol was titrated to a target dose of 25–50 mg twice a day.

Because of the negative inotropic nature of these agents, and the potential to exacerbate heart failure symptoms initially, β-blockers should be initiated when a patient is clinically euvolemic. The dose is gradually increased to target dose over several weeks. During this titration period, the clinician should remain vigilant for signs or symptoms of cardiac decompensation.

SUMMARY

Edema is a common manifestation of cardiac dysfunction and is often the symptom that brings a patient to the attention of a physician. Whereas the diagnosis of edema is often simple, differentiating cardiac from noncardiac causes of edema may be difficult and requires a thorough physical examination and patient history. Once a diagnosis of cardiac edema is made, the nature of cardiac dysfunction must be determined. This may include invasive or noninvasive testing. Therapy is then initiated and normally requires extensive patient education and lifestyle modification, in addition to pharmacologic therapy. Treatment is aimed at inhibiting the neurohormonal pathways activated in the heart failure syndrome. With this approach, a positive effect on morbidity and mortality is achieved.

REFERENCES

1. Braunwald E. Clinical aspects of heart failure: high-output heart failure; pulmonary edema. In: Braunwald E, ed. Heart Disease. WB Saunders, Philadelphia, PA: 1997.
2. Hemodynamic disorders, thrombosis, and shock. In: Robbins SL, ed. Pathologic Basis of Disease. WB Saunders, Philadelphia, PA: 1994.
3. Navas JP, Martinez-Maldonado M. Pathophysiology of edema in congestive heart failure. Heart Dis Stroke 1993;2:325–329.
4. Braunwald E. Edema. In: Fauci AS, ed. Harrison's Principles of Internal Medicine. McGraw-Hill, New York, NY: 1998.
5. Hesse B, Nielsen I, Bollerup AC, et al. Hemodynamics, compartments and the renin-aldosterone system in chronic heart failure. Eur J Cardiol 1975;3:107–115.
6. Dyckner T, Wester PO. Salt and water balance in congestive heart failure. Acta Med Scand Suppl 1986;707:27–31.
7. Schrier RW, Ecder T. Gibbs memorial lecture. Unifying hypothesis of body fluid volume regulation: implications for cardiac failure and cirrhosis. Mt Sinai J Med 2001;68(6):350–361.
8. Schrier RW, Gurevich AK, Cadnapaphomchai MA. Pathogenesis and management of sodium and water retention in cardiac failure and cirrhosis. Semin Nephrol 2001;21:157–172.
9. Abraham WT. Renal salt and water handling in congestive heart failure. In: Hosenpud JD, ed. Congestive Heart Failure. Lippincott Williams and Wilkins, Philadelphia, PA: 2000.
10. Ramires JA, Pileggi F. Diuretics in cardiac oedema. Drugs 1986;31: 68–75.
11. Moore KL. The thorax. In: Moore KL, ed. Clinically Oriented Anatomy. Williams and Wilkins, Baltimore, MD: 1980.

12. Bates B. The peripheral vascular system. In: Bates B, ed. A Guide to Physical Examination. Lippincott Company, Philadelphia, PA: 1990.
13. Ghali JK, Kadakia S, Cooper R, et al. Precipitating factors leading to decompensation of heart failure. Arch Intern Med 1988;148:2013–2016.
14. The Task Force of the Working Group on Heart Failure of the European Society of Cardiology: The treatment of Heart Failure: Guidelines. Eur Heart J 1997;18:736–753.
15. CONSENSUS Trial Study Group: Effects of enalapril on mortality in severe congestive heart failure. N Engl J Med 1987;316:1429–1435.
16. SOLVD investigators: Effect of enalapril on survival in patients with reduced left ventricular ejection fraction and congestive heart failure. N Engl J Med 1991;325:293–302.
17. The Acute Infarction Ramipril Efficacy (AIRE) study investigators: Effect of ramipril on mortality and morbidity of survivors of acute myocardial infarction with evidence of heart failure. Lancet 1993;342:821–828.
18. Packer M, Poole-Wilson PA, Armstrong PW, et al. Comparative effects of low and high doses of the angiotensin-converting enzyme inhibitor, lisinopril, on morbidity and mortality in chronic heart failure. Circulation 1999;100:2312–2318.
19. Pfeffer MA, Braunvald IU, Moie LA, et al. Effect of captopril on mortality and morbidity in patients with left ventricular dysfunction after myocardial infarction. Results of the survival and ventricular enlargement trial. The SAVE Investigators. N Engl J Med 1992;327:669–677.
20. Pitt B, Poole-Wilson PA, Segal R, et al. Effect of losartan compared with captopril on mortality in patients with symptomatic heart failure: randomized trial- the Losartan heart Failure Survival Study ELITE II. Lancet 2000;355:1582–1587.
21. Hutcheon D, Vincent ME, Sandhu RS, et al. Clinical use of diuretics in congestive heart failure. J Clin Pharmacol 1981; 21(11-12 Pt 2): 668-72.
22. Gottlieb SS. Diuretics. In: Hosenpud JD, ed. Congestive Heart Failure. Lippincott Williams and Wilkins, Philadelphia, PA: 2000.
23. Pitt B, Zannad F, Remme WJ, et al. The effect of spironolactone on morbidity and mortality in patients with severe heart failure. Randomized Aldactone Evaluation Study Investigators. N Engl J Med 1999;341:709–717.
24. Digoxin Investigation Group (DIG). The effect of digoxin on mortality and morbidity in patients with heart failure. N Engl J Med 1997;336:525–533.
25. Packer M, et al. Randomized Assessment of Effect of Digoxin on Inhibitors of ACE (RADIANCE) study. Withdrawal of digoxin from patients with chronic HF treated with ACE inhibitor. N Engl J Med 1993;329:1–7.
26. Uretsky BF, Young JB, Shahdidi FE, et al. Prospective Randomized Study of Ventricular Failure and Efficacy of Digoxin (PROVED). Randomized study assessing effect of digoxin withdrawal in patients with mild-moderate chronic CHF. J Am Coll Cardiol 1993;22:955–962.
27. Packer M, Bristow MR, Cohn JN, et al. U.S. Carvedilol Heart Failure Study Group. The effect of carvedilol on morbidity and mortality in patients with chronic heart failure. N Engl J Med 1996;334:1349–1355.
28. MERIT-HF Study Group. Effect of metoprolol CR/XL in chronic heart failure: metoprolol CR/XL randomized intervention trial in congestive heart failure (MERIT-HF). Lancet 1999;353:2001–2007.

6 Evaluation of Palpitations

Henry H. Hsia, MD, *FACC*

IMPLICATION OF PALPITATIONS IN HEART FAILURE

Disturbances in cardiac rhythm or rate are common in patients with heart failure. The symptom of palpitations can be defined as either forceful or rapid beating of the heart. This frequent complaint among patients may be associated with a variety of arrhythmias, including all forms of tachycardias (supraventricular and ventricular), ectopic beats, compensatory pauses, or alterations of cardiac outputs. The perception of "palpitations" is highly individualized and may not always suggest a diagnosis of tachycardia. In the case of premature contractions, the patient is usually more aware of the postextrasystole beat augmentation than the premature beat itself. Nonsustained ventricular tachycardia, for example, is often asymptomatic.

The prognostic significance of palpitations depends on the nature of the arrhythmia. Subjective complaint alone is generally inadequate for diagnosis and is frequently misleading. Given the high prevalence of both supraventricular and ventricular arrhythmias in the heart failure population, careful history taking, physical examination, and objective evaluations are essential for both an accurate diagnosis and determination of prognosis.

From: *Contemporary Cardiology: Heart Failure:*
A Clinician's Guide to Ambulatory Diagnosis and Treatment
Edited by: M. L. Jessup and E. Loh © Humana Press Inc., Totowa, NJ

Table 1
Differential Diagnosis of Palpitations

Symptoms of Palpitations	Differential Diagnosis	Implications
Pauses	Compensatory pauses	PACs or PVCs
Skipped beats	Extrasystoles	PACs or PVCs
Forceful, strong beats	Postextrasystole augmentation	PACs or PVCs
Rapid palpitations		
Regular	SVT > VT	SVT, A flutter, atrial tachy monomorphic VT Sinus tachycardia
Irregular	Atrial arrhythmia	AF, atrial tachy
Slow palpitations	Slow junctional, ventricular escape	AV block
	Accelerated junctional rhythm	Digitalis toxicity, reperfusion, metabolic derrangements

When episodes of palpitations are transient, they are usually described as "skipped beats" or "flip-flop," and are often a result of either atrial or ventricular extra-systoles. When a patient complains of the sensation that the heart has "stopped," it is usually correlated with the compensatory pause following a premature contraction (Table 1). Occasionally, the awareness of palpitations may accompany a slow rate. This is often associated with "forceful" heart "poundings," a sensation of "neck throbbing," and/or dyspnea. These are symptoms compatible with ventriculo-atrial (VA) dissociation and may be observed in patients with atrioventricular block (AVB) or in patients with accelerated junctional or ventricular rhythms, such as in the setting of coronary reperfusion, metabolic abnormalities, or drug-digitalis toxicity. When these symptoms accompany rapid palpitations, nonsustained or even sustained ventricular tachycardia must be excluded.

Rapid palpitations with abrupt onset and termination are characteristic features of paroxysmal tachycardia, such as reentrant supraventricular tachycardias (SVTs), atrial fibrillation/flutter, or ventricular tachycardia, whereas a gradual onset and cessation of symptoms may imply a sinus tachycardia or automatic atrial tachycardia. One of the

Onset of AV Node Reentry

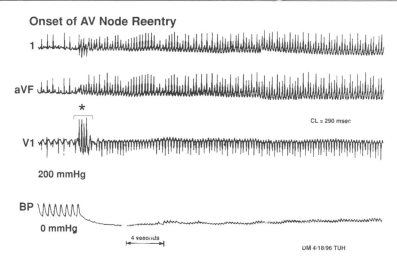

Fig. 1. Hemodynamic compromise at the onset of a SVT (AV nodal reentry) with a cycle length of 290 ms (approximately 200 beats per minute). Three surface leads were displayed along with continuous blood pressure monitoring. Systolic blood pressure dropped from 100 mm Hg to approximately 30–40 mm Hg with the initiation of the tachycardia. Patients may experience syncope or dizziness preceded by rapid palpitations. Aberrantly conducted QRS* was also noted at the onset of the tachycardia.

most common causes of palpitation in patients with heart failure is atrial fibrillation (AF). A diagnosis of AF should be entertained when the patient gives a history of chaotic rapid heartbeats. Occasionally, patients may experience syncope or dizziness preceded by rapid palpitations. Transient hemodynamic compromise may be observed at the onset of rapid tachycardia before compensatory vasoconstriction occurs. These scenarios are most commonly observed at the initiation of either reentrant SVT, rapid atrial arrhythmias, or ventricular tachycardia (Fig. 1).

DIAGNOSTIC TESTING FOR PALPITATIONS

One of the primary and most widely accepted uses of ambulatory electrocardiography is in determining whether patients' symptoms are related to cardiac arrhythmias. Unexplained palpitations is considered a Class I indication for the use of Holter monitors or event recorders (1). The yield of ambulatory electrocardiography is heavily dependent on patient selection, frequency of symptomatic palpitations, and the type of system utilized. For patients with palpitations associated with significant symptoms such as syncope, near-syncope or chest pain, a more aggressive approach with invasive electrophysiologic study should be considered *(2)*. For patients who experience palpitations daily, a continuous 24- to 48-hour Holter recording is generally sufficient for documenting the nature of patients' symptoms. However, most of the patients do not have symptoms on a daily or even weekly basis, a patient-activated, intermittent recording device coupled with the transtelephonic monitoring (TTM) capability is the diagnostic modality of choice in these patients. When episodes of palpitations are transient or are associated with incapacitating symptoms (such as syncope), a continuously recording monitor with a memory loop may be necessary.

An implantable loop recorder (ILR) should be considered in patients with recurrent palpitations and had failed multiple diagnostic modalities without echocardiographic (ECG) documentation *(3)*. The relatively nonintrusive device can be implanted in a precordial subcutaneous pocket and subsequently removed. The ILR can be activated by patients during their symptomatic episodes or can be automatically triggered by a preprogrammed tachycardia or bradycardia rate setting (Fig. 2).

In general, the sensitivity of electrophysiological studies (EPS) is low in patients with unexplained palpitations and may be considered only if long-term recording attempts fail to provide an answer. However, in patients with documented inappropriately rapid pulse rates, or in patients with palpitations preceding a syncopal episode, invasive electrophysiological evaluation is indicated *(2)*. EPS are performed to determine the mechanisms of arrhythmias, direct or provide therapy, or assess prognosis. The diagnostic yield of EPS is dependent on the underlying anatomical substrate of the individual patient. Although induction of sustained SVT, such as AV nodal reentry or AV reciprocating tachycardia, is uncommon, the induced tachyarrhythmia is distinctly abnormal and is clinically significant. In patients with structural heart disease and heart failure, induction of monomorphic ventricular tachycardia is clearly an abnormal finding and is associated with a high mortality and sudden death rate. Other abnormalities, such as sinus pause following overdrive atrial pacing or His-Purkinje AV block, also have a high degree of specificity.

Fig. 2. *(opposite page)* ECG recordings from an ILR in a patient with recurrent palpitations and near-syncope. The ILR was activated automatically during a symptomatic episode by a preprogrammed bradycardia rate setting. The patient suffered from "tachy-brady syndrome" with new onset of rapid AF followed by prolonged pauses after termination of AF.

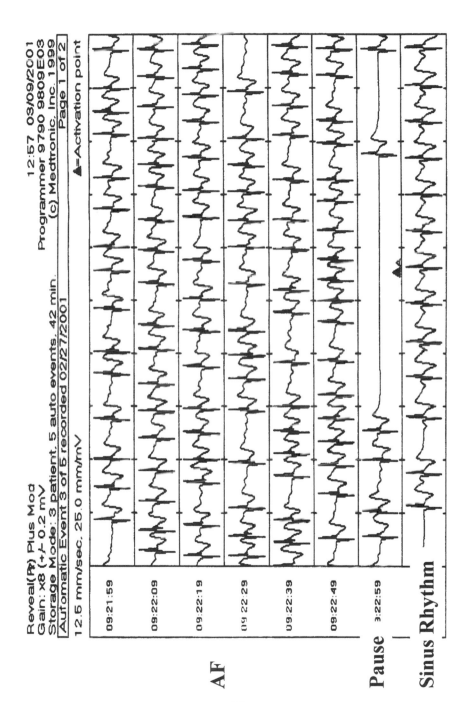

Reveal(R) Plus Mod
Gain: x8 (+/- 0.2 mV
Storage Mode: 3 patient. 5 auto events, 42 min.
Automatic Event 3 of 5 recorded 02/27/2001

12:57 03/09/2001
Programmer 9790 9809E03
(c) Medtronic, Inc. 1999
Page 1 of 2

12.5 mm/sec. 25.0 mm/mV

▲=Activation point

09:21:59
09:22:09
09:22:19
09:22:29
09:22:39
09:22:49
3:22:59

AF

Pause

Sinus Rhythm

73

Table 2
Atrial Fibrillation in Heart Failure

	N	Functional class	Mean age (years)	Incidence of AF
Consensus	253	IV	71	50%
GESICA	516	II–IV	59	29%
Stevenson, et al.	750	III–IV	51	22%
CHF-STAT	674	II–III	66	15%
V-HeFT I-II	1427	II–III	60	14%
SOLVD 1991	2569	II–II	61	10%
SOLVD 1992	4228	I	59	4%

PALPITATIONS AND ATRIAL FIBRILLATION

Atrial fibrillation is one of the most common arrhythmia management problems in patients with heart failure, occurring in 10–50% of the population (Table 2). Patients with heart failure are four times as likely to develop AF in comparison to age- and sex-matched controls, and its prevalence increases with age and severity of heart failure *(4,5)*.

There are several potential mechanisms by which AF could adversely affect the clinical course of patients with heart failure. These mechanisms include: (1) an increased hazard of thromboembolic complications, (2) hemodynamic deterioration from loss of coordinated atrial contraction to ventricular filling, (3) impaired heart-rate response to exercise, (4) tachycardia-induced ventricular dysfunction, and (5) side effects of antiarrhythmic and anticoagulation therapy *(4,6,7)*. In addition, AF may be an independent risk factor for mortality and sudden death *(5,8)*.

Unfortunately, the individual awareness of AF varies tremendously. Patients may be asymptomatic and only experience occasional palpitations, or they may present with hemodynamic decompensation, severe dyspnea, and hypotension. The symptoms may be related to the degree of ventricular filling, valvular status, underlying ventricular function, as well as influenced by R-to-R variability and heart rate. An astute clinician must suspect a diagnosis of either paroxysmal or persistent atrial arrhythmias when patients present with worsening dyspnea, intermittent palpitations, or subtle deteriorations of their exercise tolerance from the baseline status.

It is critical to recognize the presence and duration of atrial arrhythmias in patients with heart failure. The major considerations

Table 3
Risk Factors for Systemic Emboli or Strokes
in Patients with Atrial Fibrillation

Previous history of transient ischemic attack or stroke
Age
Hypertension
Heart failure
Diabetes mellitus
Coronary artery disease
Valvular heart disease
Thyrotoxicosis

Modified from ref. *12.*

include: (1) prevention of thromboembolic complications, (2) restoration and maintenance of sinus rhythm, and (3) ventricular rate control if the patient is in persistent or chronic AF.

AF greater than 48 hours in duration predisposes the development of thrombus, particularly in the left-atrial appendage *(9,10)*. It constitutes a major independent risk factor for stroke and is associated with a three- to fivefold increased risk of systemic embolism *(11,12)*. With other comorbidities that frequently exist in patients with heart failure, the threat of thromboembolic complication is significant (Table 3).

The data from several large clinical trials have clearly established the efficacy of warfarin and aspirin in reducing the risk of ischemic stroke and systemic emboli in AF (Fig. 3) *(13–18)*. The American College of Chest Physicians Consensus Conference on antithrombotic therapy has recommended warfarin therapy over aspirin in these patients with known risk factors such as heart failure (Fig. 4) *(19)*. The target INR should be at 2-3 in the absence of mechanical valvular prosthesis (Fig. 5) *(20,21)*

In patients with heart failure, hemodynamic instability and worsening of functional class is common with the development of AF. The lack of "atrial kick" may account for a significant reduction in ventricular filling and output *(22)*. In addition, AF is a progressive and self-perpetuating disease. "Electrical remodeling" with shortening of atrial refractory period is the main underlying electrophysiological change. The phenomenon of "AF begets AF" has been well demonstrated in both humans and animal models *(23–25)*. Without intervention, prolongation of arrhythmia episode duration and development of permanent AF are to be expected. It is therefore imperative to identify the presence of AF and to institute therapy early in the course of heart failure for effective arrhythmia control.

Although restoration and maintenance of sinus rhythm is desirable and should be attempted, this therapeutic goal may be difficult to achieve

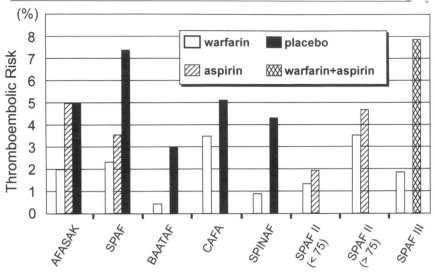

Fig. 3. Multicenter trials of primary prevention of strokes in AF. The efficacy of warfarin and aspirin in reducing the risk of ischemic stroke and systemic emboli in AF are well established. Warfarin appears to be more effective than aspirin in reducing the risk of thromboembolic complications. AFASAK, atrial fibrillation, aspirin, anticoagulation study from Copenhagen; SPAF, stroke prevention in atrial fibrillation study; BAATAF, The Boston Area Anticoagulation Trial for Atrial Fibrillation; CAFA, Canadian Atrial Fibrillation Anticoagulation study; SPINAF, stroke prevention in nonrheumatic atrial fibrillation.

in some patients. The risk and benefit ratio of long-term antiarrhythmic drug use should be carefully considered (Table 4). The type 1A and 1C antiarrhythmic agents are associated with an increased mortality, especially in patients with structural heart disease and ventricular dysfunction *(26–30)*. In addition to significant proarrhythmia, the negative inotropic effects of many antiarrhythmic drugs are poorly tolerated in this population. However, judicious use of low-dose amiodarone can be effective and is associated with an acceptable side-effect profile. It does not have a negative influence on mortality in comparison to placebo *(31,32)*. Nonpharmacologic therapies, such as implantable atrial defibrillator, multisite pacing, surgical compartmentalization, and catheter ablation, are still considered as "evolving" technologies in treating patients with AF *(33–35)*. Long-term outcomes with these therapies and appropriate patient selection have not yet been well established.

Heart rate control during AF represents an alternative approach in patients with heart failure (Table 4). The optimal strategy of either maintenance of sinus rhythm vs rate control awaits the result of a multicenter trial *(36)*. Digitalis, β-blockers, calcium-channel antago-

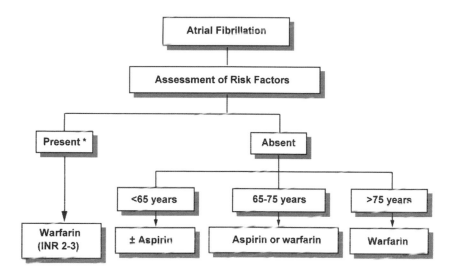

* **Heart failure is a risk factor for thrombuembolic complication in patients with atrial fibrillation**

Fig. 4. Clinical approach in patients with AF. Age, presence and absence of risk factors determine the optimal antithrombotic therapy. Risk factors include: prior transient ischemic attack or stroke, hypertension, CHF, diabetes, coronary artery disease, valvular heart disease, or thyrotoxicosis.

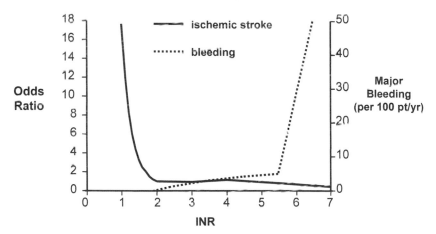

Hylek: N Engl J Med 1996; 335:540 EAFT Study Group: N Engl J Med 1995; 333:5-10

Fig. 5. The optimal range for prophylactic anticoagulation for prevention of thromboembolic complication in AF. The odds ratio for ischemic strokes decreases significantly with an INR value greater than 2. The risk of bleeding complication increases (>5%) with an INR value greater than 4. The target INR should be at 2–3 in the absence of mechanical valvular prosthesis.

Table 4
Controversies in Management of Atrial Fibrillation

	Restoration of sinus rhythm	Ventricular rate control
PROS	Eliminate symptoms, improve hemodynamic	Easier to achieve rate control than to maintain sinus rhythm
	Minimize the need for long-term anticoagulation	Lower risk of proarrhythmia
	Prevent electrophysiologic remodeling and development of permanent AF	
CONS	Difficult to maintain sinus rhythm	Reduce but not eliminate symptoms
	Frequently requires long-term antiarrhythmic drugs	Dose not prevent progression to chronic AF
	Higher risk of ventricular proarrhythmia	May cause periods of sinus bradycardia alternating with rapid AF
		Still requires long-term anticoagulation

nists, or amiodarone can attenuate the ventricular rate response during AF. However, adequate rate control with drug therapy alone may be difficult in this patient population. The negative inotropic effects often limit the use of AV blockers such as β-blockers or calcium-channel antagonists. Periods of sinus bradycardia alternating with rapid AF may result in symptomatic "tachy-brady syndrome" (37). Conversely, AV node/His-bundle catheter ablation with placement of a permanent pacemaker may provide an attractive alternative for rate control in this patient population. Furthermore, it has been shown to improve quality of life, minimize symptoms, and reduce hospital admissions (38–40).

PALPITATIONS AND VENTRICULAR ECTOPY

The major causes of death in patients with heart failure are sudden death and death from progressive pump failure (41). Although the total mortality among patients with mild heart failure is low, the relative proportion of patients dying suddenly is significant (50–70%). In patients with more advanced heart failure (Class III and IV), the major cause of death is from progressive myocardial dysfunction and hemo-dynamic deterioration. However, the relative proportion of sudden death amounts to approximately 30% of all causes of death, with the absolute

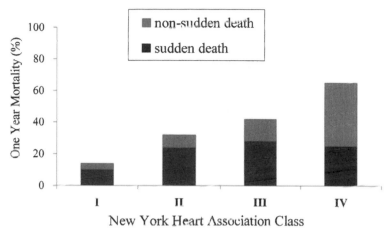

Fig. 6. The annual mortality in heart failure patients relative the New York Heart Association (NYHA) functional class. The total mortality increases with worsening heart failure. The absolute incidence of sudden death remains stable at approximately 30%. Although the total mortality in patients with mild heart failure is low, the relative proportion of sudden death is high (50–70%). In patients with advanced heart failure, the relative proportion of sudden death amounts to less than 30% of all causes of death.

incidence of sudden death remaining comparable to that of functional Class II patients *(42–44)* (Fig. 6).

Frequent ventricular ectopy and nonsustained ventricular tachycardia are prevalent (60–80%) in patients with congestive heart failure (CHF) *(45,46)*. Patients may perceive the ventricular arrhythmias as symptomatic palpitations. Although high-grade ventricular ectopy may be associated with an increased total mortality in this patient population *(46–51)*, the predictive role of spontaneous arrhythmias alone in identifying patients at risk for sudden death or sustained ventricular arrhythmias remains controversial *(45,52,53)*.

The major goals in management of patients with heart failure and ventricular ectopy are risk stratification and primary prevention of sudden cardiac death. Patients' predominant underlying heart disease is defined as either a result of coronary artery disease and prior myocardial infarction or secondary to nonischemic cardiomyopathy. Noninvasive methods such as signal-averaged ECG (SAECG) or ambulatory Holter monitoring, as well as invasive ventricular programmed stimulation are useful for risk stratification in patients with coronary artery disease *(54–57)*. Data from multicenter, randomized trials confirmed the utility of EPS in patients with ischemic heart disease and nonsustained ventricular arrhythmia *(57–59)*. Inducible sustained arrhythmia is associated

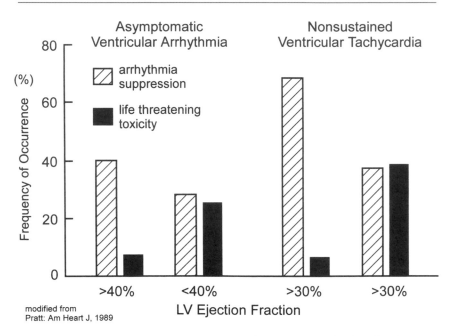

Fig. 7. The inverse relationship between left-ventricular ejection fraction and outcome of antiarrhythmic therapy. Patients with lower-ventricular ejection fractions have a lower arrhythmia suppression response with antiarrhythmic drugs in comparison to those with higher ejection fractions. Higher occurrence rate of life-threatening toxicity was also observed among patients with greater degree of ventricular dysfunction. This inverse relationship between ejection fraction and outcome of antiarrhythmic therapy was more evident in patients with higher-grade ventricular arrhythmias incomparison to those with simple premature ventricular ectopy. Modified from ref. *28.*

with a substantial risk of dying suddenly and therapy guided by EPS resulted in a significant reduction of sudden death. Importantly, this survival benefit was solely because of the use of implantable cardioverter-defibrillators (ICDs) *(58,59).*

Conversely, current methods of risk stratification are inadequate in patients with a predominantly nonischemic cardiomyopathy and palpitations. The role of SAECG is controversial *(60,61),* and ventricular programmed stimulation has proven to be of no value in this subgroup of patients *(62).* A history of unexplained syncope identifies patients with heart failure at high risk of sudden death *(63).* Empiric defibrillator therapy may be recommended in these patients, especially in those with nonischemic cardiomyopathy *(64).*

Overall, antiarrhythmic drug therapies for treatment of ventricular arrhythmias and prevention of sudden death have resulted in worsening

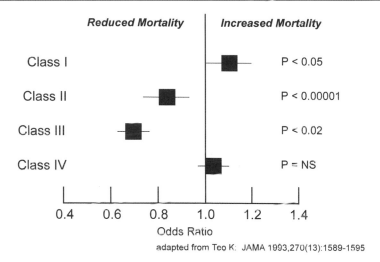

Fig. 8. A meta-analysis of randomized controlled trials on the mortality of antiarrhythmic therapy in postinfarction patients. The odds ratio was analyzed for each of the four classes of antiarrhythmic drugs. Most conventional antiarrhythmic agents (Class I: sodium-channel blockers) and (Class IV: calcium-channel blockers) are associated with an increased mortality. β-blocker (Class II) and potassium-channel blockers (Class III), such as amiodarone, are associated with a reduced mortality. Modified from ref. *31*.

outcome *(31)*, especially in patients with heart failure (Fig. 7) *(28)*. The possible exception to this rule is amiodarone that does not appear to have an adverse effect on either survival or heart failure *(65–68)*. More importantly, the only drug class that convincingly reduces total mortality, as well as the risk of sudden death, is β-blockers (Fig. 8). Relative reductions of cardiac death and sudden death in some trials ranged from 30 to 50% *(69–71)*. However, the utility of β-blockers may be limited by bradyarrhythmias or worsening heart failure in this patient population.

In summary, clinical approach of patients with heart failure and palpitations requires careful assessment of the underlying structural heart disease (ischemic vs nonischemic anatomical substrate) and the nature of potential arrhythmias. The goals of management include minimizing symptoms, reducing thromboembolic complications, and preventing sudden cardiac death. Ambulatory ECG monitors or transtelephonic event recorders should be the initial diagnostic modality. Invasive EPS evaluation is indicated in patients with palpitations associated with hemodynamically significant symptoms, such as sustained tachycardia, severe dyspnea, near-syncope, or syncope. For symptomatic atrial or ventricular premature ectopy, β-blockers should be the first line of treatment, titrated to patients' symptoms and heart rate response. In patients with documented sustained SVT or atrial flutter, aggressive nonpharmacologic approach with catheter ablation provides a curative therapy without the potential side effects and compliance issues associated with chronic drug therapy *(72)*. In heart failure patients with persistent or paroxysmal AF, low-dose amiodarone is preferred because of its low proarrhythmia potential. Furthermore, adequate anticoagulation must be maintained in patients with AF or flutter.

In patients with documented ventricular arrhythmias, EPS is indicated for risk stratification and to guide therapy, specifically in those patients with coronary artery disease and prior myocardial infarctions. In the population with nonischemic cardiomyopathy, β-blockers should be administered as tolerated. Empiric amiodarone therapy may be used for symptomatic control. In addition, empiric defibrillator implantation should be considered in high-risk patients with palpitations associated with clinically significant symptoms or syncope.

REFERENCES

1. Crawford MH, Bernstein SJ, Deedwania PC, et al. ACC/AHA Guidelines for ambulatory electrocardiography: executive summary and recommendations. A report of the American College of Cardiology/American Heart Association task force on practice guidelines (Committee to revise the guidelines for ambulatory electrocardiography). Circulation 1999;100:886–893.
2. Cheitlin MD, Garson A, Gibbons RJ, et al. ACC/AHA guidelines for clinical intracardiac electrophysiological and catheter ablation procedures. Circulation 1995;92:675–691.
3. Krahn AD, Klein GJ, Yee R, et al. Randomized assessment of syncope trial: Conventional diagnostic testing versus prolonged monitoring strategy. Circulation 2001;104:46–51.
4. Stevenson WG, Ganz LI. Atrial fibrillation in heart failure. Heart Failure 1997;13:22–29.
5. Kannel WB, Wolf PA, Benjamin EJ, et al. Prevalence, incidence, prognosis, and predisposing conditions for atrial fibrillation: Population-based estimation. Am J Cardiol 1998;82:2N–9N.
6. Saxon LA. Atrial fibrillation and dilated cardiomyopathy: therapeutic strategies when sinus rhythm cannot be maintained. PACE 1997;20:720–725.
7. Shinbane JS, Wood MA, Jensen N, et al. Tachycardia-induced cardiomyopathy: a review of animal models and clinical studies. J Am Coll Cardiol 1997;29:709–715.
8. Middlekauff HR, Stevenson WG and Stevenson LW, Prognostic significance of atrial fibrillation in advanced heart failure: a study of 390 patients. Circulation 1991;84:40–48.
9. Aberg H. Atrial fibrillation: a study of atrial thrombosis and systemic embolism in a necropsy material. Acta Med Scand 1969;185:373–379.
10. Manning WJ, Silverman DI, Keighley CS, et al. Transesophageal echocardiographically facilitated early cardioversion from atrial fibrillation suing short-term anticoagulation: final results of a prospective 4.5-year study. J Am Coll Cardiol 1995;25:1345–1361.

11. Nademanee K, Kosar EM. Long-term antithrombotic treatment for atrial fibrillation. Am J Cardiol 1998;82:37N–42N.
12. Wolf PA, Abbott RD, Kannel WB. Atrial fibrillation as an independent risk factor for stroke: the Framingham Study. Stroke 1991;22:983–988.
13. Petersen P, Boysen G, Godtfredsen J, et al. Placebo-controlled, randomised trial of warfarin and aspirin for prevention of thromboembolic complications in chronic atrial fibrillation. The Copenhagen AFASAK study. Lancet 1989;1:175–179.
14. Stroke Prevention in Atrial Fibrillation Study. Final results. Circulation 1991;84:527–539.
15. The effect of low-dose warfarin on the risk of stroke in patients with nonrheumatic atrial fibrillation. The Boston Area Anticoagulation Trial for Atrial Fibrillation Investigators. N Engl J Med 1990;323:1505–1511.
16. Connolly SJ, Laupacis A, Gent M, et al. Canadian Atrial Fibrillation Anticoagulation (CAFA) Study. J Am Coll Cardiol 18:349–355.
17. Ezekowitz MD, Bridgers SL, James KE, et al. Warfarin in the prevention of stroke associated with nonrheumatic atrial fibrillation. Veterans Affairs Stroke Prevention in Nonrheumatic Atrial Fibrillation Investigators. N Engl J Med 1992;327:1406–1412.
18. Halperin JL, Hart RG, Kronmal RA, et al. Warfarin versus aspirin for prevention of thromboembolism in atrial fibrillation: Stroke Prevention in Atrial Fibrillation II Study. Lancet 1994;343:687–691.
19. Laupacis A, Albers G, Dalen J, et al. Antithrombotic therapy in atrial fibrillation. Chest 1995;108:352S–359S.
20. Hylek EM, Skates SJ, Sheehan MA, et al. An analysis of the lowest effective intensity of prophylactic anticoagulation for patients with nonrheumatic atrial fibrillation. N Engl J Med 1996;335:540–546.
21. Koudstaal P, The European Atrial Fibrillation Trial Study. Optimal oral anticoagulation therapy in patients with nonrheumatic atrial fibrillation and recent cerebral ischemia. N Engl J Med 1995;333:5–10.
22. Tischler MD, Lee TH, McAndrew KA, et al. Clinical, echocardiographic and Doppler correlates of clinical instability with onset of atrial fibrillation. Am J Cardiol 1990;66:721–724.
23. Wijffels MC, Kirchhof CJ, Dorland R, et al. Atrial fibrillation begets atrial fibrillation. A study in awake chronically instrumented goats. Circulation 1995;92:1954–1968.
24. Daoud EG, Bogun F, Goyal R, et al. Effect of atrial fibrillation on atrial refractoriness in humans. Circulation 1996;94:1600–1606.
25. Yu WC, Chen SA, Lee SH, et al. Tachycardia-induced change in atrial refractory period in humans. Rate dependency and effects of antiarrhythmic drugs. Circulation 1998;97:2331–2337.
26. Coplen SE, Antman EM, Berlin JA, et al. Efficacy and safety of quinidine therapy for maintenance of sinus rhythm after cardioversion: a meta-analysis of randomized control trials. Circulation 1990;82:1106–1116.
27. Chatterjee K, Demarco T, Saxon LA, et al. Antiarrhythmic drug therapy for atrial fibrillation in dilated cardiomyopathy. Heart Failure 1997;13:7–21.
28. Pratt CM, Eaton T, Francis M, et al. The inverse relationship between baseline left ventricular ejection fraction and outcome of antiarrhythmic therapy: a dangerous imbalance in the risk-benefit ratio. Am Heart J 1989;118:433–440.
29. Echt DS, Liebson PR, Mitchell LB, et al. Mortality and morbidity in patients receiving encainide, flecainide, or placebo. The Cardiac Arrhythmia Suppression Trial. N Engl J Med 1991;324:781–788.
30. Flaker GC, Blackshear JL, McBride R, et al. Antiarrhythmic drug therapy and cardiac mortality in atrial fibrillation. J Am Coll Cardiol 1992l20:527–532.

31. Teo KK, Yusuf S and Furberg CD. Effects of prophylactic antiarrhythmic drug therapy in acute myocardial infarction. An overview of results from randomized controlled trials. JAMA 1993l270:1589–1595.
32. Waldo AL and Prystowsky EN. Drug treatment of atrial fibrillation in the managed care era. Am J Cardiol 1998l81:23C–29C.
33. Keane D, Zou L and Ruskin J. Non-pharmacologic therapies for atrial fibrillation. Am J Cardiol 1998l81:41C–45C.
34. Haïssaguerre M, Jaïs P, Shah DC, et al. Spontaneous initiation of atrial fibrillation by ectopic beats originating in the pulmonary veins. N Engl J Med 1998;339:659–666.
35. Chen SA, Hsieh MH, Tai CT, et al. Initiation of atrial fibrillation by ectopic beats originating from the pulmonary veins: electrophysiological characteristics, pharmacological responses, and effects of radiofrequency ablation. Circulation 1999;100:1879–1886.
36. Waldo AL. Management of atrial fibrillation: the need for AFFIRMative action. Am J Cardiol 1999;84:698–700.
37. Schumacher B, Luderitz B. Rate issues in atrial fibrillation: Consequences of tachycardia and therapy for rate control. Am J Cardiol 1998;82:29N–36N.
38. Jensen SM, Bergfeldt L, Rosenqvist M. Long-term follow-up of patients treated by radiofrequency ablation of the atrioventricular junction. PACE 1995;18:1609–1614.
39. Rodriquez LM, Smeets JL, Xie B, et al. Improvement in left ventricular function by ablation of atrioventricular nodal conduction in selected patients with lone atrial fibrillation. Am J Cardiol 1993;72:1137–1141.
40. Fitzpatrick AP. Impact on quality of life of His-Bundle catheter ablation and permanent pacing: measuring outcomes. Heart Failure 1997;13:43–46.
41. Goldman S, Johnson G, Cohn JN, et al., Mechanism of death in heart failure: the Vasodilator-Heart Failure Trial. Circulation 1993;87:VI 24–31.
42. Kjekshus J. Arrhythmias and mortality in congestive heart failure. Am J Cardiol 1990;65:42I–48I.
43. Randomized trial of low-does amiodarone in severe congestive heart failure. Lancet 1994;344:493–498.
44. Uretsky B, Sheahan RG. Primary prevention of sudden in heart failure: will the solution be shocking? J Am Coll Cardiol 1997;30:1589–1597.
45. Huang SKS, Messer JV, Denes P. Significance of ventricular tachycardia in idiopathic dilated cardiomyopathy: observation in 35 patients. Am J Cardiol 1982;51:507–512.
46. Meinertz T, Hofmann T, Kasper W, et al. Significance of ventricular arrhythmias in idiopathic dilated cardiomyopathy. Am J Cardiol 1984;53:902–907.
47. The Multi-center Post-Infarction Research Group (MPIP). Risk stratification and survival after myocardial infarction. N Engl J Med 1983;309:331–336.
48. Mukharji J, Rude RE, Poole WK, et al. Risk factors for sudden death after acute myocardial infarction: two-year follow-up. Am J Cardiol 1984;54:31–36.
49. Bigger JT, Fleiss JL, Kleiger R, et al. The relationships among ventricular arrhythmias, left ventricular dysfunction, and mortality in the 2 years after myocardial infarction. Circulation 1984;69:250–258.
50. Unverferth DV, Magorien RD, Moeschberger ML, et al. Factors influencing the one-year mortality of dilated cardiomyopathy. Am J Cardiol 1984;54:147–152.
51. Gradman A, Deedwania P, Cody R, et al. Predictors of total mortality and sudden death in mild to moderate heart failure. J Am Coll Cardiol 1989;14:564–570.
52. Olshausen KV, Stienen U, Schwarz F, et al. Long-term prognositic significance of ventricular arrhythmias in idiopathic dilated cardiomyopathy. Am J Cardiol 1988;61:146–151.

53. Packer M. Lack of relation between ventricular arrhythmias and sudden death in patients with chronic heart failure. Circulation 1992;85:I50–I56.
54. Gomes JA, Winters SL, Stewart D, et al. A new noninvasive index to predict sustained ventricular tachycardia and sudden death in the first year after myocardial infarction: based on signal-averaged electrocardiogram, radionuclide ejection fraction and Holter monitoring. J Am Coll Cardiol 1987;10:349–357.
55. Wilbur DJ, Olshansky B, Moran JF, et al. Electrophysiological testing and nonsustained ventricular tachycardia: use and limitations in patients with coronary artery disease and impaired ventricular function. Circulation 1990;82:350–358.
56. Gomes JA, Cain ME, Buxton AE, et al., Prediction of long-term outcomes by signal-averaged electrocardiography in patients with unsutained ventricular tachycardia, coronary artery disease, and left ventricular dysfunction. Circulation 2001;104:436–441.
57. Schmitt C, Barthel P, Ndrepepa G, et al. Value of programmed ventricular stimulation for prophylactic internal cardioverter-defibrillator implantation in postinfarction patients preselected by noninvasive risk stratifiers. J Am Coll Cardiol 2001;37:1901–1907.
58. Moss AJ, Hall J, Cannon DS, et al., Improved survival with an implanted defibrillator in patients with coronary artery disease at high risk for ventricular arrhythmia, N Engl J Med 1996;335:1933–1940.
59. Buxton AE, Lee KL, Fisher JD, et al. A randomized study of the prevention of sudden death in patients with coronary artery disease. N Engl J Med 1999;341:1882–1890.
60. Poll DS, Marchlinski FE, Falcone RA, et al. Abnormal signal-averaged electrocardiograms in patients with nonischemic congestive cardiomyopathy: relationship to sustained ventricular tachyarrhythmias. Circulation 1985;6:1308–1313.
61. Mancini DM, Wong KL, Simson MB. Prognostic value of an abnormal signal-averaged electrocardiogram in patients with nonischemic congestive cardiomyopathy. Circulation 1993;87:1083–1092.
62. Poll DS, Marchlinski FE, Buxton AE, et al. Usefulness of programmed stimulation in idiopathic dilated cardiomyopathy. Am J Cardiol 1986;58:992–997.
63. Middlekauff HR, Stevenson WG, Stevenson LW, et al., Syncope in advanced heart failure: high risk of sudden death regardless of origin of syncope. J Am Coll Cardiol 1993;21:110–116.
64. Knight BP, Goyal R, Pelosi F, et al. Outcome of patients with nonischemic cardiomyopathy and unexplained syncope treated with implantable defibrillator. J Am Coll Cardiol 1999;33:1964–1970.
65. Doval HC, Nul DR, Grancelli HO, et al. Randomized trial of low-does amiodarone in severe congestive heart failure. Lancet 1994;344:493–498,
66. Singh SN, Fletcher RD, Fisher SG, et al., amiodarone in patients with congestive heart failure and asymptomatic ventricular arrhythmia. N Engl J Med 1995;333:77–82.
67. Julian DG, Camm AJ, Frangin G, et al. Randomized trial of effect of amiodarone on mortality in patients with left ventricular dysfunction after recent myocardial infarction: EMIAT. Lancet 1997;349:667–674.
68. Carins JA, Connolly SJ, Roberts R, et al. Randomized trial of outcome after myocardial infarction in patients with frequent or repetitive ventricular premature depolarizations: CAMIAT. Lancet 1997;349:675–682.
69. Packer M, Bristow MR, Cohn JN, et al. The effect of carvedilol on mortality in patients with chronic heart failure. N Engl J Med 1996;334:1349–1355.
70. Hjalmarson A, Prevention of sudden cardiac death with beta blockers. Clinical Cardiology 1999;22:V11–V15.
71. Group MERIT-HF Study, Effect of metoprolol CR/XL in chronic heart failure: metoprolol CR/XL randomized intervention trial in congestive heart failure (MERIT-HF). Lancet 1999;353:2001–2007.

72. Natale A, Newby KH, Pisanó E, et al. Prospective randomized comparison of antiarrhythmic therapy versus first-line radiofrequency ablation in patients with atrial flutter. J Am Coll Cardiol 2000;35:1898–1904.

7

Examination of the Patient Suspected to Have Heart Failure

Susan C. Brozena, MD, FACC, FAHA

INTRODUCTION

The syndrome of heart failure illustrates the close correlation between the underlying pathophysiologic mechanisms and its signs and symptoms. This chapter reviews the basic pathophysiology of heart failure as it applies to the signs, symptoms, and progression of the disease. Similarities and differences are compared between heart failure with preserved and impaired systolic left-ventricular function. It then describes the initial and subsequent evaluations of a patient with heart failure.

DEFINITION OF HEART FAILURE

Heart failure is the pathophysiologic state in which the heart is unable to pump blood at a rate commensurate with the body's requirements or can do so only from an elevated filling pressure.

From: *Contemporary Cardiology: Heart Failure:*
A Clinician's Guide to Ambulatory Diagnosis and Treatment
Edited by: M. L. Jessup and E. Loh © Humana Press Inc., Totowa, NJ

Myocardial failure is the most common cause of heart failure, although other cardiac disorders can cause heart failure, such as valvular heart disease, constrictive pericarditis, and systemic disorders like thyrotoxicosis.

FRANK-STARLING MECHANISM

Nearly independent of the etiology, there are certain pathophysiologic mechanisms and adaptations that occur when a patient has myocardial failure. The most basic mechanism to understand is the Frank-Starling mechanism, as it helps describe the initial adaptation, and the progressive dysfunction of the failing heart. This mechanism illustrates how an increase in preload, reflected in elevated end-diastolic volume, can augment ventricular contraction. In the failing heart, cardiac output and ventricular performance are maintained at the expense of an elevated end-diastolic volume and pressure *(1)*.

When the perceived volume of blood delivered into the systemic vasculature is reduced, as is seen with the depressed contractile state of myocardial failure, a hallmark of heart failure, a complex sequence of compensatory mechanisms occurs, which leads ultimately to an abnormal accumulation of fluid. This expansion of blood volume also represents a very important compensatory adjustment aimed at maintaining arterial pressure and cardiac output by elevating ventricular preload, because the heart is operating on a depressed Frank-Starling pressure-function curve.

Excluding in the terminal stages of heart failure, the augmented left-ventricular end-diastolic volume can be viewed as a way to preserve cardiac forward output. Elevation of ventricular end-diastolic volume and pressure, in accordance with the Frank-Starling mechanism, increases ventricular performance, but similarly causes venous congestion and promotes the formation of pulmonary and/or peripheral edema, secondary to increased blood volume.

Clinical Correlation: Frank-Starling Mechanism

SYMPTOMS

Many of the clinical manifestations of heart failure are because of excessive volume retention. These include:
- Symptoms of pulmonary congestion such as dyspnea, cough, orthopnea, and paroxysmal nocturnal dyspnea
- Symptoms of visceral congestion such as early satiety, abdominal bloating, discomfort and swelling, and decreased appetite
- Complaints of peripheral edema

PHYSICAL EXAMINATION

- Physical manifestations of this volume overload include jugular venous distention, hepatojugular reflux, presence of gallop rhythm, hepatomegaly, peripheral edema, and in severe cases, ascites and anasarca
- Physical findings of left-ventricular dilatation include a displaced, diffuse apical impulse

NEUROHORMONAL ACTIVATION

The principal hemodynamic changes in heart failure are a reduction in cardiac output and atrial hypertension as a result of fluid retention and ventricular diastolic dysfunction. These stimulate a series of complex neurohormonal changes. For example, as a response to a decrease in arterial volume, increase in the adrenergic drive, renin-angiotensin-aldosterone activation, endothelin and vasopressin all act in concert to try to maintain organ perfusion and restore arterial volume. This would be helpful short-term, e.g., if the cause of decreased arterial volume were hemorrhage. But in chronic heart failure, the persistence of these compensatory mechanisms eventually also lead to the progression of the disease, its symptoms, signs, and outcome.

Renin-Angiotensin System

When there is a reduction in cardiac output and a decrease in perfusion, there is activation of the renin-angiotensin-aldosterone system that operates in conjunction with the adrenergic nervous system (*see* Fig. 1). For instance, release of renin from the juxtaglomerular apparatus of the kidney is stimulated by decreased renal perfusion, activation of renal baroreceptors, and also by stimulation by β-1 receptors in the kidney. Renin will cleave angiotensinogen to angiotensin-I that, in turn, is converted to the active angiotensin-II by angiotensin-converting enzyme (ACE). This is both a systemic and local phenomenon. Angiotensin-II is a very potent vasoconstrictor and participates in a cascade of events, which include increase in systemic vascular resistance along with ventricular hypertrophy.

The bradykinin system is a counter-regulatory system that results in vasodilation. Bradykinin is inactivated by ACE. Therefore, ACE inhibitors will lead to an accumulation of bradykinin that not only may contribute to hypotension, but also is the proposed mechanism for the induction of cough, often seen in patients on ACE inhibitors (*see* Fig. 1).

EFFECTS OF ALDOSTERONE

Aldosterone release is stimulated by a number of factors that include angiotensin-II. The effects of aldosterone, such as sodium retention,

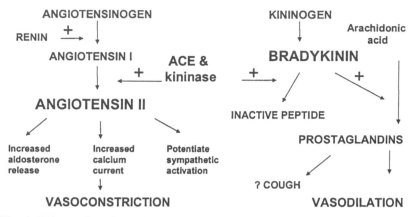

Fig. 1. Effects of angiotensin-II. Angiotensin-II has widespread effects on several organ systems as illustrated in Table 1.

Table 1
Effects of Angiotensin-II

Organ	Effect
Heart	Positive inotrope
	LV hypertrophy/remodeling
Adrenal gland	Aldosterone production and release
Brain	Potentiates sympathetic nervous system
	Stimulates thirst and sodium appetite
	Stimulates release ADH and norepinephrine
Kidney	Constricts afferent and efferent arterioles
	Stimulates proximal tubular reabsorption of sodium
Vasculature	Stimulates smooth muscle hypertrophy

potassium and magnesium loss, baroreceptor dysfunction, impaired arterial compliance, and regulation of sodium transport in colon, sweat glands, and salivary glands.

SECONDARY ALDOSTERONISM

In heart failure, secondary aldosteronism occurs with circulating levels that may reach several times normal in some individuals. There are two pathophysiologic mechanisms that are considered to be responsible for secondary aldosteronism. First, there is an increase in its production by the zona glomerulosa of the adrenal cortex related to increase in plasma angiotensin-II. Second, there is a decreased rate of hepatic clearance. One of the primary determinants of aldosterone metabolism is hepatic blood flow. In those patients with heart failure, the rate of hepatic aldosterone clearance falls by 25–50% because of reductions in hepatic perfusion *(2)*.

CLINICAL CORRELATION:
ACTIVATION OF THE RENIN-ANGIOTENSIN-ALDOSTERONE SYSTEM

Pertinent findings attributed to activation of the renin-angiotensin-aldosterone system include:

- Patients complain of thirst and in some cases, salt craving
- Signs and symptoms of fluid retention
- Increased systemic vascular resistance
- Left-ventricular hypertrophy

Sympathetic Nervous System

The level of circulating norepinephrine is increased in heart failure. The increase in adrenergic drive to maintain cardiac output serves to perpetuate increased systemic vascular resistance and tries to augment cardiac contractility. The increased levels of circulating norepinephrine in heart failure correlates with its severity and prognosis.

There are several direct effects on the myocardium that have an elevated deleterious effect. There have also been studies linking elevated norepinephrine with direct myocyte toxicity. In the β-receptor pathway, there is a decrease in the density of β-1 receptors and are "downregulated." β-2 receptors become "uncoupled" from the stimulatory G-protein. There is an increase in the density of the inhibitory G-protein that further reduces the efficiency of the system. In addition, arrhythmias may be provoked by sympathetic overdrive. Reversal of some of these abnormalities is the rationale behind the use of β-adrenergic antagonists in heart failure.

CLINICAL CORRELATION:
ACTIVATION OF THE ADRENERGIC NERVOUS SYSTEM

Pertinent findings attributed to sympathetic activation include:

- Tachycardia
- Cool, clammy extremities
- Diaphoresis
- Arrhythmias

Natriuretic Peptides

Atrial natriuretic peptide (ANP) levels are also increased in chronic heart failure. ANP is a counter-regulatory hormone that opposes many of the vasoconstrictor and salt- and water-retaining effects of the adrenergic renin-angiotensin-aldosterone and arginine vasopressin systems. ANP acts as a vasodilator agent, suppresses the formation of renin, and enhances the excretion of salt and water.

With chronic and more advanced heart failure, ventricular cells can also be recruited to secrete both ANP and brain natriuretic peptide (BNP), an analogous peptide, in response to elevated filling pressures. Initial clinical studies suggest that the plasma concentrations of BNP may be superior to those of ANP in identifying patients with severe left-ventricular dysfunction. Recombinant BNP has just recently been approved in the United States for use in patients with acute decompensated heart failure.

Cytokines

Cytokines are proteins secreted by cells in response to stress. There are two major classes: vasoconstrictive and vasodepressor or proinflammatory. The vasoconstrictive cytokine significant in heart failure is endothelin. The vasodepressor cytokines involved are TNF-β and interleukin-6. Cytokines are not considered to be causative, but rather can contribute to progression of disease by stimulating myocardial fibrosis, apoptosis or necrosis, and by their systemic effects.

CLINICAL CORRELATION: CYTOKINES

Pertinent clinical findings attributed to cytokine activation may include:

- Anorexia
- Muscle wasting
- "Cardiac cachexia"

Hypertrophy: Concentric vs Eccentric

When the heart faces a hemodynamic burden, it can compensate in several ways. It can use the Frank-Starling mechanism to increase cross-bridge formation, but this has its limits and can lead to dilatation. Muscle mass can be augmented to bear the extra load, but results in hypertrophy and remodeling. Finally, it can recruit neurohormonal mechanisms to augment contractility, but this has long-term deleterious effects.

In response to pressure overload, parallel addition of sarcomeres causes an increase in myocyte width, which, in turn, increases wall thickness, resulting in "concentric hypertrophy." For example, these types of findings would be seen in a patient with hypertensive heart disease, or aortic stenosis.

In response to volume overload, sarcomeres replicate in series that causes an increase in ventricular volume and so-called "eccentric hypertrophy." That is, cavity dilatation with a decrease in the ratio of wall thickness to chamber dimension *(3)*. These findings would be seen in a patient with idiopathic dilated cardiomyopathy or severe mitral regurgitation.

Skeletal Muscle Abnormalities

There are also many abnormalities in skeletal muscle function found to be present in heart failure patients. These include metabolic alterations considered to be related to inadequate mitochondrial oxygen utilization, change in fiber type as well as oxidative capacity that impedes endurance, and decreased strength as a result of smaller cross-sectional area *(4)*. These changes contribute to the often-heard complaints of muscle fatigue and decreased exercise tolerance in our patients.

EVALUATING THE PATIENT FOR THE CAUSE OF HEART FAILURE

Initial Evaluation

The most common "chief complaints" the patient will describe include dyspnea and fatigue. A decrease in exercise tolerance, orthopnea, paroxysmal nocturnal dyspnea, and cough are also frequent complaints, but often have to be brought out in a detailed interview of the patient and his or her family. Depending on the etiology, other symptoms may also be present, such as angina in those patients with coronary artery disease or systemic symptoms in those with infiltrative diseases.

The first step in the evaluation of a patient with heart failure, of course, is to answer the question: "What is the diagnosis?" What is the category and cause of heart failure? A useful approach that can be accomplished on the initial office visit is to determine if the patient has heart failure with a normal left-ventricular chamber size and preserved systolic function, or has a dilated heart with decreased left-ventricular systolic function. Obviously, the physical examination can be very helpful if certain findings are present.

The following compares two patients, both presenting with severe dyspnea and fatigue as a result of heart failure.

Patient 1 is a 60-year-old man. Blood pressure is 88/60 mm Hg. Pulse is 110 and regular. Jugular venous pulse is elevated with hepatojugular reflux. There are basilar rales. The left-ventricular apex is displaced laterally and there is a parasternal lift. There is paradoxical splitting of the second heart sound. There is a prominent third heart sound and a grade 2/6 apical holosystolic murmur that radiates to the axilla. The liver is enlarged and tender and there is pitting edema of the legs. The distal extremities are cool to touch. The electrocardiogram shows sinus tachycardia with complete left bundle branch block.

Patient 2 is a 78-year-old woman. Blood pressure is 160/100. Pulse is 88 and irregular. Jugular venous pulse is normal with mild hepatojugular reflux. There are basilar rales. The left-ventricular apex is not displaced. There is a prominent fourth heart sound. There is no hepatomegaly. There is peripheral edema. Extremities are warm to touch. The electrocardiogram (EG) shows atrial fibrillation and left-ventricular hypertrophy with repolarization abnormalities.

Both patients have heart failure, yet the first patient has an obvious dilated heart with systolic dysfunction, and the second patient has a normal heart size, probably with preserved systolic function and suspected hypertensive heart disease.

The differences between these two categories of heart failure are now compared.

PATIENTS WITH HEART FAILURE AND PRESERVED LEFT-VENTRICULAR SYSTOLIC FUNCTION

The most common clinical scenario in this population of patients includes complaints of dyspnea and fatigue with normal or near normal left-ventricular size on physical examination, chest X-ray, and preserved left-ventricular systolic function when measured by noninvasive or invasive testing. The definitive diagnosis of this disorder would be documentation of increased left-ventricular filling pressure with normal left-ventricular volume and systolic function. The prevalence of heart failure with preserved left-ventricular systolic function varies with age. In the older population, that is over 80 years of age, more than half of all heart failure is due to this disorder and there is a higher incidence in women (5).

When a patient is found to have heart failure symptoms with preserved left-ventricular systolic function, a differential diagnosis needs to be considered. The most common causes of this disorder include hypertension, ischemia, and possible intermittent arrhythmias. Less frequent causes include a high cardiac output state such as anemia, thyrotoxicosis, or Paget's disease. Also to be considered would be pericardial disease. If nonmyocardial causes have been excluded, then left-ventricular diastolic dysfunction is the diagnosis.

Disorders associated with left-ventricular diastolic dysfunction include systemic hypertension, coronary artery disease, hypertrophic cardiomyopathy, diabetes mellitus, chronic renal disease, aortic stenosis, atrial fibrillation, presbycardia, infiltrative cardiomyopathy, such as amyloidosis or hemochromatosis, and idiopathic restrictive cardiomyopathy (6).

Elevated Pulse Pressure. Another example of the helpfulness of the physical examination, is the fact that studies have shown that the pulse pressure increases the risk of heart failure in the elderly. In fact, for each 10 mm Hg elevation in pulse pressure, there was a 14% increase risk of heart failure ($p = 0.03$) Those patients in the highest tertile of pulse pressure (>67 mm Hg) had a 55% risk of heart failure (7).

PATIENTS WITH HEART FAILURE AND DECREASED LEFT-VENTRICULAR SYSTOLIC FUNCTION

When a patient is found to have heart failure symptoms and a decreased left-ventricular ejection fraction, by definition, there is myocardial disease. The question here is whether or not it is primary myocardial disease, or as a result of another, potentially reversible or "controllable" disorder such as coronary or valvular disease or a systemic disorder such as thyrotoxicosis. Therefore, the clinician is compelled to exclude these causes for the purpose of selecting appropriate treatment, as well as for prognosis.

The most common causes of heart failure with decreased left-ventricular systolic function are coronary artery disease, idiopathic dilated cardiomyopathy, hypertension, valvular heart disease, such as aortic or mitral regurgitation, alcohol-related cardiomyopathy, and familial cardiomyopathy. Less frequent causes include myocarditis, sarcoidosis, peripartum cardiomyopathy, and adriamycin cardiomyopathy.

AFTER THE DIAGNOSIS

Once the diagnosis has been clearly established, the patient and family have been appropriately educated, and treatment has been initiated, the clinician must decide how the patient's surveillance follow-up is to be performed. Once treatment is initiated, the serial evaluation of the patient includes the evaluation for response to treatment, as well as monitoring for possible side effects. Consideration should be given at every visit as to whether or not the patient is responding to treatment as expected. If not, why not? Careful review of compliance by the physician or the nurse should be done at each visit.

EFFECTIVENESS AND MONITORING OF TREATMENT

There are several ways to determine effectiveness of treatment. The most obvious of course is to ask if the patient feels better. The monitoring and recording at each visit of New York Heart Association (NYHA) class may also help to put the patient's progress, or lack of it, into perspective for the clinician. But all of these factors may be somewhat subjective, and the "placebo effect" is well known.

How then can we objectively measure effectiveness of treatment? There are several ways. First is by the physical examination. The second way is by following exercise capacity by either serial assessing of the ability to perform common activities, the 6-minute walk, or more formal exercise testing. Third is by monitoring changes in electrolytes and renal function. Finally, treatment effectiveness can be measured by following cardiac size and function.

The Physical Examination

The physical examination provides an objective measurement of response to treatment. Once the baseline examination is carefully recorded, serial examinations should take into consideration any changes that have occurred.

WEIGHT

What has happened to the patient's weight? The setting of a weight goal when diuretic therapy is started is important as is the response to weight reduction diets. Recent data also suggest that determining the patient's body mass index (BMI) is helpful in prognosis and often causes quite a rude awakening to some patients when they discover that their BMI is 35, officially labeling them as obese.

BLOOD PRESSURE

Has the blood pressure responded to addition of ACE inhibitors, or β-blockers? Positional changes in blood pressure should be measured at each visit to determine if orthostatic hypotension is developing, indicating that diuretic or other drug doses may need to be adjusted to avoid worsening side effects.

When is the blood pressure "too low"? Certainly if the patient has significant orthostatic symptoms, then the blood pressure is too low, regardless of the numerical value of the systolic pressure. Adjustment of diuretic dose may resolve this problem. If not, then other drug doses may need to be decreased. It is important to document any positional changes in blood pressure or pulse *before* initiating treatment to exclude any other possible cause of orthostatic hypotension.

The absolute goal for systolic blood pressure in the heart failure patient varies according to the patient, taking into consideration other comorbidities, such as renal insufficiency and cerebrovascular disease. In patients with dilated cardiomyopathy and no other comorbidity, systolic blood pressure between 80 and 90 mm Hg is often quite well tolerated. As long as the patient is asymptomatic and has adequate renal and cerebral perfusion, then it is an acceptable level.

In contrast, an elderly patient who has had a previous stroke, along with renal insufficiency, is much less likely to tolerate a low-systolic pressure. This needs to be individualized for each patient. Symptoms, monitoring of renal function with blood urea nitrogen and creatinine levels, and measuring orthostatic changes in blood pressure, are helpful in evaluating the tolerable lower range of systolic blood pressure for the individual patient.

Standard classic findings in a patient who is manifesting signs of a low-cardiac output include a low pulse pressure, as well as cool, clammy extremities. Observation of changes in this parameter should be performed.

PULSE RATE/CHARACTER

Patients with dilated cardiomyopathy may have a normal carotid upstroke but a low-carotid pulse volume because of low-cardiac output. The use of the carotid pulse character in the elderly is more difficult to assess as a result of stiffening of the arterial walls, which may affect the evaluation for volume of the arterial pulse.

The pulses in the extremities should be checked at each visit. The character of the pulse should be noted and compared. Not only does this help with a general determination of distal perfusion, but this may also provide evidence of vascular disease.

JUGULAR VENOUS PULSE

Jugular venous distention and the presence of hepatojugular reflux has been shown to have a high sensitivity and specificity for the evaluation of a patient with heart failure in regard to its correlation not only to elevated right heart pressures, but also to elevated wedge pressure (8). This is a simple, useful parameter and should be performed each time the patient is seen in the office. Proper examination of the jugular venous pulse requires that the height and character of the pulse is observed at a 30° angle of elevation with adjustment of the angle depending on the ability to observe the maximal visible oscillations of the right-internal jugular vein. The height of the external jugular vein can estimate the mean right-atrial pressure. The internal jugular vein is examined both for height and wave form. The maximum height of the oscillations is recorder in centimeters above the sternal angle (9).

Adjusting diuretics or doses of ACE inhibitors or other medications can be based on changes in this finding. The presence of a high right-atrial pressure as manifested by elevated jugular venous pulse has also been shown to have prognostic significance (10,11).

THE CARDIOPULMONARY EXAM

Of course, the cardiac examination itself is of utmost importance in the initial and serial evaluation of the patient with heart failure. Although the absence of certain findings is not always helpful in the evaluation, certainly the presence of such findings is helpful. For example, in one study of patients with documented wedge pressures >35 mm Hg, 68% of patients had a third heart sound, 42% had a displaced apical impulse, and 37% had rales. The specificity of these findings was good, but the sensitivity was not, depending on the individual parameter *(12)*. Therefore, the presence of these abnormal findings is helpful, but the absence is not.

Another study showed that rales, edema, and elevated jugular pressure were present in 58% of patients with documented wedge pressure ≥ 22 mm Hg *(13)*. The concern in this study was that reliance on physical signs alone for elevated filling pressure might result in inadequate therapy. In this population of patients who may be quite symptomatic, yet with a relatively "unremarkable" physical examination, hemodynamic monitoring may be helpful in guiding therapy.

The presence of a third heart sound may also be a prognostic indicator. Careful attention should be given to the auscultation of this finding. The third heart sound is a soft, low-frequency sound and is best heard with the bell of the stethoscope applied just lightly enough to the chest wall to form a skin seal. In some patients, the third heart sound is clearly felt during palpation even before auscultation is begun.

The presence of a third heart sound also yields prognostic information. In a study of patients with ischemic heart disease, the presence of a third heart sound and a low-maximal oxygen uptake yielded a poor prognosis *(14)*. An analysis of physical examination findings in the Study of Left-Ventricular Dysfunction (SOLVD) has shown that elevated jugular venous pressure and a third heart sound are each independently associated with adverse outcome, including progression of heart failure *(11)*.

Unfortunately, there are no studies on the significance of serial changes in physical findings as a response to treatment and a measure of prognosis. Monitoring the changes in the physical examination in a heart failure patient is an absolute necessity in objectively assessing response to treatment as well as the progression of disease. In fact, in our heart failure clinic, each patient has a physical examination flow sheet to track all of the previously mentioned physical findings. There is no question that when there is resolution of jugular venous distention and hepatojugular reflux, absence of a previously documented third heart sound, resolution of a previously heard murmur of mitral or tricuspid regurgitation, and improvement in the apical impulse, then cardiac function, and hopefully the patient, are better!

Fluid Retention/Edema

The simplest way to monitor changes in fluid retention is by monitoring body weight. There have been several studies that have shown the benefit of this simple, inexpensive way to help monitor diuretic dose. This also involves the patient in his or her care. Daily weight measurements are an integral part of the care of the symptomatic heart failure. In those patients who are stable with minimal change in diuretic dose, monitoring body weight a few times a week may suffice. Detecting edema of the extremities is fairly straightforward and can be "tracked" using the physical examination flow sheet.

Although not routine for each patient, measurement of abdominal girth in selected patients can prove to be helpful, particularly if these patients have symptoms of congestion in the absence of peripheral edema. Traditionally, these patients will note that by the end of the day they need to loosen their belts, or they may feel their clothing has become tighter. They may complain of shortness of breath when bending over, possibly because of an increase in preload that would occur in that position. Other patients know they need an extra diuretic when their rings get tight.

Measurement of Exercise Capacity/Endurance

The various methods available to measure submaximal and maximal exercise capacity in heart failure patients are reviewed in Chapter 11. In clinical practice, it is often helpful to choose one physical activity that initially caused symptoms of dyspnea or fatigue and track the patient's ability to perform that activity. For example, does the patient still get dyspnea walking up one flight of steps? Can the patient now carry grocery bags from the car into the kitchen without symptoms? Can the patient complete a day's work in the office without needing to take a nap? Submaximal exercise capacity can also be measured by the 6-minute walk and may be helpful in determining response to therapy. In addition, it does give the clinician an idea of pulse rate, and blood pressure response to submaximal exercise that may help to monitor drug therapy.

There are indications for maximal exercise testing with determination of maximal oxygen consumption. This method of quantifying maximal exercise capacity is simple, noninvasive, and provides a great deal of information with regard to cardiopulmonary response to exercise. It is helpful in determining timing for evaluation for heart transplantation and can provide information on prognosis. It is also helpful when trying to determine the individual contribution of pulmonary disease in those patients who have both cardiac and pulmonary disease.

Serial Laboratory Measurements

Results of electrolyte determinations are helpful in monitoring medication response and side effects as well as having prognostic significance, e.g., hyponatremia may be a sign of volume overload, so-called "dilutional hyponatremia," and also has prognostic significance in heart failure patients. Patients on diuretics, ACE inhibitors, aldosterone receptor antagonists, or spironolactone need to have careful monitoring of their electrolytes and renal function to monitor for potassium balance and signs of contraction alkalosis.

Other blood testing that should be serially followed includes trough digoxin levels, and lipids in selected patients. In addition, BNP has also been found to be a potentially useful marker that may aid in the diagnosis of CHF, but more research is needed to fully determine its role (15).

THE ELECTROCARDIOGRAM

The ECG is usually abnormal in those patients with heart failure. which makes the initial ECG helpful. There may be evidence of a previous infarction, a conduction defect, or low voltages, e.g., that would suggest an infiltrative process. Serial ECGs should be performed to determine if there is any increase in QRS duration that can occur as the disease progresses. In addition, in those symptomatic patients who have a wide QRS duration, either with a bundle branch block, or nonspecific ventricular conduction delay, consideration could be given for their potential candidacy for biventricular pacemaker or resynchronization therapy.

SERIAL MEASUREMENTS OF CARDIAC SIZE AND FUNCTION

All patients should have an initial measurement of left- and right-ventricular size and function. The choice of test may be individualized depending upon the clinician's preference. The most helpful is an echocardiogram with Doppler examination. This informtion includes chamber sizes, degree of hypertrophy, status of the heart valves, quantitation of valvular regurgitation or stenosis, presence or absence of thrombus, presence of regional wall-motion abnormalities, ejection fraction, presence of a pericardial effusion, Doppler indices of diastolic function, and estimation of pulmonary artery systolic pressure. The radionuclide ventriculogram also provides important information including both right- and left-ventricular ejection fractions, ventricular volume measurements, compliance curves for evaluation of diastolic function, presence of regional abnormalities.

It is helpful to monitor cardiac size and function using serial echocardiograms. Frankly, the frequency and usefulness of serial echocardiograms in patients with heart failure is somewhat controversial and is often influenced by "precertification" from the patient's insurance carrier.

It is reasonable to repeat an echocardiogram after the patient has achieved optimized, maximal medical therapy for at least 3 to 6 months. In those patients with systolic failure, "optimal" therapy would include ACE inhibitors, digoxin, β blockers, and diuretics when needed. Given the time sequence in the occurrence of favorable left-ventricular remodeling with these drugs, particularly β-blockers, a repeat echocardiogram in about 6 months after achieving target or maximally tolerated dose of the β-blocker. It has been found to be quite helpful in confirming response, as well as sharing the results with the patient. Of course, this practice at times results in having to tell the patient that there was no change in the anatomic parameters of the heart, which can be upsetting to them at times. The other benefits of the drugs need to be emphasized.

A yearly echocardiogram or radionuclide ventriculogram is not indicated in every heart failure patient. There are certain "triggers" that should alert the clinician that there may be disease progression and a change in ventricular size or function. These "triggers" include a worsening of the physical exam findings, increased symptoms, increased heart size on chest X-ray, echocardiogram changes or development of a left-bundle branch block, and new arrhythmias.

There are certain types of patients with heart failure in whom an echocardiogram should be ordered sooner than 6 months after the initial study. For example, in women with peripartum cardiomyopathy, or in patients with acute myocarditis, improvements in left-ventricular function can occur within weeks after diagnosis and should be assessed by physical examination, and in some cases, repeat echocardiogram.

SUMMARY

The signs and symptoms of heart failure, as well as its prognosis, are closely related to its pathophysiology. Regardless of the etiology, response to treatment and prognosis are based on a sound knowledge of these compensatory mechanisms. The initial and follow-up evaluation of patients with heart failure involves an understanding of these mechanisms and how they impact on the progression of disease and should include meticulous attention to the physical findings. The astute clinician will recognize those signs that indicate whether or not the medical treatment plan is effective in the particular patient and will be able to identify those patients who are responding appropriately versus those in whom the disease is progressing.

REFERENCES

1. Braunwald E. Textbook of Cardiovascular Medicine. WB Saunders, Philadelphia, PA: 1997, p. 394.
2. Weber, KT. Aldosterone and spironolactone in heart failure. N Engl J Med 1999;341:752–755.
3. Carabello BA, Lorell BH. Left ventricular hypertrophy. Pathogenesis, detection, prognosis. Circulation 2000;102:470–479.
4. Mancini DM, Wilson JR, Bolinger L, et al. In vivo magnetic resonance spectroscopy measurement of deoxymyoglobin during exercise in patients with heart failure: demonstration of abnormal muscle metabolism despite adequate oxygenation. Circulation 1994;90:500–508.
5. Vasan RS, Benjamin EJ, Levy D. Congestive heart failure with normal left ventricular systolic function: clinical approaches to the diagnosis and treatment of diastolic heart failure. Arch Int Med 1996;156(2):146–157.
6. Williams JF, Bristow MR, Fowler MB, et al. Guidelines for the evaluation and management of heart failure: report of the American College of Cardiology/American Heart Association Task Force on practice guidelines. (ACC/AHA Task Force Report) Circulation 1995;92:2764–2784.
7. Chae CU, Pfeffer MA, Glynn RJ, et al. Increased pulse pressure and risk of heart failure in the elderly. JAMA 1999;281(7):634–643.
8. Butman SM, Standen JR, Kern KB, et al. Bedside cardiovascular examination in patients with chronic heart failure: importance of rest or inducible jugular venous distention. J Am Coll Cardiol 1993;22:968–974.
9. Perloff JK. The jugular venous pulse and third heart sound in patients with heart failure. N Eng J Med 2001;345:612,613.
10. Morley D, Brozena SC. Assessing risk by hemodynamic profile in patients awaiting cardiac transplantation. Am J Cardiol 1994;73:379–383.
11. Drazner MH, Rame JE, Stevenson LW, et al. Prognostic importance of elevated jugular venous pressure and a third heart sound in patients with heart failure. N Eng J Med 2001;345:574–581.
12. Mattleman SJ, Hakki AH, Iskandrian AS, et al. Reliability of bedside evaluation in determining left ventricular function: correlation with left ventricular ejection fraction determined by radionuclide ventriculography. J Am Coll Cardiol 1983;1:417–420.
13. Stevenson LW, Perloff JK. The limited reliability of physical signs for estimating hemodynamics in chronic heart failure. JAMA 1989;261:884–888.
14. Likoff MJ, Chandler SL, Kay HR. Clinical determinants of mortality in chronic congestive heart failure secondary to idiopathic dilated or to ischemic cardiomyopathy. Am J Cardiol 1987;59:634–638.
15. Hunt SA, Baker DW, Chin MH, et al. American College of Cardiology/American Heart Association.ACC/AHA guidelines for the evaluation and management of chronic heart failure in the adult: executive summary. A report of the American College of Cardiology/ American Heart Association Task Force on Practice Guidelines (Committee to revise the 1995 Guidelines for the Evaluation and Management of Heart Failure). J Am Coll Cardiol 2001;38:2101–2113.

8 Evaluation of Ventricular Function

Craig H. Scott, MD and Victor A. Ferrari, MD

INTRODUCTION

Heart failure is the final common pathway of a number of cardiovascular diseases. Hypertension, valvular disease, coronary artery disease, congenital heart defects, and disorders of the myocytes or extracellular matrix may result in abnormalities in both systolic and diastolic function. Noninvasive imaging techniques that have the spatial and temporal resolution to assess both global and regional cardiac function, valvular function, and patterns of blood flow greatly enhance the diagnosis and management of patients with heart failure. In addition, important prognostic information may be derived from these imaging techniques.

From: *Contemporary Cardiology: Heart Failure:*
A Clinician's Guide to Ambulatory Diagnosis and Treatment
Edited by: M. L. Jessup and E. Loh © Humana Press Inc., Totowa, NJ

Echocardiography is the most commonly used imaging test for the assessment of cardiac function. It is safe, noninvasive, repeatable, does not use ionizing radiation, and can be performed adequately on the majority of patients. Other imaging techniques, such as nuclear imaging, magnetic resonance imaging (MRI), and ultrafast CT have also been used to assess cardiac function. Each technique has unique capabilities and limitations. This chapter discusses the noninvasive evaluation of ventricular function in patients with the most common causes of heart failure.

GENERAL IMAGING GOALS

The goal of noninvasive imaging methods is to provide an overall assessment of global and regional systolic function, valvular function, and when possible, diastolic function. Echocardiographic, MRI, and CT techniques can also evaluate disorders of the pericardium. Regardless of the imaging technique used, there is qualitative and quantitative information that will assist the clinician in evaluating and treating heart failure.

As a global measure of left-ventricular function, the ejection fraction (LVEF) provides a useful assessment of overall cardiac performance and has important prognostic information. The ejection fraction is given as the percentage of blood ejected from the heart per beat:

$$EF = (EDV - ESV)/EDV$$

where EDV = end diastolic volume, and ESV = end systolic volume.

The normal range for LVEF is 55–75% *(1)*. Patients with an LVEF less than 40% by any mechanism have been shown to have an increased mortality in comparison to those with greater ejection fractions. This has been shown in multiple studies examining infarction *(2,3)*, valvular disease, and idiopathic cardiomyopathy *(4)*.

However, the ejection fraction does not correlate well with overall patient status, and specifically, ejection fraction correlates poorly with functional status *(5)*. For example, some patients with an ejection fraction of 10% can still exercise with minimal symptoms, whereas others with an ejection fraction of 45% become symptomatic walking only short distances. Clearly, there are other important factors that affect patients' exercise capacity beyond this simple functional measurement, however, ejection fraction retains an important clinical role.

There are also other parameters that imaging techniques measure that can help assess patient status, prognosis, and assist in management. Noninvasive imaging provides specific information about the causes of heart failure. Measurements of wall thickness and abnormal diastolic filling suggest hypertension, hypertrophic cardiomyopathy, or aortic stenosis. Regional wall motion abnormalities at rest or with stress testing, or combined with assessments of rest and stress perfusion, may indicate coronary artery disease as the etiology for congestive heart failure (CHF). Valvular stenosis or regurgitation can result in pressure or volume overload states, which may lead to heart failure or worsen existing heart failure should they develop. Abnormal diastolic filling patterns can suggest infiltrative processes or pericardial constriction. Currently, echocardiography provides the most comprehensive assessment of left-ventricular function of all of the available techniques. It provides a rapid evaluation of the size and overall shape of the left-ventricle, regional-wall thicknesses and segmental function, and depicts the overall left-ventricular diastolic function.

ECHOCARDIOGRAPHY

The echocardiogram is an excellent technique to assess cardiac function. It is portable, allowing even the most ill intensive care unit patients to be imaged. It is safe, using ultrasound instead of ionizing radiation and avoiding intravenous contrast-related adverse effects. Chest-wall echocardiography has no known important side effects. Transesophageal echocardiography is somewhat more invasive, requiring intubation of the esophagus, but in experienced hands and with appropriate patient screening, has a low complication rate.

Echocardiography can assess global and regional LV function both qualitatively and semiquantitatively. It can assess valvular stenosis and regurgitation, measure wall thickness, and in conjunction with either treadmill or pharmacologic stress testing, can aid in the diagnosis of coronary artery disease.

GLOBAL AND REGIONAL FUNCTION

Global LVEF and regional-wall motion can be assessed with echocardiography. Whereas a number of quantitative techniques exist, the most accurate is the biplane Simpson's rule test (Fig. 1). Orthogonal left-ventricular long-axis views are obtained in systole and diastole. Their contours are traced and the long axis of the left ventricle is determined. The two contours are considered to be the greater and lesser axes of an ellipse normal to the long axis. The area of these stacked ellipses can be determined and their spacing is known, such that each individual ellipse has an associated volume. The summation of these individual slice volumes is the volume of the chamber.

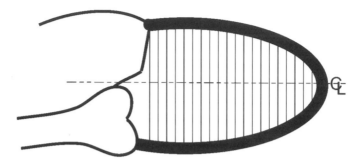

Fig. 1. Determination of the volume using the long axis Simpson's rule method. The left-ventricular volume is the summation of a series of equal height stacked disks of varying radii, where the radius of the disk is based on the distance from the ventricular long axis to multiple locations along the left-ventricular endocardial edge. The method can also be used to estimate mass by applying the same technique to the epicardial edge and subtracting the determined endocardial (blood pool) volume.

Clinically, more straightforward measurements of chamber dimensions and wall thickness are employed. M-mode and two-dimensional (2D) techniques are generally used to determine the thickness of the anterior septum and posterior wall in diastole, as well as the left-ventricular chamber diameter near the mid-ventricle in both systole and diastole. The diameters of the left atrium and aortic root are also measured. Qualitative assessments of ejection fraction by experienced interpreters have been validated against quantitative techniques with excellent correlation (6,7).

Regional-wall motion can be evaluated at rest and with stress to assess for the presence of coronary artery disease. Resting-wall motion variation suggests infarction, or stunned or hibernating myocardium, but can also be seen in global cardiomyopathies, patients with intraventricular conduction delays, or with right-ventricular pressure and/or volume overload. However, a significant number of patients with nonischemic cardiomyopathies can have regional-wall motion abnormalities at initial presentation (8), presumably as a result of heterogeneity of the disease process. The pattern of the regional abnormality can be helpful in differentiating ischemic from nonischemic disease. Coronary artery occlusions typically cause regional-wall motion abnormalities and/or wall thinning distal to the occlusion. Therefore, it would be unlikely that a basal anterior-wall motion abnormality with preserved anterior apical function would be consistent with an infarction in the mid-left-anterior descending coronary distribution. However, coronary anatomy varies—10% of patients have the posterior descending artery supplied by the circumflex artery, the remainder supplied by the right coronary, with a few having both coronaries supplying the posterior wall. Nevertheless, there are occasional echocardiograms that can clearly show thinned, akinetic segments surrounded by normally functioning myocardium that are consistent with infarction rather than a cardiomyopathic process.

Because resting-wall motion can be misleading in difficult cases, stress testing has been used in patients with suspected coronary artery disease. Standard stress testing by echocardiography has an approximately 85% sensitivity and specificity for the detection of coronary artery disease (9). Specifically, the sensitivity of stress echocardiography for the diagnosis of coronary artery disease is 58% for single-vessel disease, 86% for two-vessel disease and 94% for three- vessel disease (10). Stress testing in patients with low-ejection fraction using any technique is not as sensitive or specific as those with normal function. This may be a result of a greater incidence of conduction system abnormalities, more difficulty assessing changes in resting-wall motion, or wall thinning and distortion of the normal anatomy. Some physicians believe that stress testing in this low ejection fraction patient group has insufficient accuracy to exclude the presence of coronary artery disease and opt to perform cardiac catheterization directly.

Pharmacologic stress testing with dobutamine has been shown to be specific for the detection of hibernating myocardium (11,12). This is a condition in patients with severe coronary artery disease where the myocytes are chronically deprived of sufficient blood flow to contract, but remain alive. Low-dose dobutamine infusion causes an increase in wall thickening in hibernating myocardium, which may decrease at higher dobutamine infusion rates. Nuclear perfusion techniques are more sensitive for the detection of hibernation, but are less specific, likely because they identify isolated myocytes that cannot regain function even if revascularized (13). Echocardiography can also assess wall thickness, which is important in hibernation. If the left-ventricular wall is thinned to less than 5mm, it is unlikely to regain function after revascularization.

VISUAL APPEARANCE

The most striking echocardiograms are those of patients with dilated cardiomyopathies (Fig. 2). The left ventricle appears markedly enlarged with relatively symmetric wall thickness. In the most severe cases, all cardiac chambers are enlarged with thinning of the left-ventricular wall, a change in the relationship of the right-ventricular moderator band to

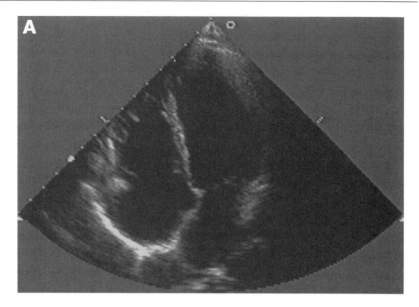

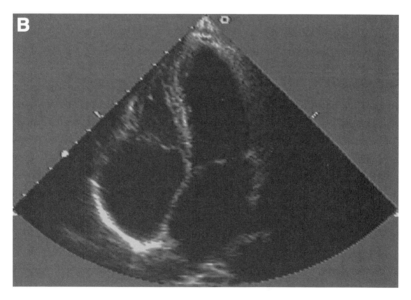

Fig. 2. Apical 4 chamber echocardiographic view of a normal heart and one with a dilated cardiomyopathy (DCM): (A) normal end-diastole, (B) Normal end-systole, (C) DCM end-diastole, (D) DCM end-systole. Note that the calibration marks along the edge of the image are 1 cm. The normal heart is smaller and contracts more vigorously than the DCM heart.

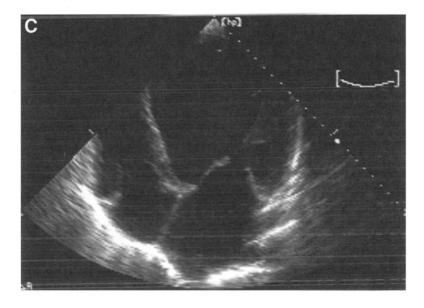

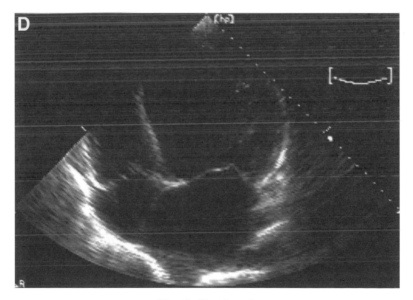

Fig. 2. Continued.

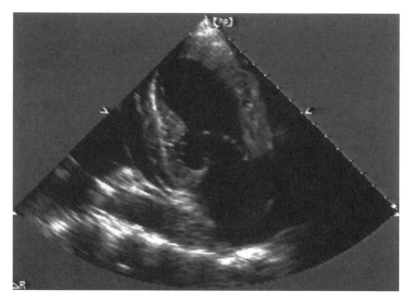

Fig. 3. Echocardiogram—apical 2 chamber view of the left ventricle. The myocardium is grainy, the mitral valve is thickened, and there is a small pericardial effusion.

the ventricular septum and RV free wall, and severely depressed ventricular function.

Certain infiltrative cardiomyopathies have a distinct appearance on 2D echocardiography. Amyloidosis is suspected in patients with a constellation of findings, which include a pericardial effusion, atrial and ventricular wall hypertrophy plus valvular thickening. There is also biventricular dysfunction without cavity dilatation and thickening of all valve leaflets, as well as the interatrial septum. The classic description is that the ventricular walls have a ground glass appearance on 2D echocardiography (Fig. 3).

Hypertrophic cardiomyopathies can have asymmetric markedly thickened and frequently hypokinetic walls. Wall thickness and function can be assessed by echocardiography. A ratio of 1.4:1 between the thickness of the septum and the posterior wall suggests asymmetric hypertrophy of the septum, one of the hallmarks of the septal variant of hypertrophic cardiomyopathy.

DOPPLER IMAGING AND BLOOD FLOW

The frequency of sound is changed when it reflects off a moving object. The change in frequency is linearly dependent on the velocity of the object, which is the Doppler effect. The change in frequency of an ultrasound beam can be used to determine the velocity of flowing blood. This velocity information can be color-coded and overlayed onto the 2D image in real-time and is called color Doppler. This technique allows visualization of stenotic and regurgitant valvular abnormalities (Fig. 4). The Doppler information can also be displayed as a graph of velocity with time (Fig. 5) known as spectral Doppler. With this technique, the velocities of stenotic or regurgitant jets can be measured. The Bernoulli equation allows for the estimation of pressure based on velocity information in certain circumstances. If a small orifice separates two chambers at different pressures, the velocity of fluid flowing between them is dependent only on the pressure difference between the two chambers using the equation:

$$\Delta P = 4V^2$$

where ΔP is the difference in pressure between the two chambers, and V is the maximum velocity measured by continuous wave Doppler ultrasound at the orifice.

This equation makes it possible to noninvasively estimate pressure gradients across stenotic valves and to use the peak velocity of the tricuspid regurgitation (TR) jet to estimate the pulmonary artery systolic pressure (Fig. 6).

Doppler imaging therefore allows for the assessment of the severity of aortic, mitral, and tricuspid regurgitation, all of which are important in the evaluation of both the causes and effects of cardiomyopathy. Severe tricuspid regurgitation can cause peripheral edema and hepatic congestion. Severe mitral regurgitation (MR) can cause shortness of breath, pulmonary edema, and pulmonary hypertension. Severe MR increases the volume load to the left ventricle, resulting in chamber dilatation. A vicious cycle can begin as MR caused by cardiomyopathic chamber dilatation increases preload, thereby worsening chamber dilatation and promoting worsening of MR. Both end-systolic diameter and LVEF are important predictors of outcome in chronic MR (14,15). Poorer postoperative outcomes are seen in patients with end-systolic diameters of 52 mm or greater, or with an LVEF less than 50%. Long-standing aortic regurgitation (AR) will cause chamber dilatation and hypertrophy from increased preload and afterload. Eventually, heart failure can result. The timing of aortic valve repair is a clinically challenging problem, and echocardiography plays an important role in managing AR patients. Echocardiography can help assess changes in the degree of AR, as well as in the diameter of the left ventricle, and was useful in clinical trials examining the use of afterload reducing agents

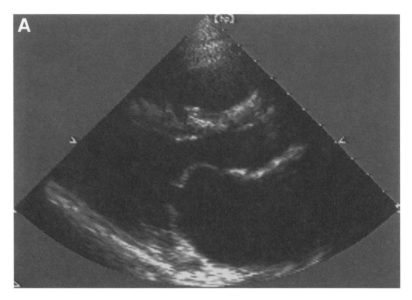

Fig. 4A. Echocardiogram—parasternal long axis view with diastolic doming of the mitral valve consistent with rheumatic mitral stenosis.

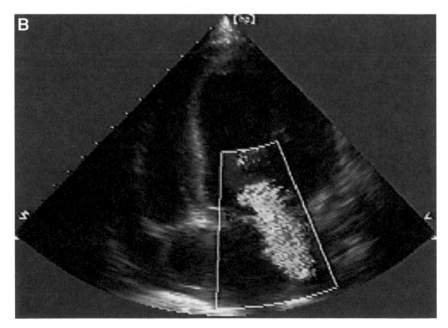

Fig. 4B. Echocardiogram—apical chamber view of severe MR displayed with color Doppler. The direction of the jet is color coded wih blue, implying flow away from the transducer (vertex of the sector at the top of the image).

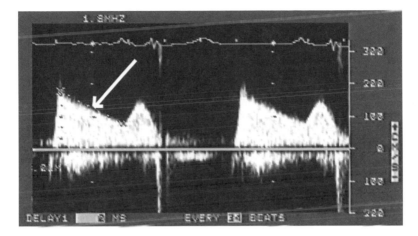

Fig. 5. Spectral Doppler echocardiographic image: Velocity vs time of blood flow through a stenotic mitral valve. Pressure half time, a validated method used to calculate mitral valve area, can be determined by the slope of the passive diastolic filling portion of the curve (arrow). The flatter the slope, the more severe the stenosis.

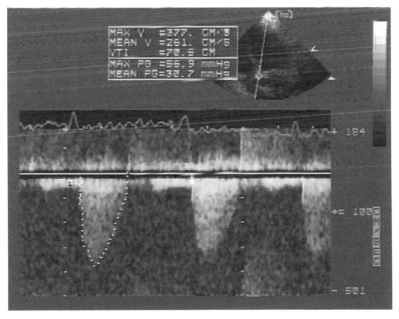

Fig. 6. Continuous wave spectral Doppler display: The peak and mean velocity of blood flow determined from this image allows calculation of pressure gradients when used in conjunction with the modified Bernoulli equation. This image displays peak velocity through a stenotic aortic valve.

to forestall AVR *(16,17)*. Other studies have shown that patients with severe AR and an left-ventricular end-systolic diameter of less than 40 mm will remain stable and do not require urgent surgery. However, those patients with an end-systolic diameter of greater than 55 mm or an EF of less than 50% and AR have an increased risk of death because of complications of left-ventricular dysfunction if not repaired *(18)*.

Spectral Doppler can be used to determine the presence of pulmonary hypertension, which can indicate pulmonary vascular disease or elevations in the left-atrial pressure associated with a noncompliant left-ventricle or the presence of MR. There are limitations to this measurement. If there is severe TR, the orifice is too large to accurately apply the Bernoulli equation, resulting in an underestimate of the pulmonary pressure. Also, the technique calculates the pressure difference between the right ventricle and the right atrium, but the right atrial pressure is not known and must be estimated using variation in the inferior vena cava size with respiration. Despite these limitations, estimation of PA pressure with Doppler echocardiography is reasonably accurate, noninvasive, and repeatable.

VENTRICULOGRAPHY

The left-ventricular chamber can be imaged during cardiac catheterization. A pigtail catheter with multiple end-holes is guided up the aorta from the femoral artery, across the aortic valve, and positioned in the mid-left-ventricular cavity. A power injector loaded with an ionic or nonionic iodinated contrast agent quickly injects 30–50 cc of dye into the left-ventricle, allowing X-ray cineangiography to image the left-ventricular chamber. The image is typically composed so that the anterior and inferior walls are viewed (Fig. 7). Some laboratories use a biplane technique, with two imaging cameras that allow a second view, typically along the short axis of the heart. This type of injection can also assist in the diagnosis of MR as the dye will be seen filling the left atrium. Injections in the aortic root can be used to assess the presence and severity of AR.

Ventriculography is invasive, requiring an arterial puncture. It also requires a fairly large contrast injection, which usually causes some patient discomfort and can worsen existing renal function, even if the newer nonhyperosmolar contrast agents are used. Because of these limitations, ventriculography is infrequently used as a primary modality to assess left-ventricular function unless the patient is already undergoing a cardiac catheterization for assessment of coronary artery disease.

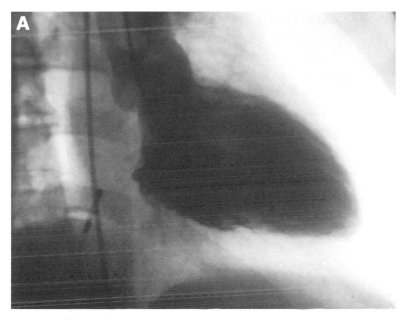

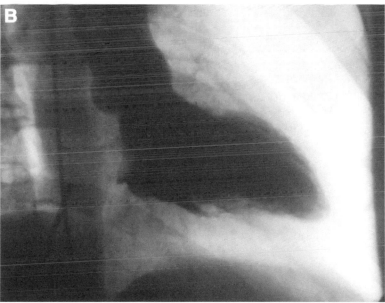

Fig. 7. Ventriculogram using the right anterior oblique (RAO) view during a cardiac catheterization: **(A)** end-diastole, **(B)** end-systole. A catheter is placed in the left ventricle and dye is injected continuously, while cine X-ray images are acquired. The anterior/anterolateral and inferior walls are best seen in this view.

MUGA

The MUltiply Gated Acquisition (MUGA) scan is a nuclear test that measures differences in LV tracer agent counts detected by a gamma camera between systole and diastole. The gamma camera acquires images over multiple heartbeats and averages them together to create an image of the left-ventricular blood pool. The tracer agent typically used for this study is technetium-99 (^{99}Tc).

The MUGA scan or radionuclide angiocardiogram does not directly quantify volumes, but uses the ratio of counts acquired during systole and diastole to calculate the ejection fraction. The test is highly repeatable with repeat tests varying by only about 4% (19) and is most useful when accurate reassessment of ejection fraction is necessary. A common use of MUGA scanning is in patients about to receive cardiotoxic chemotherapeutic agents, such as adriamycin (20). The study can be repeated as necessary to assess small changes in global function as a result of the chemotherapy. There are two different types of MUGA study: first pass and equilibrium. Each has advantages and disadvantages. First pass techniques require less time to gather images (a few heartbeats) so are better suited to peak exercise assessments of ejection fraction, but may have difficult with poor mixing in the right-ventricular chamber, making right-ventricular ejection fraction (RVEF) estimates less reliable. Equilibrium studies must use arrhythmia rejection techniques to optimize the results, but RVEF calculations may be falsely low from overlap of the left-ventricular chamber in the imaging plane. Overall, therefore, an estimate of right-ventricular performance by MUGA is not optimal, but is best performed using first pass techniques (21). Gated MUGA produces images of the left-ventricular blood pool at multiple points through the cardiac cycle. Reconstruction of these images enables the interpreter to assess regional wall motion.

The drawbacks to MUGA scanning are its use of ionizing radiation and its low spatial resolution. Essentially, it can determine ejection fraction accurately and repeatably, but cannot as easily assess subtle-wall motion abnormalities, wall thickness, valvular function, regurgitation, or ischemia.

MRI

Magnetic resonance imaging is the newest imaging modality to be used for assessment of cardiac function. Like MUGA, MRI are acquired over multiple heartbeats and averaged together to produce a clearer image. The spatial and temporal resolution of MRI can be greater than echocardiography depending on the hardware and software available on the scanner. Many parameters need to be adjusted to optimize the images. With MRI, the scanner must be gated to the QRS signal. This can be challenging because the monitoring has to take place in a strong magnetic field with substantial electromagnetic interference. Filtering and fiber optic systems improve gating, which is essential for proper imaging. Respiratory motion must also be accounted for. There are multiple techniques available for dynamic cardiac imaging: breath-hold imaging, respiratory gating that suspends acquisition during free breathing, or navigator techniques that track the motion of the diaphragm and adjust the imaging planes accordingly during acquisition.

Cine MRI produces an image with good contrast, and high resolution (Fig. 8). MRI is a tomographic technique, so that the location of each imaging plane and its relation to the other images is known. This is important because any three-dimensional (3D) reconstruction requires knowledge of the image locations, and it is especially useful for quantitative imaging of left-ventricular volumes, mass, and ejection fraction. Cine techniques can also display turbulent flow. Normally blood is bright, but turbulence causes dephasing of the MRI signal, which turns the displayed turbulent areas from bright to black. Phase-contrast methods can calculate the velocity of flowing blood in any direction, making them useful for assessing gradients. However, the time to acquire these images is more lengthy.

Fast gradient recall techniques (GRE) have slightly lower contrast and resolution, but permit more rapid acquisition. A single slice image can be acquired in as few as 15 heartbeats—well within a single breath hold.

Echo planar imaging and hybrid sequences provide the most rapid imaging, but are sensitive to any metal or noncardiac motion in or near the imaging plane that disturb the homogeneity of the MRI field.

VOLUMETRIC AND FUNCTIONAL ASSESSMENT

Three-dimensional information can be gathered in one image acquisition or by using multiple 2D acquisitions in both the long and short axes. Because MRI collects images in a tomographic manner, the location of each imaging plane and its relation to the other images is known. Also, the cine technique has good contrast between the blood and myocardium allowing accurate determination of the endocardial border (Fig. 8). Once the endocardial borders are determined for all slices, a computer can reassemble these into a 3D image of the left-ventricular chamber. Images acquired at end diastole can be compared to end systole so both volumes can be obtained. This allows calculation of stroke volume and ejection fraction. This technique for determining volumes and mass

End Diastole   End Systole

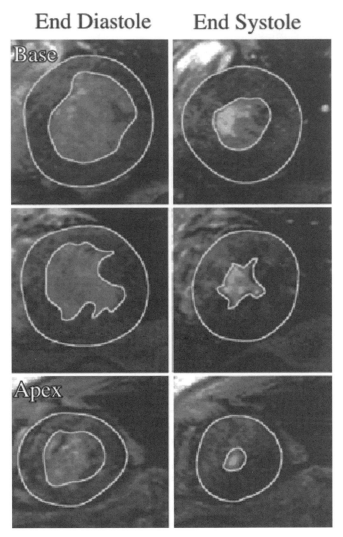

Fig. 8. Cine MRI acquired at multiple cardiac short-axis levels: The epi- and endocardial contours can be determined using a semiautomated algorithm that locates the high-contrast edge of the bright blood signal and the darker myocardium. A series of these images acquired orthogonal to the left-ventricular long axis allow precise reconstruction of left-ventricular volume and mass.

is likely the most accurate method available *(22)* and has been shown to be more precise than echocardiography in determining mass in disease states *(23)*. One limitation is that it is somewhat time-consuming to acquire and process the images. Further advancement in automated algorithms will accelerate the use of this test.

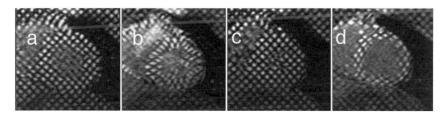

Fig. 9. Tagged cardiac MRI (**A**) end diastole, (**B**) end systole, (**C**) retagged end-systole, (**D**) retagged end diastole. Note: (A) and (D) are the same time in the cardiac cycle, (B) and (C) are also the same time. The retagging allows visualization of diastolic filling. Often, the tags begin to fade about 400 msec into the cardiac cycle. Retagging sharpens the images, allowing quantitative evaluation of global and regional left-ventricular diastolic function.

Regional wall motion can also be assessed with MRI. Cine MRI can be used to qualitatively determine wall motion, as well as global function and chamber by experienced readers. Wall thickening, which is defined as a change in the thickness of any left-ventricular wall in the direction of the center of the left-ventricular cavity, can be quickly and accurately measured. Myocardial tissue tagging allows placement of a grid of noninvasive markers on the myocardium at the beginning of systole that persist to at least early diastole (Fig. 9). These tags move and deform with the myocardium as it contracts. Quantification of the motion of these tags can yield an observer independent measure of local cardiac function at rest and with pharmacologic stress *(24)*. Tagging has been studied in patients with idiopathic hypertrophic subaortic stenosis (IHSS), ischemia, and infarction. The technique is a useful research tool and may become clinically relevant when analysis becomes more straightforward.

ASSESSMENT OF DIASTOLIC FUNCTION

It has been estimated that between 20 and 40% of patients with heart failure symptoms have isolated diastolic dysfunction with no concomitant valvular disease *(25,26)*. The primary mechanism related to development of CHF symptoms appears to be an impairment of ventricular relaxation with an upward shift in the diastolic pressure-volume curve, resulting in decreased ventricular compliance *(27)* (Fig. 10). Although disorders such as restrictive or hypertrophic cardiomyopathies exhibit significantly impaired diastolic filling, most patients with isolated diastolic dysfunction have no known myocardial diseases. Elderly women with hypertension make up the largest subset of this population *(28)*.

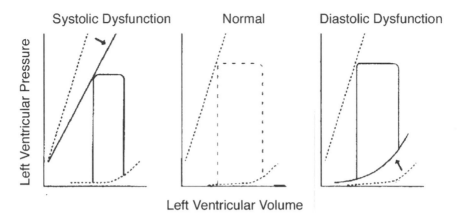

Fig. 10. Diastolic dysfunction: Representative left-ventricular pressure-volume loops in a patient with left-ventricular systolic dysfunction (left), and diastolic dysfunction (right), compared with normal (center). Note the smaller left-ventricular end-diastolic volume in diastolic dysfunction vs systolic dysfunction, however, there is a significant increase in left-ventricular end-diastolic pressure in comparison to normal, related to abnormal diastolic relaxation properties (arrow). Modified from ref. 27.

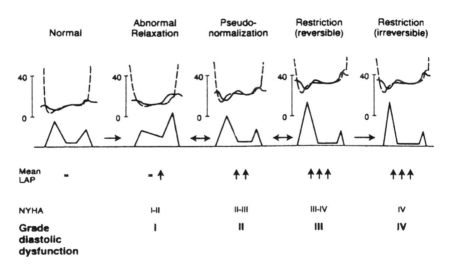

Fig. 11. Four phases of diastolic dysfunction—The progressive increase in left atrial and left-ventricular end-diastolic pressures is seen as the grade of diastolic dysfunction increases (upper panel). The left-ventricular inflow pattern is seen just below these curves, as well as the mean left-atrial pressure (LAP) and the New York Heart Association (NYHA) Class, as related to symptomatic CHF. Modified from ref. 30.

Left-ventricular hypertrophy and an age-related decrease in left-ventricular compliance are importantly related to the development of this clinical syndrome. Early studies reported a smaller mortality rate in comparison to patients with systolic dysfunction, however, more recent series in elderly populations with CHF symptoms demonstrate a poor prognosis regardless of the LVEF *(29)*. Associated cardiovascular disorders such as diabetes and coronary artery disease can further impair diastolic relaxation. Whereas MUGA and MRI scans can measure early diastolic filling rates, a larger number of echocardiographic parameters have been developed to aid in assessing diastolic function. The mitral valve filling pattern, as measured by pulsed-wave Doppler technique, is an important guide to the general state of diastolic dysfunction, which has four phases (Fig. 11). The E to A wave ratio is a straightforward parameter that compares the peak velocity of the early and late diastolic filling waves. A ratio of less than 1 indicates the earliest phase of diastolic dysfunction, known as impaired relaxation (Fig. 12). A ratio of greater than 2 is seen in restrictive disorders. In restriction, the shorter the early left-ventricular filling deceleration time (EDT), the worse the prognosis. Normal ratios are generally between 1 and 2, however, pseudonormalized or restrictive patterns may also fall into this range, and additional data are needed to specify the disease state *(30)*. The irreversible restrictive state is defined as a restrictive filling pattern which does not respond to intensive therapy.

One additional parameter that helps to distinguish pseudonormalized from normal patterns is the pulmonary vein flow pattern *(31,32)*. Figure 13 shows the normal pattern of pulmonary vein (PV) flow. The relative amplitudes of the second phase of the systolic component of PV flow (PV_{S2}) and the diastolic filling wave amplitude (PV_d) are related to the left atrial pressure (LAp). Normally in the pulmonic veins, there is systolic forward flow, diastolic forward flow, and a small reversal of flow during atrial systole. In a patient with elevated LAp, there is reduced forward flow during systole, and a pattern that resembles the E:A wave reversal in the mitral filling Doppler measurement. Table 1 shows the values for these parameters and their correspondence to various states of diastolic dysfunction.

These filling patterns and their response to changes in therapy provide the basis for the serial evaluation of diastolic dysfunction in CHF. Changes in filling patterns over the course of the respiratory cycle as observed in the hepatic veins, in concert with mitral and tricuspid filling patterns aid in the diagnosis of constrictive pericarditis (Fig. 14).

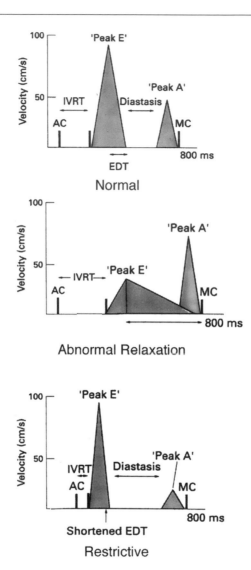

Fig. 12. Mitral inflow patterns as recorded by pulsed-wave Doppler echocardiography show normal early EDT and a normal isovolumic relaxation time (IVRT). Aortic and mitral closure events are seen. Note the reversal of the E and A wave peak velocities in the impaired relaxation phase of diastolic dysfunction, with a prolonged IVRT. In the restrictive phase, there is an increase in the peak E wave amplitude and a diminutive A wave, with shortening of the IVRT. Modified from ref. *32a.*

Newer approaches such as color M-mode Doppler and echo-cardiography myocardial strain rate analyses may prove to be less load-dependent than conventional Doppler methods *(33).*

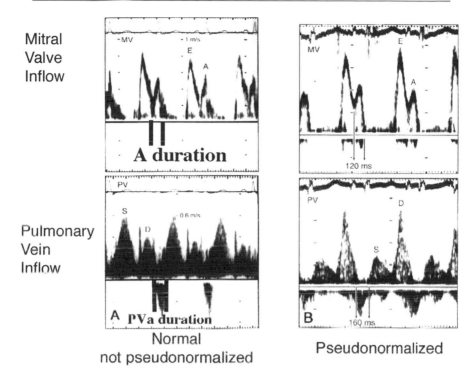

Fig. 13. PV normal filling patterns—The typical pattern of a normal PV pulsed-wave Doppler velocity profile is shown. The second systolic (PVs2) and the diastolic (PVd) velocity components are used to assess diastolic function. The amplitude and duration of the PVa component (during atrial systole), relative to the mitral A wave, are additional components to aid in characterizing diastolic function.

Table 1
Assessment: Interpretation of Filling Patterns

Filling	DT/PV	Mitral A/ Pva dur.	Pva vel.
Normal	160–240 ms PVs2 > PVd	MAd > Pva	<35 cm/s
Pseudonormal	160–200 ms PVs2 < PVd	MAd < Pva	>35 cm/s
Restrictive	<160 ms PVs2 << PVd	MAd < Pva	>35 cm/s

Quantitative assessment of diastolic dysfunction and ranges for normal, pseudonormal, and restrictive patterns. DT, decleration time; PV, pulmonary vein velocity components; MAd, Mitral A-wave duration; PVa dur, PV atrial component duration; PVa vel., velocity of PVa component.

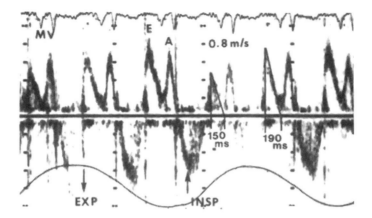

Fig. 14. Constrictive pericarditis—Pulsed wave Doppler patterns associated with constrictive physiology. There is a reciprocal relationship between mitral and tricuspid filling patterns, with a decrease in mitral E wave velocity on inspiration (INSP) and a shortening of deceleration time 150 vs 190 ms). Modified from ref. *32*.

A comparison of all techniques discussed in this chapter is summarized in Table 2.

LIMITATIONS OF IMAGING TECHNIQUES

In general, conduction system disease modifies the activation sequence of the left ventricle thereby affecting some forms of imaging. Left-bundle branch block (LBBB) can affect perfusion assessment by nuclear techniques, causing false positive septal-wall perfusion defects that can mimic ischemia or infarction *(34)*. LBBB can also affect the interpretation of regional-wall motion as a result of dyssynchrony of contraction.

Gated images perform best with regular R-R intervals on the ECG monitor. Signal averaging must be performed. A variation in the R-R interval as seen in atrial fibrillation or frequent atrial and/or ventricular ectopy changes filling times, thus a beat-to-beat fluctuation in volume is present. Unfortunately, atrial arrhythmias are very common in patients with cardiomyopathy. Single-photon emission computed tomographic (SPECT) perfusion imaging, with its low temporal and spatial resolution, is not as affected by these slight changes in volume, but MRI images can become blurred. More rapid MRI data acquisition and more sophisticated gating models that reject aberrant beats may reduce the effect of arrhythmias on image quality. It can even be more difficult to assess global function using echocardiography in patients with atrial fibrillation, especially with poorly controlled heart rates.

Table 2
Comparison of Imaging Techniques for the Assessment of Left-Ventricular Function

	Echocardiography			Nuclear imaging		
		Stress		Stress		
	Routine	Treadmill	Pharmacologic	Treadmill	Pharmacologic	MUGA
Invasive	No	No	No	No	No	No
Volume assessment accuracy	Very good	Low	Low	Low	Low	Repeatable
Qualitative global function	Excellent	Excellent	Excellent	Fair	Fair	Excellent
Quantitative global function	Good	Good	Good	Fair	Fair	Excellent
Detection of coronary artery disease	Good	Very good	Very good	Very good	Very good	Good for detecting infarction
Assess regional perfusion	Destructive harmonic imaging	Can infer from wall motion	Can infer from wall motion	Excellent	Excellent	N/A
Detect valvular disease	Excellent	N/A[a]	N/A[a]	N/A	N/A	N/A

125

Invasive	Yes	Yes	Yes	No	No	No
Volume assessment accuracy	Accurate in some circumstances	N/A	N/A	Excellent	N/A	N/A
Qualitative global function	Good	N/A	N/A	N/A	Excellent	Excellent
Quantitative global function	Good	N/A	N/A	N/A	Excellent	N/A
Detection of coronary artery disease	Good	Excellent	N/A	Very good	Very good	Very good
Assess regional perfusion	N/A	Only with Doppler flow wire	N/A	N/A	Can infer from wall motion	Excellent
Detect valvular disease	Good	N/A	Good	N/A	Good	N/A

[a]Can be used to assess hemodynamic effect of stress.

MRI studies cannot be performed on patients with cerebral aneurysm clips, pacemakers, or claustrophobia, thereby limiting its usefulness in these patients. Open MRI scanners and adequate sedation can help claustrophobic patients. Prosthetic valves, sternal wires, and other embedded chest metal can disrupt the magnetic field and degrade image quality, though these tend to be only local disturbances.

Transthoracic echocardiographic images are importantly affected by patient anatomy. Approximately 10% of studies have poor endocardial border definition (35). Obesity, poststernotomy state, pulmonary disease (especially obstructive disease), breast implants, prosthetic material, and chest wall deformities limit acoustic windows. Transesophageal echocardiography (TEE) or the use of echocardiographic contrast agents (35) can overcome many of these limitations. Patients with known esophageal disease, gastric ulcer, or history of gastric/esophageal surgery, as well as patients with tenuous respiratory status must be evaluated carefully before TEE is attempted.

LONG-TERM FOLLOW-UP

Patient status in cardiomyopathy, or in any disease process, is not static. In the course of the disease, physicians initiate therapy that may affect cardiac function, or a new process, such as endocarditis, transplantation with rejection, postinfarction remodeling or a subsequent infarction may occur. Once a cardiomyopathy is identified, cardiac status often needs to be evaluated serially. Noninvasive techniques are essential for serial evaluation. Echocardiography is the most commonly used technique for serial evaluation. Patients with known cardiomyopathy and stable symptoms can be assessed yearly. Any worsening of existing symptoms or new clinical findings may prompt more frequent assessment.

Often, it is important to assess the efficacy of a specific therapy, such as afterload reduction or the use of β-blockers. Symptoms, examination and blood tests are invaluable in assessing efficacy of therapy. Serial echocardiography can provide additional or corroborative evidence of beneficial or detrimental effects of treatment.

Some patients with cardiomyopathy may eventually undergo cardiac transplantation. TEE is frequently used intraoperatively to evaluate graft function both global and local anastamosis patency, along with the presence of valvular abnormalities. Patients who have had cardiac transplantation undergo frequent echocardiography to assess for evidence of acute and chronic rejection. Many institutions have protocols that determine when echocardiography is performed, in conjunction with endomyocardial biopsy. Patients can develop TR as a result of trienspid valve or subvalvular trauma during right-ventricular biopsy, and this can be serially assessed. Chronic cardiac transplant rejection results in accelerated atherosclerosis. Stress testing, specifically with echocardiography, is used to detect variations in wall motion that would indicate focal atherosclerosis *(36)*.

CONCLUSION

Noninvasive imaging is an essential component in determining diagnosis, prognosis, and therapeutic efficacy in patients with cardiomyopathy. Echocardiography is a very useful modality owing to its portability, accuracy, ubiquity, and the wealth of information it can provide about all aspects of cardiac conditions, including regional and global function and chamber size, valvular disease, pericardial disease, and assessment for the presence of left-ventricular thrombus, among others. Nuclear assessments of ejection fraction and perfusion are widely available and are also useful. MRI is a technique not yet widely available, but is very promising as a unified test that can assess systolic and diastolic function, perfusion, and perhaps even coronary anatomy.

All clinically important noninvasive imaging techniques are dependent on the skills of the interpreter and the available equipment, thus there may be some variability among individual interpreters and institutions. The selection of imaging modality by the clinician is therefore dependent on the clinical question, and the availability and reliability of the test at any given institution.

REFERENCES

1. Kennedy JW, Baxley WA, Figley MM. Dodge HT. Blackmon JR. Quantitative angiocardiography. I. The normal left ventricle in man. Circulation 1966;34:272–278.
2. The Multicenter Postinfarction Research Group. Risk stratification and survival after acute myocardial infarction. N Engl J Med 1983;309:331–336.
3. Ong L, Green S, Reiser P, Morrison J. Early prediction of mortality in patients with acute myocardial infarction: a prospective study of clinical and radionuclide risk factors. Am J Cardiol 1986;57:33–38.
4. Goodwin, JF. Prospects and predictions for the cardiomyopathies. Circulation 1974;50:210–219.
5. Benedict CR, Johnstone DE, Weiner DH, et al. Relation of neurohumoral activation to clinical variables and degree of ventricular dysfunction: a report from the Registry of Studies of Left Ventricular Dysfunction. SOLVD Investigators. J Am College Cardiol 1994;23:1410–1420.

6. Stamm RD, Carabello BA, Mayers DL, Martin RP. Two-dimensional echocardiographic measurement of left ventricular ejection fraction: prospective analysis of what constitutes an adequate determination. Am Heart J 1982;104:136–144.

7. Amico AF, Lichtenberg GS, Reisner SA, et al. Superiority of visual versus computerized echocardiographic estimation of radionuclide left ventricular ejection fraction. Am Heart J 1989;118:1259–1265.

8. Wallis DE, O'Connell JB, Henkin RE, et al. Segmental wall motion abnormalities in dilated cardiomyopathy: a common finding and good prognostic sign. J Am College Cardiol 1984;4:674–679.

9. Segar DS, Ryan T. Stress Echocardiography in Textbook of Echocardiography and Doppler in Adults and Children, St. John Sutton MG ed. Blackwell Sci 1996, p. 543.

10. Quinones MA, Verani MS, Haichin RM, et al. Exercise echocardiography versus 201Tl single-photon emission computed tomography in evaluation of coronary artery disease. Analysis of 292 patients. Circulation 1992;85:1026–1031.

11. Smart SC, Sawada S, Ryan T, et al. Feigenbaum H. Low-dose dobutamine echocardiography detects reversible dysfunction after thrombolytic therapy of acute myocardial infarction. Circulation 1993;88:405–415.

12. Barilla F, Gheorghiade M, Alam M, et al. Low-dose dobutamine in patients with acute myocardial infarction identifies viable but not contractile myocardium and predicts the magnitude of improvement in wall motion abnormalities in response to coronary revascularization. Am Heart J 1991;122:1522 1531.

13. Pasquet A, Lauer MS, Williams MJ, et al. Prediction of global left ventricular function after bypass surgery in patients with severe left ventricular dysfunction. Impact of pre-operative myocardial function, perfusion, and metabolism. Eur Heart J 2000;21:125–136.

14. Wisenbaugh T, et al. Prediction of outcome after valve replacement for rheumatic mitral regurgitation in the era of chordal preservation. Circulation 1994;89:191.

15. Enriquez-Sarano M, et al. Echocardiographic prediction of survival after surgical correction of organic mitral regurgitation. Circulation 1994;90:833.

16. Rothlisberger C, Sareli P, Wisenbugh T. Comparison of single dose nifedipine and captopril for chronic severe aortic regurgitation. Am J Cardiol 1993;71:799.

17. Scognamiglio R, Rahimtoola SH, Fasoli G, et al. Nifedipine in asymptomatic patients with severe aortic regurgitation and normal left ventricular function. N Engl J Med 1994;331:689.

18. Borow KM. Surgical outcome in chronic aortic regurgitation: a physiologic framework for assessing preoperative predictors. J Am Coll Cardiol 1987;10:1165.

19. Marshall RC, Berger HJ, Reduto LA, et al. Variability in sequential measures of left ventricular performance assessed with radionuclide angiocardiography. Am J Cardiol 1978;41:531–536.

20. Alexander J, Dainiak N, Berger HJ, et al. Serial assessment of doxorubicin cardiotoxicity with quantitative radionuclide angiocardiography. N Engl J Med 1979;300:278–283.

21. Winzelberg GG, Boucher CA, Pohost GM, et al. Right Ventricular function in aortic and mitral valve disease. Chest 1981;79:520–528.

22. Weiss JL, Shapiro EP, Buchalter MB, Beyar R. Magnetic resonance imaging as a noninvasive standard for the quantitative evaluation of left ventricular mass, ischemia, and infarction. Ann NY Acad Sci 1990;601:95–106.

23. Bottini PB, Carr AA, Prisant LM, et al. Magnetic resonance imaging compared to echocardiography to assess left ventricular mass in the hypertensive patient. Am J Hyperten 1995;8:221–228.

24. Scott CH, Sutton MS, Gusani N, et al. Effect of dobutamine on regional left ventricular function measured by tagged magnetic resonance imaging in normal subjects. Am J Cardiol 1999;83:412–417.

25. Aronow WS, Ahn C, Kronzon I. Prognosis of congestive heart failure in elderly patients with normal versus abnormal left ventricular systolic function associated with coronary artery disease. Am J Cardiol 1990;66:1257–1259.

26. Davie AP, Francis CM, Caruana L, et al. The prevalence of left ventricular diastolic filling abnormalities in patients with suspected heart failure. Eur Heart J 1997;18:981–984.

27. Gaasch WH. Diagnosis and treatment of heart failure based on left ventricular systolic or diastolic dysfunction. JAMA 1994;271:1276–1280.

28. Dougherty AH, Naccarelli GV, Gray EL, et al. Congestive heart failure with normal systolic function. Am J Cardiol 1984;54:778–782.

29. Senni M, Redfield MM. Heart failure with preserved systolic function: A different natural history? J Am Coll Cardiol 2001;38:1277–1282.

30. Nishimura RA, Tajik AJ. Evaluation of diastolic filling of the left ventricle in health and disease: Doppler echocardiography is the clinician's Rosetta stone. J Am Coll Cardiol 1997;30:8–18.

31. Rossvoll O, Hatle LK. Pulmonary venous flow velocities recorded by transthoracic Doppler ultrasound: relation to left ventricular diastolic pressures. J Am Coll Cardiol 1993;21:1687–1696.

32. Oh JK, Appleton CP, Hatle LK, et al. The noninvasive assessment of left ventricular diastolic function with two-dimensional and Doppler echocardiography. J Am Soc Echocardiogr 1997;10:246.

32a. Shiels P, MacDonald TM. Isolated diastolic heart failure—what is it? Postgrad Med J 1998; 74:451–454.

33. Garcia MJ, Thomas JD, Klein AL. New Doppler echocardiographic applications for the study of diastolic function. J Am Coll Cardiol 1998;32:865–875.

34. Hirzel HO, Senn M, Nuesch K, et al. Thallium-201 scintigraphy in complete left bundle branch block. Am J Cardiol 1984;53:764–769.

35. Crouse LJ, Cheirif J, Hanly DE, et al. Opacification and border delineation improvement in patients with suboptimal endocardial border definition in routine echocardiography: results of the Phase III Albunex Multicenter Trial. J Am Coll Cardiol 1993;22:1494–500.

36. Verhoeven PP, Lee FA, Ramahi TM, et al. Prognostic value of noninvasive testing one year after orthotopic cardiac transplantation. J Am Coll Cardiol 1996;28:183–189.

9

Coronary Artery Disease and Congestive Heart Failure

Robert L. Wilensky, MD
and Bruce D. Klugherz, MD

OVERVIEW OF MYOCARDIAL ISCHEMIA AND CONGESTIVE HEART FAILURE

Myocardial ischemia is a result of myocardial oxygen demand exceeding available supply. In nonatherosclerotic canine coronary vessels, resting distal coronary blood flow can be maintained until the arterial diameter is constricted by 85%. Myocardial contractile function is lost by 75% following reduction of blood flow. However, *maximal* coronary artery blood flow declines when arterial diameter is constricted

From: *Contemporary Cardiology: Heart Failure:*
A Clinician's Guide to Ambulatory Diagnosis and Treatment
Edited by: M. L. Jessup and E. Loh © Humana Press Inc., Totowa, NJ

by 30–45% *(1)*, a circumstance clinically analogous to conditions of increased oxygen demand such as anemia, fever, hypertension, or exercise in the setting of mild atherosclerosis. The human condition differs from experimental nonatherosclerotic animals as to the presence of paradoxical vasoconstriction, resulting from endothelial dysfunction and diffuse atherosclerosis that leads to long-narrowed segments of coronary arteries. Although autoregulatory range in humans with single vessel coronary artery disease and normal left-ventricular function is similar to experimental animals, in the setting elevated venous pressure (i.e., congestive heart failure [CHF]), left-ventricular hypertrophy (i.e., diastolic dysfunction), diabetes or chronic hypertension, microvascular autoregulation is impaired, and subendocardial ischemia results *(2,3)*. Therefore, a lesser severity of stenosis may cause ischemia at minimal exertion. With left-ventricular hypertrophy, an increased myocardial muscle mass requires increased oxygen, and ischemia may result in the absence of underlying atherosclerosis.

Regardless of the underlying mechanism of ischemia in these conditions, the resultant changes at the subcellular level remain uniform. Because cardiac muscle relies primarily on aerobic metabolism for normal functioning, a shift to anaerobic metabolism may result in a variety of cellular biochemical, electrical, and structural changes. Experimental evidence suggests that the shift from aerobic to anaerobic metabolism following coronary ligation occurs within seconds. Although resultant biochemical changes, such as loss of high-energy phosphates and increased tissue acidity, as well as ultrastructural changes including cellular edema and mitochondrial and sarcolemmal disruption do not occur until nearly an hour after ligation *(4)*.

Myocardial segments subtended by stenotic coronary arteries manifest regional diastolic dysfunction. Acute augmentation of diastolic filling rates and reduced diastolic filling duration has been observed following restoration of vessel caliber among patients with single vessel coronary artery disease and normal *systolic* function *(5)*. Serial balloon inflations lasting 15–75 seconds impair diastolic relaxation, which may last up to 12 minutes after the final inflation, thereby indicating persistent dysfunction *(6)*. Although the precise mechanism underlying diastolic impairment because of ischemia remains uncertain, cellular calcium overload or decreased calcium uptake by the sarcoplasmic reticulum may contribute.

Deterioration of cardiac systolic performance occurs when more than 20% of the myocardial mass is nonfunctional as a result of ischemia or infarction. Left-ventricular systolic function is reduced and symptoms of CHF result. Over time, the loss of functioning myocardium increases end-diastolic volume, thereby increasing wall stress and potential for ischemia. Replacement of cardiomyocytes with fibrotic tissue following either multiple small myocardial infarctions or a single large infarct will result in increased left-ventricular stiffness that, in turn, leads to diastolic dysfunction either acutely or chronically. The nonischemic myocardium compensates for the loss of ischemic myocardium to maintain cardiac output, but by so doing, may result in increased myocardial cell loss from increased oxygen demand *(7)*. In the setting of diffuse atherosclerosis, the remaining myocardium may be unable to adequately compensate for the loss of myocardium, leading to worsening myocardial dysfunction.

INCIDENCE OF CORONARY ARTERY DISEASE IN PATIENTS WITH CHF

The incidence of coronary artery disease in patients with CHF is difficult to determine, given the inherent selection bias in referral patterns reflected in the published patient series. However, the incidence appears to be about 50% *(8)*. Documented coronary artery disease was present in 32% of patients with heart failure in three general practices in northwest London and 45% of patients in two general practices in Liverpool *(9,10)*. A review of 673 patients referred to a tertiary referral center for CHF revealed that only 11% of patients had coronary artery disease as the etiology of CHF *(11)*. This percentage may be abnormally low, reflecting referral bias. In the Study of Left-Ventricular Dysfunction (SOLVD) trials, 71% of patients in the treatment study and 83% in the prevention study had ischemic heart disease. In total, 75% had experienced a previous myocardial infarction, and 35% had ongoing symptoms of angina pectoris at the time of entry into the study *(12)*. At the University of Pennsylvania, of our patients evaluated for cardiac transplantation between 1997 and 2001($n = 197$), 54% had coronary artery disease as the etiology of their severe left-ventricular failure, whereas 46% had left-ventricular failure attributable to idiopathic dilated cardiomyopathy or congenital heart disease.

MYOCARDIAL STUNNING, HIBERNATION, AND VIABILITY

Systolic dysfunction owing to infarction results from myocardial cell loss and increased left ventricular stiffness. However, myocardial function can also be decreased with preserved viability in the setting of persistent ischemia, resulting from repetitive ischemic insults (stunning) or decreased baseline blood flow (hibernation). Recognition of these states has particular significance for patients with CHF because timely revascularization may result in restoration of cardiac function. Characteristics of stunned myocardium include the presence of a regional contractile abnormality in the setting of normal coronary perfusion in the absence of myocellular necrosis, and the ability of this segment to recover function (such as following successful coronary reperfusion for acute myocardial infarction) and retention of the ability to contract under positive inotropic stimulation or postextrasystole *(13,14)*. Myocardial stunning may also develop following repetitive episodes of ischemia including repetitive stress-induced injury, such as stable angina *(15)*. Stunning also appears to be an age-related response to ischemia because a more prolonged recovery of myocardial function is observed senescent hearts *(16)*.

Unlike stunning, "hibernation" is felt to reflect a physiologic adaptation to chronic hypoperfusion *(17)*, such that the myocardium downregulates or depresses mechanical function to match reduced oxygen supply. Hibernation was initially noted in patients with coronary artery disease but without ongoing myocardial ischemia who had an improvement in left-ventricular function following coronary artery bypass surgery. Myocardial hibernation may be present with diffuse atherosclerosis or multiple high-grade lesions in one or more coronary arteries (Fig. 1). Recent data, however, has suggested that hibernating myocardium can result from decreased vasodilatory reserve even with normal myocardial resting blood flow *(18)*. The characteristics of myocardial hibernation include decreased myocardial perfusion in the setting of decreased myocardial contraction (perfusion-contraction matching), recovery of myocardial substrate and energy metabolism during ischemia and maintenance of inotropic reserve in the absence of myocardial necrosis *(19)*. Experimental evidence for this pathopysiologic process comes from nuclear magnetic resonance spectroscopic studies of isolated perfused rat hearts; in these studies, modest reductions in coronary blood flow significantly reduced oxygen consumption and systolic function in the absence of decreased ATP or myocardial pH, and before significant production of lactic acid. Myonecrosis or biochemical alterations are absent and angina with ST segment displacement on the electrocardiogram (ECG) are not typically present. As hibernation may be present in up to one-third of patients with left-ventricular dysfunction *(20–22)*, its detection is clinically important because the symptoms of heart failure can be reversed with adequate revascularization.

Although it was originally thought that hibernation and stunning represent separate pathophysiologic processes, more recent studies have

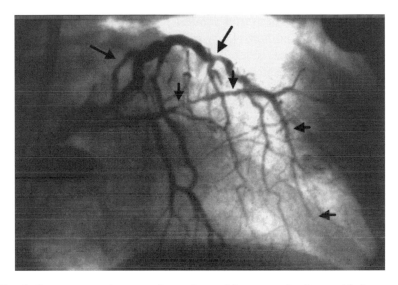

Fig. 1. Coronary angiogram of a patient with a severely diseased left-anterior descending coronary artery (arrowheads) and moderate disease in the diagonal and left circumflex arteries (arrows). The patient had decreased left-ventricular systolic function in the myocardium perfused by the diseased left-anterior descending artery. Upon revascularization a return of function was observed.

shown that the two may co-exist. Indeed, reversible contractile dysfunction in the setting of coronary artery disease can result from repetitive stunning without a reduction in resting blood flow *(23)*. In the porcine model of chronic ischemia and myocardial dysfunction, hibernation and stunning were frequently present in similar myocardial regions fed by a stenotic coronary artery. The hibernating regions were associated with greater ischemia and greater resting ventricular dysfunction *(24)*. In the human condition, many patients may have both repetitive ischemic insults and decreased resting myocardial blood flow.

EVALUATION OF THE PATIENT WITH CHF AND POSSIBLE ISCHEMIC HEART DISEASE

Although CHF resulting from the myocardial infarction is easily identified, heart failure resulting from active coronary artery disease may be more difficult to ascertain in the setting of either subclinical myocardial ischemia or multiple small myocardial infarctions. It has been recognized for some 20 years that unstable atherosclerotic plaques are associated with platelet aggregation and disaggregation, resulting in embolization of the platelet aggregates *(25)*. These aggregates may result in a myocardial infarction limited in size and escaping clinical detection. However, a multiplicity of these myocardial infarctlets results in considerable myocardial cell death, decreased left-ventricular function, CHF, or death and often the diagnosis is entertained only when the patient presents with CHF.

The clinical scenario of decreased left-ventricular function owing to multiple small infarcts may be confused with myocardial hibernation, resulting from progressive narrowing or occlusion of coronary arteries, leading to myocardial ischemia or stunning. Idiopathic-dilated cardiomyopathy with co-incident coronary artery disease is also manifested as decreased left-ventricular functions. Also, ischemia may be subclinical but results in decreased systolic function and CHF. Because the decreased left-ventricular systolic function can be a result of any of these mechanisms, the clinician must utilize multiple diagnostic tests to establish myocardial viability and the presence of coronary artery disease and determine whether revascularization is warranted (Table 1) because severe coronary artery disease is one of the few potentially remediable causes of left-ventricular dysfunction. Over the past decade-and-a-half, a variety of noninvasive imaging modalities have evolved to determine the presence of myocardial viability, and often evaluation of ischemia and determination of myocardial hibernation is undertaken simultaneously. Accepted clinical methods include thallium or technecium-based scintigraphy to assess myocardial perfusion and cell membrane integrity, dobutamine stress echocardiography to evaluate myocardial contractile reserve, and positron emission tomography (PET) to assess myocardial glucose metabolism. Other techniques, such as magnetic resonance imaging (MRI), and electromechanical endocardial mapping remain investigational.

Thallium Imaging

Thallium-201 is a radioactive cationic element transported across the myocyte sacrolemmal membrane by the Na+/K+ ATPase transporter. Cellular uptake of thallium is maintained as long as sufficient blood flow is present, and the myocardial cell is viable (i.e., has a functioning Na/K transporter). When used to detect ischemia and flow-limiting lesions in the coronary arteries, the thallium nuclide is administered following exercise or stress and after 3–4 hours of rest. Initial uptake of thallium into cardiac myocytes is directly proportional to regional blood flow, and hence, reduced thallium uptake will be observed in the presence of blood flow-limiting epicardial coronary stenosis in comparison to the rest study. However, the tracer is retained in the cell only as long as the electrochemical gradient exists across the cell membrane. There-

Table 1

Clinical Differences Between Various Disease States That Are Clinically Manifested as Decreased Left-Ventricular Function and Co-Existent Coronary Artery Disease

Diagnostic test	Multiple myocardial infarctions	Myocardial hibernation	Myocardial stunning	Idiopathic cardiomyopathy with co-incident coronary artery disease
ECG	Segmental wall-motion abnormalities	Segmental wall-motion abnormalities	Segmental wall-motion abnormalities	Global hypokinesia
Stress test	Possible inducible ischemia	Probable inducible ischemia	May or may not have inducible ischemia	May or may not have inducible ischemia
Viability study	No viability	Viability	Viability	No viability
Cardiac catheterization	Severe coronary artery disease	Severe coronary artery disease	Severe coronary artery disease	Minimal coronary artery disease in relation to extent of myocardial damage

after, the tracer back-diffuses into the circulating blood pool and redistributes to previously ischemic areas. As such, perfusion defects present following stress imaging may vanish after redistribution; such defects are termed "reversible," and indicate the presence of flow-limiting coronary artery lesions. If used for the detection of both ischemia and myocardial viability, thallium scintigraphy is best applied as a triple-phase study, e.g., imaging after stress, then after 3–4 hours of rest, and again after an additional 24 hours of rest. In patients with decreased left-ventricular function, some perfusion defects that persist after 3–4 hours rest imaging show reversibility after reinjection of radiotracer at 24 hours. In one study, more than 20% of perfusion defects that initially appeared irreversible demonstrated improvement 18–24 hours later (26). The implication of such an observation is that these areas represent regional myocardial "hibernation" rather than scarring. These segments are more likely to recover contractile function following revascularization (27).

Technetium-99m-Sestamibi

Technetium-99m-sestamibi is another radionuclide flow tracer. It is commonly used in a similar manner to thallium-201 for the determination of stress-induced myocardial ischemia. However, because Tc-99m-sestamibi redistributes slower than thallium, it is not routinely used for viability assessment. When applied to determine the presence of viable myocardium, use is made of the observation that viable but dysfunctional tissue will take up the nuclide but to a lesser degree than normal tissue. The nuclide is not taken up by nonviable tissue. In the setting of decreased uptake, a threshold of 50–60% of normal nondysfunctional tissue indicates viable myocardium (28).

Dobutamine Stress Echocardiography

Dobutamine stress echocardiography detects inotropic reserve that is present in viable but hypocontractile segments. This modality evolved after several experimental observations that impaired regional function because of myocardial stunning could be reverted by pharmacologic adrenergic stimulation (29). Four potential responses to infusion of dobutamine may be observed and include: (1) no change, indicating the absence of myocardial viability, (2) biphasic response, characterized by an improvement of wall motion during low-dose dobutamine, followed by worsening regional wall motion at higher dose, thereby implying the presence of viable but likely ischemic myocardium; (3) sustained improvement, which suggests the presence of viability in the absence of concomitant ischemia; and (4) deterioration of wall motion, which also suggests viability. In a recent study, low-dose dobutamine infusion correctly predicted 75% of akinetic regions that had impaired contractility after revascularization and 86% of regions that remained hypocontractile after revascularization *(30)*.

Positron Emission Tomography

PET for the detection of myocardial viability typically utilizes two radiotracers, one for assessing regional myocardial blood flow (nitrogen-13-ammonia), and the other for identifying preserved metabolic activity (fluorodeoxyglucose [FDG]). FDG is a glucose analog that is incorporated into the glucose metabolic pathways. Becuase both hibernating and stunned myocardium exhibit a change in oxidative metabolism from fatty acids to glucose, FDG utilization is increased in these settings. One of three scan patterns is typically observed: (1) normal blood flow and normal glucose utilization, indicating viable myocardium; (2) reduced blood flow and glucose utilization (matched pattern), implying nonviability; or (3) reduced blood flow accompanied by increased glucose utilization, again indicating viability. Although PET and dobutamine echocardiography have similar positive predictive values in patients with severe ischemic heart failure (66 vs 68%) the negative predictive value of dobutamine stress echocardiography is significantly lower (54 vs 96%) *(31)*. The highest positive predictive accuracy of PET may be in those patients with ejection fractions less than 30% *(32)*.

PET is also the least prevalent of the aforementioned testing modalities because tracer generation requires the presence of a cyclotron facility. Hence, most practitioners must choose between thallium scintigraphy and dobutamine echocardiography for clinical evaluation. Although there are many studies comparing the predictive accuracy of these two modalities, it remains uncertain which is superior because of methodologic considerations. It must also be borne in mind that these two techniques quantitate different variables (cell membrane function vs inotropic reserve); hence, the value of the test depends on how myocardial viability is defined.

CATHETERIZATION IN PATIENTS WITH CHF
AND CORONARY ARTERY DISEASE

Although nuclear stress testing may be utilized to diagnose coronary artery disease in patients with CHF, the accuracy of this modality is impaired in the setting of significant left main or multivessel coronary disease, owing to a state of balanced hypoperfusion. Unfortunately, such are the anatomic scenarios that often occur in conjunction with significant left-ventricular systolic dysfunction. Coronary angiography circumvents this weakness. Although many patients with cardiomyopathy do not have underlying ischemic heart disease, exclusion of coronary artery disease as the etiology can usually be accomplished with limited morbidity. Conversely, finding critical stenoses of all three epicardial coronary arteries may be sufficient evidence to consider ischemia as the underlying cause of the cardiomyopathy. Therefore, many clinicians advocate cardiac catheterization to establish the etiology in patients with an increased likelihood of coronary artery disease and newly diagnosed left-ventricular dysfunction. An increased likelihood is noted in patients with cardiac risk factors, known coronary artery disease, or age greater than 40 years in men and 50 years in women. The 1995 American College of Cardiology/American Heart Association (ACC/AHA) Task Force on Heart Failure made cardiac catheterization a Class I indication (usually indicated, always acceptable) in patients with angina or large areas of ischemic or hibernating myocardium, along with those patients with CHF and coronary artery disease who are to undergo surgical correction of noncoronary cardiac lesions *(33)*.

The objectives of cardiac catheterization in patients with CHF are fourfold: (1) to document the presence of coronary artery disease using selective coronary angiography; (2) to correlate coronary artery disease to the accompanying systolic dysfunction; (3) to diagnose or confirm segmental wall-motion abnormalities that reflect the physiologic significance of coronary stenoses; and (4) to determine the suitability of the diseased vessels for percutaneous or surgical revascularization.

Left ventriculography is often performed in conjunction with coronary arteriography. The left ventriculogram indicates a possible ischemic etiology of decreased left-ventricular function when multiple wall-motion abnormalities are present. Specifically, segmental variation in myocardial contractile performance, with poor contractility of some regions and hypercontractility of others, confirms the physiologic significance of underlying coronary artery disease. Performance of ventriculography in two projections yields information regarding wall motion of all four major walls (anterior, septal, lateral, and inferior) and basal to apical segments (Fig. 2). Idiopathic or nonischemic etiology is considered when there is global left-ventricular dysfunction and decreased function without specific segmental wall-motion abnormalities. However, myocarditis or even idiopathic-dilated cardiomyopathy can result in segmental wall-motion abnormalities, thereby giving the impression of an ischemic origin.

Often, moderate (noncritical) coronary artery disease is encountered in patients with systolic dysfunction, the relevance of which is uncertain.

Diastole   Systole

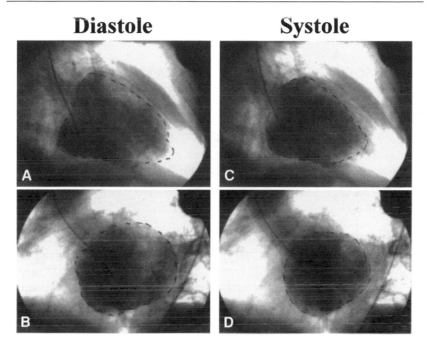

Fig. 2. Left ventriculography in two views of a patient with severely depressed left-ventricular function (ejection fraction 20%). Comparing the ventriculograms in diastole and systole, one appreciates decreased left-ventricular systolic function and regional wall-motion abnormalities. This patient had severe three-vessel coronary disease, and surgical revascularization resulted in a partial return of systolic function. Ventriculograms were obtained in the right-anterior oblique (panels a and c) and left-anterior oblique views (panels b and d). The left ventriculogram in diastole is shown in panels (a) and (b) and systole in panels (c) and (d).

In such cases, the physiologic signficance of such stenoses can be further assessed using either adjunctive catheterization laboratory-based techniques developed to estimate the coronary flow reserve in the diseased vessels. Flow reserve may be estimated by measuring coronary blood flow velocity, using a steerable small caliber wire with a miniaturized Doppler flow transducer at its tip, or by measuring the trans-lesional pressure gradient proximal and distal to the stenosis, using a wire with a pressure transducer near its tip. Both techniques have been shown to correlate with nuclear stress tests' assessments of stenosis significance *(34)*. The Doppler wire and pressure wire measurements are typically obtained under conditions of maximal coronary hyperemia, induced with intracoronary injections of adenosine. With either technique, observation of limited coronary flow reserve in a vessel containing a lesion of intermediate severity by angiographic assessment implies the potential for prolonged or repetitive ischemia, which may promote regional myocardial dysfunction.

REVASCULARIZATION OF THE PATIENT WITH CHF AND CORONARY ARTERY DISEASE

Revascularization is warranted in those patients with angina and decreased left-ventricular function, as revascularization may result in dramatic increases in ejection fraction and left-ventricular function when ventricular dysfunction is attributable to hibernation or stunning *(35)*. In fact, several multicenter randomized studies have shown that patients with double- or triple-vessel disease and decreased left-ventricular function are most likely to enjoy the benefit of bypass surgery compared to patients treated by medications alone. Although, in-hospital mortality and morbidity is increased in patients with decreased left-ventricular function, these patients (even those with frank CHF) have decreased *long-term* mortality rates *(36)*. As a result, a decreased left-ventricular ejection fraction (LVEF) is no longer a contraindication to bypass surgery and approximately 10% of patients undergoing coronary artery bypass surgery have ejection fractions < 35–40% *(37–39)*. In contrast, patients with left-ventricular dysfunction but without active ischemia do not have a mortality benefit following revascularization *(36)*. The benefit of revascularization correlates with the extent of ischemic myocardium not infracted, which can be successfully revascularized *(33)* thereby reflecting the presence of stunned or hibernating myocardium.

There have been no randomized trials comparing percutaneous coronary intervention or coronary artery bypass surgery for treatment of patients with decreased left-ventricular function and angina, but it is assumed that the two approaches are similar when controlled for degree of total revascularization. Patients with decreased left-ventricular function undergoing percutaneous coronary interventions are at increased risk of peri-procedural death. In patients with a clinical history of CHF the 30-day (2 vs < 1%) and 6-month (5 vs 1%) mortality rates were higher than patients without congestive heart failure *(40)*. Heart failure was an independent predictor of 6-month mortality. In patients undergoing coronary artery bypass surgery, a decreased preoperative LVEF (< 40%) infers a greater risk of in-hospital death and increased mortality for at least 5 years following the operation compared with patients with normal LVEF *(37)*. Multivariate correlates of long-term mortality in patients undergoing revascularization, either percutaneous or surgical, indicate that the presence of CHF is an important predictor of death *(41)*.

Improvement in systolic function following revascularization translates to a reduction in death or nonfatal cardiac events. In a recent study of 318 patients with ischemic cardiomyopathy, the 18-month mortality rate was 6% for revascularized patients with preoperative evidence of myocardial viability vs 20% for those with viability treated medically, and 17% for those without viability who underwent revascularization *(42)*. Similar observations have been made using PET. In a retrospective analysis of 76 patients with coronary artery disease and left-ventricular dysfunction, the 35 patients selected for surgical revascularization on the basis of clinical and angiographic data only suffered an 11.4% in-hospital mortality and a 79% 1-year survival rate. In the 34 patients (of the remaining 41) with viable tissue determined by PET, the in-hospital mortality was 0% and 1-year survival was 97% *(43)*. Similarly, using thallium scintigraphy, others have shown a significant reduction in the frequency of cardiac death or transplant among patients with ischemic cardiomyopathy who had greater than the median viability index, based on the number of asynergic segments with more than 50% thallium-201 uptake *(44)*.

In patients with regional wall-motion abnormalities and coronary artery disease but no electrocardiographic evidence of myocardial infarction, 85% of myocardial wall-motion abnormalities improved function following revascularization *(22)*. In patients with a previous myocardial infarction up to 50% may have areas of hibernating myocardium interspersed with areas of scar tissue *(45)*. In one retrospective study of patients with ischemic heart disease and decreased left-ventricular function (mean ejection fraction of 26%), over half had viable myocardium with enough functionally significant viability to result in improved left-ventricular function in 27% *(21)*. Improvement in overall systolic function following coronary artery bypass grafting correlates with the number of asynergic segments judged to be viable by more than 50% thallium-201 uptake *(46,47)*. In one study *(46)*, LVEF improved from 29% to 41% among patients with greater than 7 (of 15) viable asynergic segments, but was unchanged among patients fewer than 7 viable segments. In 30 patients undergoing percutaneous revascularization or bypass surgery and having abnormal myocardial segments, 59% of hibernating segments improved following revascularization, whereas the remaining 41% did not. The global left-ventricular ejection fraction improved from 30 to 37%, with virtually all the improvement in the patients undergoing bypass surgery *(31)*. There have been no prospective studies designed to evaluate the implications of performing revascularization to reverse hibernating myocardium.

Revascularization of stunned myocardium may be associated with greater return of myocardial function than revascularization of hibernating myocardium. In 29 patients with severe coronary artery disease and reduced left-ventricular function, ventricular biopsy from the dysfunctional area at the time of coronary artery bypass grafting revealed that 70% of the dysfunctional areas were stunned, whereas only 24% were hibernating. Of the stunned segments, 31% demonstrated complete functional restoration, whereas only 18% of hibernating segments demonstrated restoration of function *(48)*. In a noninvasive study using dual isotope, gated single-photon emission computed tomographic (SPECT) imaging severe regional dysfunction was observed in 584 of 1080 myocardial segments from 54 patients. Of the 584 segments, 24% were hibernating, 23% were stunned, and 22% were scarred and nonviable. Improvement in wall motion was observed in 83% of stunned areas, 59% of hibernating segments, and only 13% of scarred segments *(49)*. Hence, varying degrees of myocardial injury attributable to ischemia can co-exist and stunned myocardium may predict an increased likelihood of functional recovery. These observations may, in part, explain the favorable effects of revascularization in patients with decreased ventricular function in the presence of angina as opposed to the generally disappointing results observed in patients without angina.

In the setting of diastolic dysfunction, myocardial ischemia may be present during periods of myocardial stress. These periods include increased heart rate, increased blood pressure, increased afterload (such as in the setting of aortic stenosis), or when left-ventricular hypertrophy is present. Because myocardial blood flow occurs during diastole, ischemia can occur in the setting of tachycardia when the diastolic filling period is inadequate to perfuse the myocardium. When left-ventricular hypertrophy is present, subendocardial ischemia results from increased myocardial tension, leading to occlusion of subendocardial arterioles. In these cases, no epicardial ischemia can be documented by either cardiac catheterization or stress testing, although ischemia, occasionally with electrocardiographic changes, is present during such episodes. The treatment is designed to decrease the underlying causes of the ischemia, either left-ventricular myocardial cell mass, afterload, or heart rate. In this setting, rarely does myocardial ischemia result in myocardial infarction.

Percutaneous revascularization and coronary artery bypass grafting are the only two techniques commonly used to revascularize the myocardium in patients with CHF. Additional strategies that remain largely experimental include transmyocardial laser revascularization and angiogenic gene or protein administration. For some patients with CHF and multivessel disease not suitable for percutaneous or surgical revascularization, therapeutic angiogenesis may offer a benefit. Angiogenic growth factors administered as recombinant protein or via gene transfer include fibroblast growth factor (FGF), vascular endothelial growth factor (VEGF), and hepatocyte growth factor (HGF). These agents have been shown to accelerate and/or increase collateral vessel

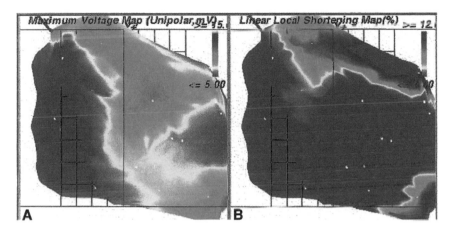

Fig. 3. Electromechanical map of the patient in Fig. 2. The left panel shows the electrical activity of the left-ventricle in the right-anterior oblique view. Colors pertain to the extent of normal mechanical function (purple-blue), decreased electrical activity (green), and severely depressed electrical activity (red). The right panel is a mechanical map of the left ventricle obtained simultaneously with the electrical activity. Similar colors denote presence of normal mechanical activity (purple-blue), decreased mechanical activity (green) and severely depressed mechanical activity (red). Areas of myocardium demonstrating depressed mechanical activity, but normal electrical activity represent hibernating myocardium, whereas the presence of depressed mechanical and electrical activity indicates myocardial necrosis. Note the large area of hibernating myocardium.

development in myocardial or ischemic hindlimb animal models *(50)*. Application of this strategy for the treatment of human myocardial ischemia was first reported in 1998. Among 24 patients treated with direct intramyocardial injection of DNA-encoding VEGF, anginal frequency was reduced, exercise time doubled, and improved myocardial blood flow was suggested by increased tracer uptake on both stress and rest nuclear perfusion scans *(51)*. Restoration of electromechanical concordance, an invasive measure of segmental myocardial viability, has been used to predict resolution of myocardial hibernation (Fig. 3).

CONCLUSION

Myocardial ischemia can cause both reversible or irreversible myocardial damage and eventually CHF. By the timely identification of those patients with impaired left-ventricular function secondary to ischemia, subsequent revascularization can result in return of left-ventricular function and increased ejection fraction. The identification of hibernating or stunned myocardium is necessary to identify those patients with a high likelihood of functional recovery, as well as avoiding coronary bypass grafting in high-risk patients with little chance of functional recovery.

REFERENCES

1. Gould KL, Lipscomb L. Effects of coronary stenoses on coronary flow reserve and resistance. Am J Cardiol 1974;34:50.
2. De Bruyne B, Melvin J, Heyndrickx G, Wijns W. Autoregulatory plateau in patients with coronary artery disease. Circulation 1994;90:113.
3. Harrison D, Florentine M, Brooks L, et al. The effect of hypertension and left ventricular hypertrophy on the lower range of autoregulation. Circulation 1988;77:1108.
4. Jennings RB, Murry CE, Steenbergen C, Reimer KA. Development of cell injury in sustained acute ischemia. Circulation 1990;82:II.2–II.12.
5. Bonow RO, Vitale DF, Bacharach SL, et al. Asynchronous left ventricular regional function and impaired global diastolic filling in patients with coronary artery disease: reversal after coronary angioplasty. Circulation 1985;71:297–307.
6. Wijns W, Serruys PW, Slager CJ, et al. Effect of coronary occlusion during percutaneous transluminal angioplasty in humans on left ventricular chamber stiffness and regional diastolic pressure-radius relations. J Am Coll Cardiol 1986; 7:455–463.
7. Pantely GA, Bristow JD. Ischemic cardiomyopathy. Prog Cardiovasc Dis 1984;37:95–114.
8. Haber RH, LeJemel T, Sonnenblick EH. The pathophysiologic profile of congestive heart failure. Cardiovasc Drugs Ther 1988;2:397–400.
9. Parameshwar J, Shackell MM, Richardson A, et al. Prevalence of heart failure in three general practices in north London. Br J Gen Pract 1992;42:287–289.
10. Mair FS, Crowley TS, Bundred PE. Prevalence, aetiology and management of heart failure in general practice. Br J Gen Pract 1996;46:77–79.
11. Kasper EK, Agema WRP, Hutchins GM, et al. The causes of dilated cardiomyopathy: a clinicopathologic review of 673 consecutive patients. J Am Coll Cardiol 1994;23:586–590.
12. Johnstone D, Limacher M, Rousseau M, et al. Clinical characteristics of patients in studies of left ventricular dysfunction (SOLVD). Amer J Cardiol 1992;70:894–900.
13. Stack RS, Phillips HR III, Grierson DS, et al. Functional improvement of jeopardized myocardium following intracoronary streptokinase infusion in acute myocardial infarction. J Clin Invest 1983;72:84–95.
14. Patel B, Kloner RA, Przyklenk K, Braunwald E. Post-ischemic myocardial "stunning." A clinically relevant phenomenon. Ann Intern Med 1988;108:626–628.
15. Nixon JV, Brown CN, Smitherman TC. Identification of transient and persistent segmental wall motion abnormalities in patients with unstable angina by 2-dimensional echocardiography. Circulation 1982;65:1497–1503.
16. Abete P, Cioppa A, Calabrese C, et al. Ischemic threshold and myocardial stunning in the aging heart. Exp Gerontol 1999;34:875–884.
17. Rahimtoola SH. The hibernating myocardium. Am Heart J 1989;117:211–221.
18. Pagano D, Fath-Ordoubadi F, Beatt KJ, et al. Effects of coronary revascularization on myocardial blood flow and coronary vasodilator reserve in hibernating myocardium. Heart 2001;85:208–212.
19. Heusch G, Schulz R. The biology of myocardial hibernation. Trends Cardiovasc Med 2000;10:108–114.

20. Afridi I, Qureshi U, Kopelen HA, Winters WL, Zoghbi WA. Serial changes in response of hibernating myocardium to inotropic stimulation after revascularization: a dobutamine echocardiographic study. J Am Coll Cardiol 1997;30:1233–1240.
21. Auerbach MA, Schoder H, Hoh C, et al. Prevalence of myocardial viability as detected by positron emission tomography in patients with ischemic cardiomyopathy. Circulation 1999;99:2921–2926.
22. Lewis SJ, Sawada SG, Ryan T, et al. Segmental wall motion abnormalities in the absence of clinically documented myocardial infarction: clinical significance and evidence of hibernating myocardium. Am Heart J. 1991;121:1088–1094.
23. Bolli R. Myocardial "stunning" in man. Circulation 1992;86:1671–1691.
24. Hughes GC, Landolfo CK, Yin B, et al Is chronically dysfunctional yet viable myocardium distal to a severe coronary stenosis hypoperfused? Ann Thorac Surg 2001;72:163–168.
25. Falk E. Unstable angina with fatal outcome: Dynamic coronary thrombosis leading to infarction and/or sudden death. Circulation 1985;71:699–708.
26. Gutman J, Berman D, Freeman M, et al. time to complete redistribution of thallium-201 in exercise myocardial scintigraphy: relationship to the degree of coronary stenosis. Am Heart J 1983; 106:989–995.
27. Kiat H, Berman D, Maddahi J, et al. Late reversibility of tomographic myocardial thallium-201 defects: an accurate marker of myocardial viability. J Am Coll Cardiol 1988;12:1456–1463.
28. Udelson JE, Coleman PS, Metherall J, et al. Predicting recovery of severe regional ventricular dysfunction: comparison of resting scintigraphy with 201 TL and 99m Tc-sestamibi. Circulation 1994;89:2552–2361.
29. Bolli R, Zhu W, Myers M, Hartley C, Robert R. Beta-adrenergic stimulation reverses postischemic myocardial dysfunction without producing subsequent functional deterioration. Am J Cardiol 1985;56:964–968.
30. Vanoverschelde JJ, D'Hondt AM, Gerber BL, et al. Head-to-head comparison of exercise-redistribution-reinjection thallium SPECT and low dose dobutamine echocardiography for prediction of the reversibility of chronic left ventricular dysfunction. JACC 1996;28:432–442.
31. Pagano D, Bonser RS, Townsend JN, et al. Predictive value of dobutamine echocardiography and positron emission tomography in identifying hibernating myocardium in patients with postischemic heart failure. Heart 1998;79:281–288.
32. Ordoubadi F, Pagano D, Mainho NV, et al. Coronary revascularization in the treatment of moderate and severe postischemic left ventricular dysfunction. Am J Cardiol 1998;82:26–31.
33. Guidelines for the evaluation and management of heart failure. Report of the American College of Cardiology/American Heart Association Taks Force on Practice Guidelines (Committee on Evaluation and Management of Heart Failure). Circulation 1995;92:2764–2784.
34. Kern MJ, de Bruyne B, Pijls NH. From research to clinical practice: current role of intracoronary physiologically based decision making in the cardiac catheterization laboratory. J Am Coll Cardiol 1997;30:613–620.
35. Elefteriades JA, Tolis G Jr., Levi E, Mills LK, Zaret BL. Coronary artery bypass grafting in severe left ventricular dysfunction: excellent survival with improved ejection fraction and functional state. J Am Coll Cardiol 1993;22:1411–1417.
36. Baker DW, Jones R, Hodges J, et al. Management of heart failure. III. The role of revascularization in the treatment of patients with moderate or severe left ventricular systolic function. JAMA 1994;272:1528–1534.

37. Herlitz J, Karlson BW, Sjoland H, et al. Long term prognosis after CABG in relation to preoperative left ventricular ejection fraction. Int J Cardiology 2000;72:163–171.
38. Higgins TL, Estafanous FG, Loop FD, et al. Stratification of morbidity and mortality by preoperative risk factors in coronary artery bypass patients. A clinical severity score. J Am Med Assoc 1992;267:2344–2347.
39. Trachiotis GD, Weintraub WS, Johnston TS, et al. Coronary artery bypass grafting in patients with advanced left ventricular dysfunction. Ann Thorac Surg 1998;66:1632–1639.
40. Anderson RD, Ohman EM, Holmes DR Jr, et al. Prognostic value of congestive heart failure history in patients undergoing percutaneous coronary interventions. J Am Coll Cardiol 1998;32:936–941.
41. Brooks MM, Jones RH, Bach RG, et al. Predictors of mortality and morbidity from cardiac causes in the bypass angioplasty revascularization investigation (BARI) randomized trial and registry. Circulation 2000;101:2682–2689.
42. Alfridi I, Grayburn PA, Panza JA, et al. Myocardial viability during dobutamine echocardiography predicts survival in patients with coronary artery disease and severe left ventricular systolic dysfunction. J Am Coll Cardiol 1998;32:921–926.
43. Haas F, Haehnel CJ, Picker W, et al. Preoperative positron emission tomographic viability assessment and perioperative and postoperative risk in patients with advanced ischemic heart disease. J Am Coll Cardiol 1997;30:1693–1700.
44. Pagley PR, Beller GA, Watson DD, et al. Improved outcome after coronary bypass surgery in patients with ischemic cardiomyopathy and residual myocardial viability. Circulation 1997;96:793–800.
45. Brunken R, Tillisch J, Schwaiger M, et al. Regional perfusion, glucose metabolism, and wall motion in patients with chronic electrocardiographic Q wave infarctions: evidence for persistence of viable tissue in some infarct regions by postitron emission tomography. Criculation 1986;73:951–963.
46. Ragosta M, Beller GA, Watson DD, et al. Quantitative planar rest-redistribution 201-Tl imaging in detection of myocardial viability and prediction of improvement in left ventricular function after coronary bypass surgery in patients with severely depressed left ventricular function. Circulation 1993;87:1630–1641.
47. Perrone-Filardi P, Pace L, Prastaro M, et al. Assessment of myocardial viability in patients with chronic coronary artery disease. Rest-4 hour-24 hour 201-Tl tomography versus dobutamine echocardiography. Circulation 1996;94:2712–2719.
48. Haas F, Jennen L, Heinzmann U, et al. Ischemically compromised myocardium displays different time-course of functional recovery: correlation with morphological alterations? Eur J Cardio-Thor Surgery 2001;20:290–298.
49. Narula J, Dawson MS, Singh BK, et al. Noninvasive characterization of stunned, hibernating, remodeled and nonviable myocardium ischemic cardiomyopathy. J Am Coll Cardiol 2000;36:1913–1919.
50. Ware JA, Simons M. Angiogenesis in ischemic heart disease. Nature Med 1997;3:158–164.
51. Losordo DW, Vale P, Symes J, et al. Gene therapy for myocardial angiogenesis: Initial clinical results with direct myocardial injection of phVEGF165 as sole therapy for myocardial ischemia. Circulation 1998;98:2800–2804.

10 Hemodynamic Evaluation of Patients with Heart Failure

Ruchira Glaser, MD
and Daniel M. Kolansky, MD

Contents

INTRODUCTION

In the proper setting, the use of a pulmonary artery catheter to measure hemodynamic parameters in the patient with chronic heart failure may be extremely helpful. During the management of the patient with chronic heart failure, it often becomes difficult to accurately define the patient's hemodynamic status by physical exam and chest radiograph alone. The radiographic appearance of pulmonary edema is neither sensitive nor specific for the diagnosis of pulmonary venous hypertension. In patients who have chronic elevations in the pulmonary capillary wedge pressure (PCWP), especially, compensatory mechanisms may make physical and radiographic exam findings unreliable (1–4). Invasive monitoring is particularly useful when the response to therapy is not adequate because it may help to better understand the underlying pathophysiology and, in turn, guide therapy.

From: *Contemporary Cardiology: Heart Failure:*
A Clinician's Guide to Ambulatory Diagnosis and Treatment
Edited by: M. L. Jessup and E. Loh © Humana Press Inc., Totowa, NJ

WHICH PATIENTS SHOULD BE EVALUATED?

In a review of the use of right-heart catheterization (RHC), the American College of Cardiology (ACC) reassessed the role of RHC in patients with cardiac disease and provided recommendations, as outlined here *(5)*.

There are five general categories of information that may be obtained in the hemodynamic evaluation of the heart failure patient (Table 1). First, RHC allows for assessment of hemodynamic status. RHC may be used to distinguish between a hemodynamic and permeability mechanism in patients with pulmonary edema. In many patients with dyspnea, pulmonary edema, or both, an initial trial of diuretic and/or vasodilator therapy may be attempted empirically. In those patients who have symptoms of dyspnea or fatigue, despite this trial, RHC may be warranted. In addition, there are many patients who have co-existing manifestations of both "forward" and "backward" heart failure, e.g., a patient may have dyspnea, abdominal bloating, and peripheral edema, but may be relatively hypotensive and have significantly impaired renal function. In this type of patient, an empiric trial of vasodilators and diuretics may decrease preload with adverse effects. Furthermore, RHC may be useful in determining the hemodynamic contribution to respiratory failure in patients with both pulmonary and cardiac disease *(5)*. Similarly, there may be co-existing cardiac conditions that contribute significantly to the hemodynamic picture in patients with heart failure, e.g., the role of right-ventricular dysfunction, valvular disease, especially mitral regurgitation, intracardiac shunt, outflow tract obstruction, and constrictive and restrictive disease may be delineated with RHC. Finally, RHC may be especially useful in distinguishing between a cardiogenic and noncardiogenic (hypovolemic or distributive) mechanism in patients with shock- and left-ventricular dysfunction. This is true in those patients in whom empiric volume expansion potentially may be harmful *(5)*.

Second, RHC is helpful in the management of severe heart failure. Despite careful empiric adjustment of therapy, this is most beneficial in those patients who have continued symptoms of and clinical evidence of hypoperfusion and congestion. Hemodynamic information help the clinician more effectively titrate the dosages of medications in patients with shock or severe decompensated heart failure. In contrast, it is not indicated in the routine management of pulmonary edema *(5)*.

Third, those heart failure patients with decompensated heart failure undergoing intermediate- or high-risk noncardiac surgery may benefit from RHC *(5)*. High-risk operations include certain vascular, emergency or prolonged procedures. An assessment of the hemodynamic

Table 1
Recommendations for the Use of RHC in Heart Failure[a]

1. Differentiation between hemodynamic and permeability pulmonary edema or dyspnea (or determination of contribution of left heart failure to respiratory insufficiency in patients with concurrent cardiac and pulmonary disease) when a trial of diuretic and/or vasodilator therapy has failed or is associated with high risk
2. Differentiation between cardiogenic and noncardiogenic shock when a trial of intravascular volume expansion has failed or is associated with high risk; guidance of pharmacologic and/or mechanical support
3. Guidance of therapy in patients with concomitant manifestations of "forward" (hypotension, oligouria and/or azotemia) and "backward" (dyspnea and/or hypoxemia) heart failure
4. Determination of whether pericardial tamponade is present when clinical assessment is inconclusive and echocardiography unavailable, technically inadequate or nondiagnostic
5. Guidance of perioperative management in selected patients with decompensated heart failure undergoing intermediate or high-risk noncardiac surgery
6. Detection of presence of pulmonary vasoconstriction and determination of its reversibility in patients being considered for heart transplantation

[a]Modified from ref. 5.

status of the patient often enables a better risk assessment for the anticipated surgery. More importantly, it allows the patient's perioperative therapies to be directed toward optimization of hemodynamics. If necessary and if possible, surgery may be delayed for a short time while the patient's heart failure is managed in the intensive care unit using hemodynamic monitoring. Postoperatively, RHC may continue for a short duration to further guide management.

Fourth, RHC helps to risk-stratify patients who are evaluated for orthotopic heart transplantation The degree and reversibility of pulmonary vasoconstriction impacts on outcome after heart transplantation. During preoperative RHC, the clinician may identify patients with high pulmonary vascular resistance and measure the response to vasodilators.

Finally, tamponade is a clinical condition in which RHC is occasionally indicated. It should be emphasized that cardiac tamponade is a diagnosis suspected on clinical grounds and further confirmed by echocardiography. In cases when both the clinical and echocardiographic features are equivocal, RHC may be helpful (5). However, therapy should never be delayed in the unstable patient for a formal hemodynamic assessment.

HOW TO PERFORM AND INTERPRET AN EVALUATION

Performance of RHC

The pulmonary artery (PA) catheter is a fluid-filled catheter that is connected to a pressure transducer via noncompliant pressure tubing. Intracardiac pressure events are transmitted from the heart through the catheter to a transducer, which then converts mechanical events into electrical signals. The proximal lumen of the catheter in most patients allows for measurement of right atrial pressure and oxygen saturation. The distal lumen, located at the catheter tip, allows for measurement of the PA pressure and saturation. The PCWP is obtained by inflating the balloon at the catheter tip and occluding that pulmonary artery segment. The PCWP is an indirect measurement of the left-atrial pressure *(6)*.

Central venous access sites for introduction of the catheter most commonly include the internal jugular, femoral, and subclavian veins. Fluoroscopic guidance is often used in the cardiac catheterization laboratory and should be considered in RHCs involving femoral venous approach, right-ventricular dilatation, severe tricuspid regurgitation, the presence of a temporary or recently placed permanent pacer wire, or the presence of baseline left-bundle branch block. In the case of left-bundle branch block, the use of fluoroscopy helps to minimize catheter manipulation in the right heart, and thus reduces the chance of concurrent right- and left-bundle branch block leading to complete heart block. If complete heart block does occur, fluoroscopy additionally aids in more rapid placement of a temporary pacemaker *(5)*.

The potential complications related to RHC are associated with "establishment of venous access, the procedure itself, and catheter residence" *(5)*. Complications related to venous access include arterial puncture, bleeding at the insertion site, nerve injury, pneumothorax, and air embolism. The primary complications related to the procedure itself are arrhythmias. These are usually minor, consisting of premature ventricular or atrial contractions, and transient as the catheter traverses the right heart. Sustained ventricular arrhythmias are much less common and generally occur in those with pre-existing arrhythmogenic disturbances or underlying myocardial ischemia. As mentioned previously, RHC may also cause temporary right-bundle branch block, which may lead to complete heart block in those patients with pre-existing left-bundle branch block. Knotting of the catheter, especially if not advanced under fluoroscopy, rarely may occur. Finally, those complications that usually occur as a result of catheter residence include PA rupture, which may also rarely occur during placement, thrombophlebitis, venous or intracardiac thrombus formation, pulmonary infarction, endocarditis, and other catheter-related infections. Risk factors for pulmonary artery rupture include pulmonary hypertension and recent cardiopulmonary bypass. The rate of infection and thrombosis is usually related to the duration of catheter residence *(5)*.

Interpretation of Hemodynamic Data

RHC allows for the measurement and derivation of central venous or right-atrial pressure, pulmonary artery pressure, PCWP, cardiac output, and vascular resistance *(5)*.

Measurement of the intracardiac pressure is fundamental to hemodynamic monitoring (Fig. 1) *(7)*. The right-atrial pressure is used clinically to assess the adequacy of right-ventricular filling volume, and to determine the hydrostatic pressure in the systemic veins. The latter is an important variable in the formation of peripheral edema and visceral congestion, e.g., abdominal bloating and pain in the heart failure patient are often the result of hepatic and intestinal edema; elevated right-atrial pressures can confirm that suspicion in a patient *(6)*. Normal right-atrial pressure is 2–8 mm Hg *(7)*.

The pulmonary artery pressure reflects both cardiac and pulmonary processes. In patients with normal pulmonary vascular resistance and no mitral valve obstruction, the pulmonary artery diastolic pressure is very close to both the mean PCWP and to the left-ventricular end diastolic pressure *(8)*. When the PA diastolic pressure is greater than the mean PCWP pressure by more than 5 mm Hg, conditions that increase pulmonary vascular resistance should be considered. Normal PA systolic pressure is 15–30 mm Hg, and normal PA diastolic pressure is 4–12 mm Hg *(6)*.

The PCWP is used to assess the adequacy of left-ventricular filling and the hydrostatic pressure in the pulmonary veins *(6)*. Though not a perfect measure, in most circumstances, it approximates left-atrial pressure, which, in turn, is indicative of left-ventricular diastolic pressure (in the absence of significant mitral stenosis or regurgitation). The Frank-Starling principle allows the clinician to adjust therapy and thereby manipulate the PCWP for optimal cardiac performance *(5)*. The Frank-Starling relationship states that the degree of stretching of myocardial fiber or, by extension, the end diastolic volume, determines the degree of myocardial shortening. In abnormal hearts, the response of stroke volume to an increase in the left-ventricular EDP is diminished. Cardiac disease usually causes a decrease in compliance, resulting in higher filling pressures needed to achieve the same degree of filling volume *(9)*. It is important, however, to note that there are increasing data that, whereas this concept may hold true in acute left-ventricular dysfunction, such as that seen with acute myocardial infarction, it often

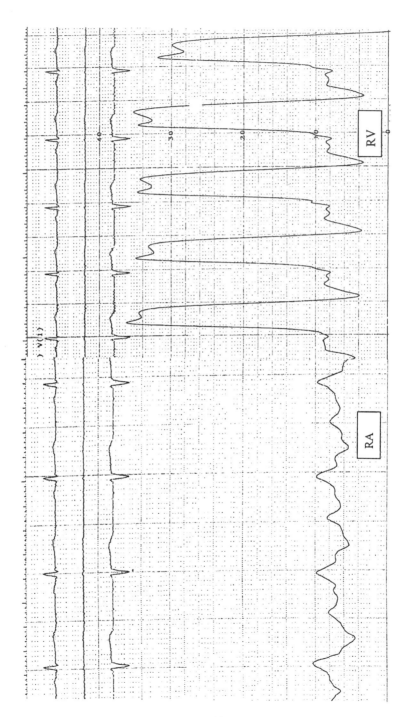

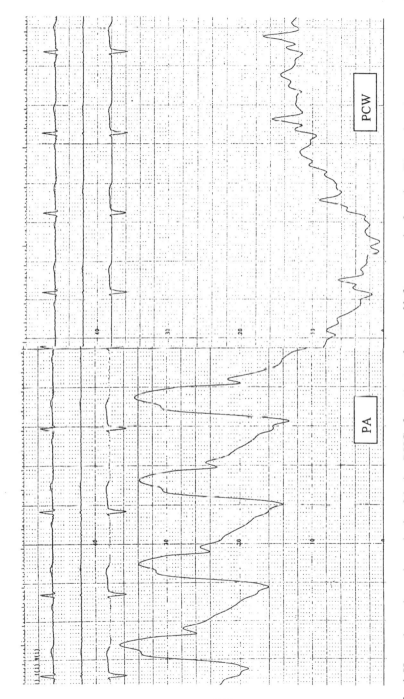

155

Fig. 1. Hemodynamic tracings obtained during RHC of a patient with normal left-ventricular function. The patient demonstrates normal right atrial (RA), right ventricular (RV), pulmonary artery (PA), and pulmonary capillary wedge (PCW) pressure.

is not the case in chronic heart failure. In the latter case especially, it has been demonstrated that with effective vasodilator therapy, patients achieve higher cardiac output and lower PCWP, with no lower limit or "optimal" PCWP *(10)*. Thus, it is more likely that the "optimal" PCWP varies tremendously among patients, and requires a more empiric, individualized approach that assesses clinical status and cardiac output at various filling pressures in each patient *(5)*.

The PCWP is also a measure of the hydrostatic pressure in the pulmonary capillaries, and thus can be useful in the diagnosis and management of pulmonary edema. In the absence of lung injury or hypoalbuminemia, the threshold for hydrostatic pulmonary edema occurs at a mean PCWP of ≥24–25 mm Hg. If there is a history of chronic heart failure, this may be as high as 30 mm Hg prior to the development of pulmonary edema because of increased lymphatic drainage of the lung *(5,11,12)*. Hence, in patients with values that are this elevated, pulmonary edema is most often cardiogenic in origin. Conversely, if there is radiographic or physical exam evidence of pulmonary edema in the presence of a low PCWP, noncardiogenic causes of pulmonary edema, including infection, toxins, high altitude, and neurogenic pulmonary edema, should be considered *(9)*.

In the chronic heart failure patient with impaired left-ventricular systolic function, often all intracardiac pressures are elevated to varying degrees *(6,13)*. As mentioned previously, patients with chronic heart failure generally tolerate higher intracardiac pressures than do patients with acute heart failure. In some patients, right-sided heart failure may predominate, resulting in an elevated right-atrial pressure out of proportion to the PCWP pressure. However, it is rare for the mean right-atrial pressure to exceed the mean PCWP pressure unless a complication such as pulmonary embolism has occurred. Moderate pulmonary hypertension is also a common finding. The PA pulse pressure may be narrow in the presence of a low-stroke volume. The PCWP tracing often has large *v* waves, which may result from both noncompliance of the left ventricle and secondary mitral regurgitation *(6)*.

The cardiac output is an extremely useful finding in the overall assessment of left-ventricular function. The clinician can confirm a low value in a patient suspected to have significant congestive heart failure. In addition, the cardiac output may be used to quantitate the degree of hemodynamic impairment and to evaluate the response to therapy. Measurement of the cardiac output over time can be used to gauge the effects of therapy. Finally, the cardiac output is essential in calculation of multiple-derived variables, including vascular resistance *(13,14)*.

The cardiac output is the product of heart rate and stroke volume. It is measured in the cardiac catheterization laboratory by one of two methods. The Fick principle, described in 1870, assumes that pulmonary and systemic blood flow are equal. Fluid containing a known concentration of indicator enters a chamber at a flow rate. If an additional indicator is added at a constant rate, the concentration of the indicator at outflow increases. The rate at which the indicator leaves the system must equal the rate at which it enters, plus the rate at which it is added. In the case of cardiac output, the indicator is oxygen *(14)*. Cardiac output is oxygen consumption divided by the arteriovenous oxygen difference. The arteriovenous difference is the amount of oxygen extracted by tissues from each liter of blood circulated *(6)*. Ideally, oxygen consumption is measured directly, especially in critically ill patients who may consume more oxygen. However, it can also be assumed as a basal value. The second method for determining cardiac output is the thermodilution technique, which uses cold solution injected into the right atrium as an indicator. A thermistor at the catheter tip measures PA temperature continuously. After injection of the cold solution into the right atrium, PA temperature drops transiently. The cardiac output is calculated by plotting the temperature change over time and measuring the area under that curve. The thermodilution method is unreliable in tricuspid regurgitation, in which there is loss of indicator into the right heart, left to right shunt, in which there is recirculation of indicator, and in the case of extremely low cardiac output *(14)*.

Cardiac output may be used to assess both the degree of hemodynamic impairment and the response to therapy. Cardiac output is usually corrected for body size and expressed as the cardiac index (cardiac output per square meter of body surface area). In heart failure, the cardiac output and index are usually reduced (Table 2). It is important to note that there is a wide range of what is considered a normal cardiac index. Consequently, when the cardiac index falls to values <2.5 L/min/m^2, it usually indicates a severe disturbance in left-ventricular function. In acute heart failure, patients with cardiac index <1.8 L/min/m^2 manifest clinical cardiogenic shock. In contrast, chronic heart failure patients often adapt to low cardiac index values. This is achieved primarily by extracting increased amounts of oxygen from hemoglobin in peripheral tissue *(15)*. The effects of vasodilator therapy, ionotropes, and diuretics may all be determined by repeat measurement of the cardiac index during or after therapy.

Measurement of cardiac output allows for the calculation of the systemic and vascular resistance. Although these are derived values, they offer important information about the interaction between the cardiac pumping function and the systemic and pulmonary circulation *(14)*. The

Table 2
Most Typical Hemodynamic Patterns of the Most Common Causes of Low Cardiac Output[a]

	Right atrial pressure	PA pressure	PA balloon occluded pressure	Cardiac index
Left-ventricular failure	Normal	Elevated	Elevated	Reduced
Mitral stenosis	Normal	Elevated	Elevated	Normal or reduced
RV failure (RV infarction)	Elevated	Elevated	Normal	Reduced
Pulmonary embolism	Elevated	Elevated	Elevated	Reduced
Tamponade	Elevated	Elevated (diastolic more than systolic)	Elevated	Reduced
Hypovolemia	Normal or reduced	Normal or reduced	Normal or reduced	Reduced

[a]Modified from ref. 13.

systemic vascular resistance (SVR) is a function of the mean arterial pressure and the cardiac output. The SVR is calculated as the difference between the mean arterial pressure and the right-atrial pressure, which is then divided by the cardiac output. The patient with left-ventricular dysfunction, especially acutely, typically manifests elevated SVR. Careful arterial vasodilatation to decrease the SVR may improve cardiac performance. Similarly, the pulmonary vascular resistance (PVR) measures the resistance to flow imposed by the lung vessels without the influence of left-atrial pressure. The PVR is calculated as the difference between the mean PA pressure and mean PCWP pressure, which is then divided by the cardiac output. Elevated PVR may develop after long-standing heart failure. The reversibility of this is measured during assessment for heart transplantation. Vasodilator agents, such as oxygen, nitroprusside, and nitric oxide may be given to determine if elevated PVR is fixed *(16)*. Those who have substantial fixed preoperative elevation of PVR have a high incidence of postoperative right-heart failure *(17)*. Elevated PVR may also signify pulmonary disease independent of cardiac impairment, and thus the PVR may be useful in patients with both pulmonary and cardiac disease.

Finally, a careful analysis of pressure waveforms and measurement of filling pressures may delineate the relative hemodynamic contributions of concomitant cardiac pathology. The most common related findings are mitral and tricuspid regurgitation. Functional mitral regurgitation develops secondary to left-ventricular dilatation, and, similarly, tricuspid regurgitation occurs with right-ventricular dilatation. This may subsequently play a significant hemodynamic role in the patient's heart failure. The regurgitation is a result of two mechanisms. First, papillary muscles and chordae tendinae may fail to anchor or constrain the valve leaflets in the dilated ventricle. Second, there may be dilation of the valve annulus. In the case of severe mitral or tricuspid regurgitation, the pulmonary capillary wedge and right-atrial tracings respectively will often have large *v* waves *(9)*.

The diagnosis of cardiac tamponade is supported by "equalization" of right atrial, right-ventricular diastolic, PA diastolic and PCWPs. In addition, there is often absence or blunting of the *y* descent in the right atrial tracing. Other clinical conditions such as right-ventricular infarction and pericardial constriction also may cause equalization of pressures. Although restrictive cardiomyopathy is a different entity than constriction, it shares many of the same hemodynamic properties, including usual elevation of the right atrial and PCWP pressures. The careful analysis of pressure waveforms and measurements may help to distinguish tamponade, constriction, and restriction.

Other cardiac conditions that may be identified in the RHC include cardiac shunt and dynamic outflow tract obstruction. Intracardiac shunt is important to recognize, not only for its contribution to symptoms, but also because the presence of shunt potentially decreases the accuracy of the Fick measurement of cardiac output. The degree of shunt can be calculated once the mixed venous oxygen saturation, PA oxygen saturation and arterial oxygen saturation (assumed to be equal to the pulmonary venous oxygen saturation) are measured. Finally, hypertrophic cardiomyopathy is a condition usually diagnosed using history, exam, and echocardiography. The degree of dynamic outflow tract obstruction may be further quantified by left-heart catheterization and provocative maneuvers. This may determine whether surgical- or catheter-based therapies to relieve the obstruction, such as myomectomy or ethanol septal ablation, are indicated. Measurement of left ventricular end-diastolic pressure also helps to assess the role of diminished compliance and diastolic dysfunction in the patient.

USING RHC DATA TO GUIDE MANAGEMENT

The information obtained during RHC often allows for further efficient management of the patient. The clinician can use therapy directed at the specific hemodynamic derangements seen, as well as assess the efficacy of the empiric therapy that was already in place, e.g., the filling pressures may be used to determine the degree of diuresis, or conversely, volume, that a patient requires. The measurement of SVR may help to determine how much further vasodilator therapy, such as angiotensin-converting enzyme (ACE) inhibition, a patient requires and/or will tolerate. The presence of a low-cardiac index in the setting of relatively low mean arterial pressures and elevated filling pressures may lead the clinician to choose ionotropic therapy.

The concept of "tailored therapy" for heart failure, introduced by Stevenson et al., addresses the use of the right-heart catheter in severe CHF. In their first study, they examined 50 patients who underwent evaluation for urgent heart transplantation. Using hemodynamic data, nitroprusside and intravenous diuretics were given to reduce the mean PCWP to 15–20 mm Hg, and maintain a SVR of 1200 dynes s/cm^5, whereas maintaining a systolic blood pressure of ≥80 mm Hg. As the intravenous medications were decreased, oral vasodilators were added. Of the 50 patients, 40 could be discharged from the hospital without transplantation (18). In a subsequent study of 150 patients, those patients who survived to discharge had continued hemodynamic efficacy of therapy at a mean follow-up of 8 months (19).

Finally, by using the PA diastolic pressure and the mean PCWP, together with cardiac output, the contribution of pulmonary pathology in patients with both left-ventricular dysfunction and pulmonary disease can be evaluated. In those patients who have primary pulmonary hypertension, a mean PA pressure of >85 mm Hg, right-atrial pressure >20 mm Hg, and cardiac index <2.0 L/min/m^2, are hemodynamic variables predictive of poor survival (20–23). The hemodynamic response to vasodilator agents is usually determined prior to initiation of long-term pharmacologic vasodilator therapy for primary pulmonary hypertension (5).

CONCLUSION

In the patient with significant left-ventricular dysfunction and heart failure, RHC may prove an invaluable tool. It allows the clinician to better understand the patient's hemodynamic status and use therapy targeted toward that patient's specific hemodynamic derangements. The role of concomitant disease is also better delineated with invasive hemodynamic monitoring. The dynamic hemodynamic data obtained allow the clinician to optimize care of an often complex and challenging clinical condition.

REFERENCES

1. Stevenson LW, Perloff JK. The limited reliability of physical signs for estimating hemodynamics in chronic heart failure. JAMA 1989;261;884–888.
2. Chakko S, Woska D, Martinez H, et al. Clinical, radiographic, and hemodynamic correlations in chronic congestive heart failure: Conflicting results may lead to inappropriate care. Am J Med 1991;90.353–359.
3. Butman SM, Ewy G, Standen JR, Kern KB, Hahn E. Bedside cardiovascular examination in patients with severe chronic heart failure: importance of rest or inducible jugular venous distension. J Am Coll Cardiol 1993;22:968–974.
4. Dash II, Lipton MJ, Chatterjee K. Estimation of pulmonary artery wedge pressure from chest radiograph in patients with chronic congestive cardiomyopathy. Br Heart J 1980;12:143–148.
5. Meuller HS. Present Use of Bedside Right Heart Catheterization in Patients with Cardiac Disease. J Am Coll Cardiol 1998;32:840–864.
6. Sharkey SW. A Guide to Interpretation of Hemodynamic Data in the Coronary Care Unit. Lippincott-Raven, Philadelphia, PA: 1997.
7. Grossman W, Barry WH. Cardiac catheterization. In: Braunwald E, ed. Heart Disease. WB Saunders, Philadelphia, PA: 1988, pp. 247–252.
8. Jenkins BS, Bradley RD, Branthwaite MA. Evaluation of pulmonary arterial end diastolic pressure as an indirect estimate of left atrial mean pressure. Circulation 1970;42:75–78.
9. Schlant RC, Sonnenblick EH, Katz AM. Pathophysiology of heart failure. In: Hurst JW, ed. The Heart: Arteries and Veins. McGraw-Hill, New York: 1998, pp. 687–726.

10. Stevenson LW, Tillisch JH. Maintenance of cardiac output with normal filling pressures in patients with dilated heart failure. Circulation 1986;74:1303–1308.
11. Sprung CL, Rackow EC, Fein IA, Jacob AI, Isikoff SK. The spectrum of pulmonary edema: Differentiation of cardiogenic, intermediate, and noncardiogenic forms of pulmonary edema. Am Rev Resp Dis 1981;124:718–722.
12. McHugh TJ, Forrester JS, Alder L, Zion D, Swan HJC. Pulmonary and vascular congestion in acute myocardial infarction: hemodynamics and radiologic correlates. Ann Int Med 1972;76:29–33.
13. Vincent JL. Hemodynamic monitoring, pharmacologic therapy, and arrhythmia management in acute congestive heart failure. In: Hosenpud JD, Greenberg BH, eds. Congestive Heart Failure. Pathophysiology, Diagnosis, and Comprehensive Approach to Management. Springer-Verlag, New York: 1994, pp. 509–521.
14. Winniford MD, Kern MJ, Lambert CR. Blood flow measurement and quantification of vascular stenoses. In: Pepine CJ, ed. Diagnostic and Therapeutic Cardiac Catheterization. Williams & Wilkins, Baltimore, MD: 1998, pp. 399–441.
15. Finch CA, Lenfant C. Oxygen transport in man. N Engl J Med 1972;286:407–414.
16. Costard-Jackle A, Fowler MB. Influence of preoperative pulmonary artery pressure on mortality after heart transplantation: testing of potential reversibility of pulmonary hypertension with nitroprusside is useful in defining a high risk group. J Am Coll Cardiol 1992;19:48–54.
17. Addonizio LJ, Gersony WM, Robbins RC. Elevated pulmonary vascular resistance and cardiac transplantation. Circulation 1987;76:52–55.
18. Stevenson LW, Dracup KA, Tillisch JH. Efficacy of medical therapy tailored for severe congestive heart failure in patients transferred for urgent cardiac transplantation. Am J Cardiol 1989;63:461–464.
19. Steimle AE, Stevenson LW, Chelimsky-Fallick C, et al. Sustained hemodynamic efficacy of therapy tailored to reduce filling pressures in survivors with advanced heart failure. Circulation 1997;96:1165–1172.
20. D' Alonzo GE, Barst RJ, Ayres SM, et al. Survival in patients with primary pulmonary hypertension: results from a national prospective registry. Ann Int Med 1991;115:343–349.
21. Rubin LJ. Primary Pulmonary Hypertension. N Engl J Med 1997;336:111–117.
22. Sandoval J, Bauerle O, Palomar A, et al. Survival in primary pulmonary hypertension. Validation of a prognostic equation. Circulation 1994;89:1733–1744.
23. Rich S, Dantzker DR, Ayres SM, et al. Primary pulmonary hypertension: a national prospective study. Ann Int Med 1987;107:216–223.

11 Exercise Performance Evaluation in Patients with Heart Failure

Andrew Kao, MD, FACC

Contents

INTRODUCTION

One of the hallmarks of the congestive heart failure (CHF) syndrome is exercise intolerance. This chapter discusses the reasons why heart failure patients cannot exercise normally, and the various tests available to objectively assess this exercise intolerance. These objective measurements can provide prognostic information about heart failure and can also be utilized to assess the efficacy of new treatment modalities for heart failure.

From: *Contemporary Cardiology: Heart Failure:*
A Clinician's Guide to Ambulatory Diagnosis and Treatment
Edited by: M. L. Jessup and E. Loh © Humana Press Inc., Totowa, NJ

Table 1
Five Body Systems Involved in the Performance of Excercise

Organ system	Normal physiology	Potential abnormalities in CHF
Respiratory	Normal alveolar O_2/ CO_2 exchange	Pulmonary edema with abnormal gas exchange, dyspnea/hypoxia
Hematologic	Normal amount of hemoglobin with normal O_2 binding	Anemia of chronic disease with decreased O_2 binding capacity
Cardiac	Increase in stroke volume, followed by heart rate	Inadequate stroke response; chronotropic incompetence
Vascular	Peripheral vasodilation to augment exercise muscle flow	Inappropriate peripheral vasoconstriction
Skeletomuscular	Appropriate O_2 extraction by exercising muscle	Abnormal peripheral O_2 extraction/ high energy phosphate turnover; deconditioning

O_2 = oxygen; CO_2 = carbon dioxide

DETERMINANTS OF EXERCISE PERFORMANCE IN THE HEART FAILURE PATIENT

In order to understand the determinants of exercise performance in a heart failure patient, we need to briefly review normal exercise physiology.

All forms of exercise require skeletal muscle contraction with the binding and release of actin and myosin fibers. This actin–myosin binding and release is an energy-dependent process. Thus, in order for skeletal muscles to perform exercise, it needs to receive adequate blood and oxygen supply to regenerate adenosine triphosphate (ATP) molecules used for the actin–myosin binding. ATP molecules can be generated in two ways. The most efficient method of ATP generation comes from aerobic metabolism, where the breakdown of glucose yields 38 ATP molecules via the citric acid cycle *(1)*. In contrast, anaerobic metabolism yields only 2 ATP molecules via glycolysis *(2)*.

The successful performance of exercise requires the normal coordination of five body systems: respiratory, hematologic, cardiac, vascular, and skeletomuscular (Table 1). The respiratory system needs to have normal alveolar physiology to allow adequate oxygen saturation of hemoglobin and for adequate release of carbon dioxide accumulated during both aerobic and anaerobic metabolism. The hematologic sys-

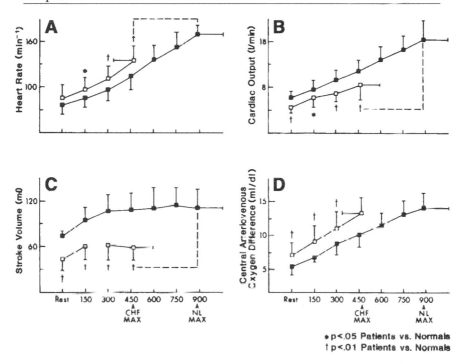

Fig. 1. Resting and exercise heart rate in 30 heart failure patients (open squares) and 12 normal subjects (closed squares), and resting and exercise cardiac output, stroke volume, and arteriovenous oxygen difference in patients with heart failure ($n = 25$) and normal subjects ($n = 10$); (*) indicates $p < 0.05$, (+) indicates $p < 0.01$ patients vs normal subjects. Dashed lines indicate intergroup comparison of maximal data. Reproduced with permission from Sullivan et al. (3).

tem must carry normal amounts of hemoglobin for oxygen binding. The hemoglobin molecules must have normal oxygen binding and release characteristics, so that it can bind oxygen normally in the lungs and release oxygen normally in the tissues. The heart needs to pump an adequate amount of blood to the working skeletal muscle to meet its metabolic demand. There are two mechanisms for the heart to augment cardiac output, namely, heart rate and stroke volume. During the early phase of exercise, the rise in cardiac output is primarily because of a rapid rise of stroke volume, with a gradual increase in heart rate (3) (Fig. 1). During the latter phase of exercise, stroke volume plateaus, and further increase in cardiac output results entirely from a linear increase in heart rate (Fig. 1). Under normal circumstances, the heart always limits exercise capacity, because the lungs have more than enough ventilatory capacity to adequately exchange oxygen and carbon dioxide to

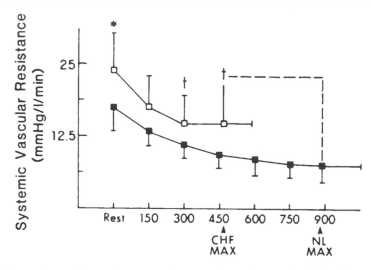

Fig. 2. Resting and exercise systemic vascular resistance in 25 patients with heart failure (open squares) and 10 normal subjects (closed squares). (*) indicates $p < 0.05$, (+) indicates $p < 0.01$ patients versus normal subjects. Dashed lines indicate intergroup comparison of maximal data. Reprinted with permission from Sullivan et al. *(3)*.

meet the skeletal muscle's metabolic demands. With the increase of cardiac output during exercise, the autoregulatory segments of the vasculature need to vasodilate normally to allow adequate delivery of blood and oxygen to the working skeletal muscles. Whereas this vasodilatation cannot be measured directly, it is represented by a gradual decrease of systemic vascular resistance with exercise, as seen in Fig. 2 *(3)*. Finally, after receiving adequate blood and oxygen supply, the skeletal muscle needs to have normal metabolic capacity to utilize and regenerate high-energy phosphates in order to maintain the process of muscular contractions.

In a heart failure patient, any alterations in or abnormalities of the five systems previously mentioned can contribute to exercise intolerance (Table 1). Pulmonary edema results in abnormal gas exchange with resultant hypoxia and sensation of dyspnea. This reduces the binding of oxygen to hemoglobin, and thus limits the delivery of oxygen to the skeletal muscles. Chronic heart failure is often associated with anemia with decreased oxygen binding capacity and reduced oxygen delivery to the working skeletal muscle. Cardiac insufficiency is manifested in two manners: inadequate stroke volume response and chronotropic incompetence. Given the reduced ejection fraction, stroke volume is reduced at rest, and the early rise of stroke volume in response to exercise is significantly blunted (Fig. 1) *(3)*. In addition, the heart failure patient often has resting tachycardia to compensate for the reduced stroke volume at rest. However, the elevated sympathetic drive results in downregulation of the β receptors with decreased peak exercise heart rate (Fig. 1) *(3,4)*. Thus, both components of the cardiac output response to exercise are reduced, resulting in significantly blunted cardiac output response to exercise. This reduces the delivery of oxygen and nutrients to the working skeletal muscle, again limiting its ability to contract repeatedly. The elevated sympathetic tone in heart failure is associated with vasoconstriction at rest, and endothelial dysfunction contributes to blunted vasodilation during exercise (Fig. 2) *(3,5)*. This further restricts the delivery of oxygen and nutrients to the skeletal musculature. Finally, there are significant changes of the skeletal muscle in heart failure, which are reminiscent of changes seen in deconditioning. These changes include a reduction of muscle fiber size and a change of the muscle fiber type, along with a reduction of the endurance type I fibers and an increase of the fast-twitch, easily fatigable type II fibers (Fig. 3) *(6)*. This pattern of change in muscle fiber type is also observed in muscle biopsies of healthy volunteers after a period of immobilization *(7)*, as well as in the muscle biopsies of rats after a period of hind limb immobilization *(8)*. In addition, there are significant reductions in the number of mitochondrial-based oxidative enzymes in the heart failure skeletal musculature *(6)*, with a reduced ability for aerobic metabolism *(6,9–11)*. In addition, this reduction of oxidative capacity is not primarily a result of muscle atrophy or impaired blood flow, suggesting that it is a primary defect in the skeletal muscle's metabolic machinery *(12)*. Thus, there are multiple etiologies of exercise intolerance in heart failure with derangements in all five body systems involved in the performance of exercise.

SERIAL ASSESSMENTS OF EXERCISE PERFORMANCE IN THE HEART FAILURE PATIENT

In order to more accurately assess a heart failure patient's exercise performance, several methods have been developed to standardize this assessment. This allows accurate communication between practitioners, helps to evaluate prognosis, and helps to evaluate the utility of conventional and experimental therapies of heart failure. There are two types of assessments: subjective and objective. The subjective methods include New York Heart Association (NYHA) classification, various activity scales, and quality of life questionnaires. The objective methods include various modes of exercise testing to document submaximal exercise capacity (6-minute corridor walk test and anaerobic threshold

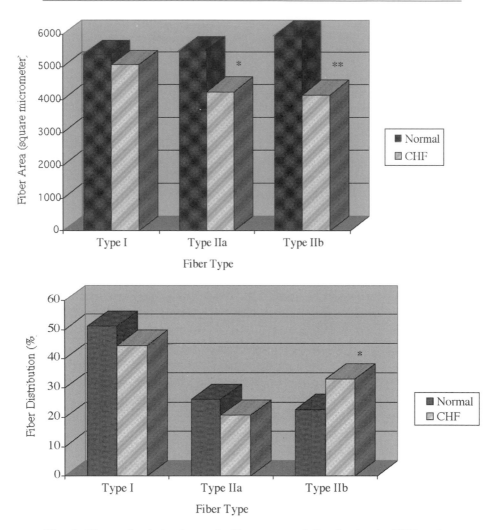

Fig. 3. Change in skeletal muscle fiber type and distribution in CHF patients compared to normal volunteers. (*) indicates $p < 0.05$ and (**) indicates $p < 0.01$. Adapted from Mancini et al. *(6)*.

analysis), as well as maximal exercise capacity (exercise time and maximal oxygen consumption measurement). This section describes each of these assessment methods.

NYHA classification is the most widely used method of describing a heart failure patient's exercise capacity (Table 2) *(13)*. The advantage of this classification is that it does not require any specialized training or equipment to use or interpret. However, it is often difficult to be accurate in this form of assessment. There is no question that different

Table 2
Definition of NYHA Functional Class

NYHA class	Definition
I	No symptoms with ordinary exertion
II	Symptoms with ordinary exertion
III	Symptoms with less than ordinary exertion
IV	Symptoms at rest

Note. Class I includes the highest functioning patients, and Class IV are the sickest patients. Used with permission from The Criteria Committee of the NYHA (13).

practitioners would agree on the Class IV patients, as these patients have symptoms at rest. There is also general agreement about the Class I patients, because these patients have no symptoms with ordinary exertion. However, the definition of "ordinary" will be different for a young athlete and an elderly sedentary patient. Thus, it is important to ascertain the normal level of exertion prior to a patient becoming diagnosed with heart failure in order to determine whether that patient is truly asymptomatic with normal level of exertion. Finally, the definition of "symptoms with less than ordinary exertion" is even more difficult, and there is often disagreement between practitioners as to whether a patient is functional Class II or III. To further complicate matters, some practitioners will use "Class IIIb" to describe a patient who has advanced heart failure, but does not have symptoms at rest. Smith and colleagues (14) studied 804 patients with heart failure in the Vasodilator-Heart Failure Trial (V-HeFT)-II. Patients were subjectively classified according to NYHA class and were also separated into three groups based on objective exercise testing. Whereas exercise performance tended to decrease with advancing NYHA class, there was a significant overlap in classes at each of the three levels of objective exercise capacity. Of the patients with the worst objective exercise capacity, 28% were classified as NYHA Class I or II, whereas 27% of NYHA Class III and IV patients had the highest level of exercise performance.

In order to circumvent the subjectivity of NYHA classification, various activity scales have been developed to more objectively document a patient's exercise capacity. However, these scales still rely on a patient's self-report of symptoms and may not truly reflect a patient's exercise capability. One of the more commonly used scales is the specific activity scale (SAS) (15). This scale categorizes various activities as Classes I, II, III, or IV (Table 3). The original study asked two physicians to categorize patients according to the NYHA classification, and there was only a 56% correlation on the patients' functional status. On

Table 3
Heart Failure Functional Classes According to the Specific Activity Scale

Class I (≥7 METs)	A patient can perform any of the following activities: Carrying 24 pounds up eight steps Carrying an 80-pound object Shoveling snow, spade soil Skiing Playing basketball, touch football, squash, or handball Jogging/walking 5 mph
Class II (≥5 METs)	A patient does not meet Class I criteria but can perform any of the following activities to completion without stopping: Carrying anything up eight steps Having sexual intercourse Gardening, raking, weeding Walking 4 mph, rollerskate, dance foxtrot
Class III (≥2 METs)	A patient does not meet Class I or Class II criteria but can perform any of the following activities to completion without stopping: Walking down eight steps Taking a shower Changing bedsheets Mopping floors, cleaning windows Walking 2.5 mph Pushing a power lawnmower Bowling, playing golf Dressing without stopping
Class IV (≤2 METs)	None of the above

Note. METs is a measure of the basal oxygen usage and is the amount of oxygen required to maintain life at rest. Used with permission from Goldman et al. *(15)*.

the other hand, the SAS had a 73% interobserver agreement, much better than the NYHA class, and can be used just as accurately by nonmedical personnel. In addition, when the SAS and NYHA classes were compared to treadmill exercise time, the SAS had a 68% concordance, whereas the NYHA class only had a 51% validity. In addition, the SAS was significantly better for classifying Class II patients than the NYHA class (70 vs 31%). Finally, NYHA classification underestimated true exercise capacity more frequently than SAS. The advantage of SAS is that it gives concrete activities that can be answered quickly and easily. It can be administered as a questionnaire to patients before the practitioner's evaluation. This questionnaire can be completed at the time of each clinic visit, and the results can be accurately communicated between practitioners. Unfortunately, by using a rigid set of activities to define functional class, some sedentary patients without cardiovascular

Table 4
Duke Activity Status Index (DASI)

Activity	Weight
Can you:	
1. Take care of yourself, that is, eating, dressing, bathing, or using the toilet?	2.75
2. Walk indoors, such as around your house?	1.75
3. Walk a block or two on level ground?	2.75
4. Climb a flight of stairs or walk up a hill?	5.50
5. Run a short distance?	8.00
6. Do light work around the house like dusting or washing dishes?	2.70
7. Do moderate work around the house like vacuuming, sweeping floors, or carrying groceries?	3.50
8. Do heavy work around the house like scrubbing floors or lifting or moving heavy furniture?	8.00
9. Do yardwork like raking leaves, weeding, or pushing a power mower?	4.50
10. Have sexual relations?	5.25
11. Participate in moderate recreational activities like golf, bowling, dancing, doubles tennis, or throwing a basketball or football?	6.00
12. Participate in strenuous sports like swimming, singles tennis, football, basketball, or skiing?	7.50

DASI = total of weights for "yes" replies. Peak oxygen uptake = $0.43 \times DASI + 9.6$. Used with permission from Hlatky et al. (16).

disease could be classified as Class II or III functional status, and elderly patients who are performing at the expected capacity would not be classifed as NYHA Class I (no symptoms with ordinary exertion).

The Duke Activity Status Index (DASI) is another self-administered questionnaire developed by Hlatky and colleagues (16) to accurately measure functional capacity. Fifty patients underwent stress testing with measured peak oxygen uptake (see p. 176), and answered questions about their ability to perform various activities of daily living. Based on these answers, a 12-item questionnaire was developed (Table 4) to correlate with the oxygen uptake measurements. The Spearman correlation between the DASI and peak oxygen uptake is 0.81. The investigators then used this scale to score another 50 patients, then performed exercise testing. There was still a significant correlation (Spearman correlation coefficient 0.58, $p < 0.0001$) between the DASI score and the peak oxygen uptake. Unfortunately, this scale is more cumbersome to use because it involves calculation, and oxygen uptake measurements as well as DASI scores will have little meaning to most practitioners. Although this is a well-constructed questionnaire, it may not be as useful clinically.

Table 5
Minnesota Living with Heart Failure Questionnaire

These questions concern how your heart failure (heart condition) has prevented you from living as you wanted during the last month. These items listed below describe different ways some people are affected. If you are sure an item does not apply to you or is not related to your heart failure, then circle 0 (No) and go on to the next item. If an item does apply to you, then circle the number rating of how much it prevented you from living as you wanted. Remember to think about ONLY THE LAST MONTH.

Did your heart failure prevent you from living as you wanted during the last month by:

	No	Very little			Very much	
1. Causing swelling in your ankles, legs, etc?	0	1	2	3	4	5
2. Making your working around the house or yard difficult?	0	1	2	3	4	5
3. Making your relating to or doing things with your friends or family difficult?	0	1	2	3	4	5
4. Making you sit or lie down to rest during the day?	0	1	2	3	4	5
5. Making you tired, fatigued, or low on energy?	0	1	2	3	4	5
6. Making your working to earn a living difficult?	0	1	2	3	4	5
7. Making your walking about or climbing stairs difficult?	0	1	2	3	4	5
8. Making you short of breath?	0	1	2	3	4	5
9. Making your sleeping well at night difficult?	0	1	2	3	4	5
10. Making you eat less of the foods you like?	0	1	2	3	4	5
11. Making your going places away from home difficult?	0	1	2	3	4	5
12. Making your sexual activities difficult?	0	1	2	3	4	5
13. Making your recreational pastimes, sports, or hobbies difficult?	0	1	2	3	4	5
14. Making it difficult for you to concentrate or remember things?	0	1	2	3	4	5
15. Giving you side effects from medications?	0	1	2	3	4	5
16. Making you worry?	0	1	2	3	4	5
17. Making you feel depressed?	0	1	2	3	4	5
18. Costing you money for medical care?	0	1	2	3	4	5
19. Making you feel a loss of self-control in your life?	0	1	2	3	4	5
20. Making you stay in a hospital?	0	1	2	3	4	5
21. Making you feel you are a burden to your family or friend?	0	1	2	3	4	5

There are six possible responses to each question, with "0" being no limitations at all to "5" being severely limited. The response to each question is summed to obtain the total score. Used with permission from Rector et al. *(17)*.

Table 6
Scores of Patients in the Initial Study
Using the Minnesota LHFQ

Group	Score	Range
Asymptomatic	10	4–24
Conventional therapy	31	21–51
Investigational drug therapy	52	35–63
NYHA I	13	5–27
NYHA II	36	28–60
NYHA III	53	34–64

Note. The 83 patients in the study were categorized as NYHA Classes I, II, and III, as well as those who are asymptomatic, those who have symtoms but are stable on conventional therapy, as well as those who have heart failure symptoms severe enough to warrant investigational drug therapy. These three groups roughly correspond to the subjective NYHA Classes I, II, and III. Used with permission from Rector et al. (17).

The quality-of-life questionnaire is another potentially useful way of assessing a patient's functional capacity. Again, by asking the same set of questions, the scoring can be standardized, and the results can be compared more meaningfully between patients. The most commonly used heart failure-related quality of-life questionnaire is the Minnesota Living With Heart Failure Questionnaire (LHFQ) (17). This is a 21-item survey that asks patients whether certain symptoms limit their functional capacity, and whether their ability to perform certain activities is limited by heart failure (Table 5). Each question has a score from 0 (no symptoms or no limitation in that activity) to 5 (severe symptoms or severe limitation in that activity). The individual scores are then added with a possible total score of 105. In addition, the sum of the responses to questions 2–7, 12, and 13 comprise the physical score of this questionnaire, and the sum of the responses to questions 17–21 comprise the emotional score (18).

This questionnaire was initially utilized in 83 patients, and was found to be reproducible on repeat testing. These 83 patients were separated into NYHA Class I, II, and III, as well as patients who are asymptomatic, on conventional heart failure therapy, and those symptomatic enough to warrant participation in an investigational drug study. The results of this initial report are outlined in Table 6. As can be seen from this table, the asymptomatic patients have the lowest scores (10–13), and the sickest patients (the investigational drug therapy group or the NYHA Class III group) have the highest score (52–53), whereas the Class II and stable conventional therapy group have intermediate scores (31–36). However, these groups have large overlap of scores, especially between the

NYHA Class II and III patients, and between those who are stable on conventional therapy and those who required investigational therapy. Thus, for each individual patient, it is difficult to ascertain Class II vs Class III status, which is precisely the difficulty of utilizing the NYHA classification. The value of this questionnaire lies in the change in score over time. It has been found to detect improvements in investigational drug studies *(18–20)*. Thus, if a therapy lowers the LHFQ score, it indicates an improvement of that patient's quality of life with reduced symptoms or improved ability to perform activities.

However, more recent studies of β-blocker use in heart failure revealed that the LHFQ is not as responsive to clinical change as previously demonstrated *(21,22)*. Therefore, investigators in Kansas City developed a more comprehensive questionnaire for heart failure patients, the Kansas City Cardiomyopathy Questionnaire (KCCQ) *(23)*. The KCCQ is a 23-item questionnaire designed to quantify disease-specific physical limitations, symptom frequency and severity, quality of life, social interference and self-efficacy (Appendix A) *(23)*. The KCCQ was found to yield reproducible scores on 3-month follow-up testing, and it was more sensitive to improvement in heart failure status than the LHFQ. There are eight domains of the KCCQ (physical limitation, symptoms, symptom stability, social limitation, self-efficacy, quality of life, functional status, and clinical summary), and each domain has been validated. In addition, patients who died or were rehospitalized during this initial study had significantly lower (worse) scores on the functional status and clinical summary domains than the other patients in this study, suggesting that these scores may have prognostic indications. However, this obviously needs to be confirmed in a larger study. Although the KCCQ is much more comprehensive than the LHFQ, it has not been tested in larger populations of heart failure patients. Its ultimate utility in the assessment of a heart failure patient's quality of life remains to be seen.

Given the subjective nature of the assessment tools mentioned previously, it is often necessary to objectively measure a heart failure patient's functional capacity. These objective methods either assess the submaximal or maximal exercise capacity. Although assessment of a patient's maximal exercise capacity is useful, it may not be as applicable to a patient's daily life. When aerobic metabolism is no longer adequate to supply ATPs for skeletal muscular contractions, anaerobic metabolism is then utilized to produce additional ATPs for energy. This process produces lactic acid, the buildup of which leads to muscle soreness. This is an uncomfortable feeling; thus, most patients will perform activities that do not require anaerobic metabolism. Therefore, assessment of submaximal exercise capacity may indicate how easily a patient can perform activities of daily living.

The most commonly used assessment of submaximal exercise capacity is the 6-minute corridor walk test. This was originally developed as a 12-minute walk test for the assessment of chronic bronchitis by McGavin and colleagues *(24)*. Lipkin and colleagues *(25)* adopted and modified this test for heart failure using 26 patients and 10 normal volunteers. All participants were asked to walk in a level enclosed 20-m long corridor. Each participant was instructed to walk continuously if tolerated and to cover as much ground as possible in 6 minutes. Stopping or slowing down was allowed if necessary. All participants should believe that they could not have covered any more ground at the end of the 6-minute test. Participants were encouraged as needed and were advised when they had walked 3 and 5 minutes. There were significant differences in the distance walked between normal volunteers (683 m), Class II patients (559 m), and Class III patients (402 m). Thus, this test provides good discrimination between various functional classes of patients. Encouragement of the subject resulted in a significant improvement in 6-minute walk distance, but as long as encouragement is given or withheld in the same fashion, serial testing results are consistent *(26)*. Patients do experience a "practice effect," an increase in the 6-minute walk distance between the first, second, and third tests *(24,26)*. However, another study suggested that the improvement in the 6-minute walk distance occurs only between the first and second tests and remains stable thereafter *(27)*. The advantages of the 6-minute corridor walk test is that it can be performed easily in a practitioner's office without any special equipment, as long as there is the required space available in the office. It can be performed by medical office personnel after minimal training. After the first two or three tests, any change in walk test distance should represent a true change in functional capacity. The University of Pennsylvania worksheet for the recording and calculation of 6-minute walk distance is shown in Appendix B.

The other assessment of submaximal exercise capacity is the analysis of the lactate or anaerobic threshold (AT). This method takes advantage of the fact that as anaerobic metabolism occurs, lactate is produced. The detection in an abrupt change in arterial *(28–30)* or mixed venous *(31)* lactate levels indicates the onset of anaerobic metabolism. Unfortunately, this method is cumbersome and relies on serial sampling of arterial or mixed venous lactate levels. Because sampling can only occur every 30 seconds *(28)* to 3 minutes *(31)*, it would be quite easy to "miss" the actual onset of anaerobic metabolism, and serial measurements of AT using this method may not be as useful. With the advent of oxygen uptake measurements, the detection of AT is easier and less cumbersome (*see* p. 178). Because the AT remains stable over time *(28)*, such detection can ascertain whether a patient's submaximal exercise capacity has improved or deteriorated.

By far the most powerful method of documenting a patient's exercise capacity is the measurement of oxygen uptake during maximal exercise testing. In order to understand this concept, we need to briefly review the Fick concept of cardiac output *(32)*. This concept states that the uptake or release of a substance by an organ is equal to the product of the blood flow to the organ and the difference in the arterial and venous concentrations of that substance. For the pulmonary circuit, this substance is oxygen. The uptake of oxygen by the lungs from the environment is equal to the product of the pulmonary blood flow and the difference in the concentration of oxygen in the pulmonary artery (venous) and left ventricle or aorta (arterial), because pulmonary venous blood is difficult to sample. If there are no intracardiac shunts, the flow of blood through the pulmonary circuit would be the same as the flow of blood through the systemic circulation *(33)*. This concept is expressed by the formula:

$$VO_2 = CO \times AVO_2D$$

where VO_2 is the oxygen uptake (or more commonly known as oxygen consumption; mL/minute), CO is the cardiac output (L/minute), and AVO_2D is the arteriovenous oxygen difference (mL/dL). Because AVO_2D increases linearly with exercise (Fig. 1) *(3)*, VO_2 is directly proportional to cardiac output. Thus, measurement of VO_2 during exercise is a noninvasive indicator of cardiac output reserve. In clinical practice, the units for VO_2 is divided by a patient's weight (mL/kg/minute) to standardize the measurements between patients.

Harrison and colleagues were the first investigators known to have used this principle to assess exercise capacity in heart failure patients *(34,35)*. The measurements were made intermittently by collecting expired gas in Douglas bags. Unfortunately, this precluded the measurement of "steady-state" VO_2. Measurement of VO_2 had been a tedious procedure until the development of breath-by-breath analysis techniques and sophisticated computer software *(36)*. This technology yields ventilatory and gas exchange information, which are helpful in the clinical evaluation of a patient. Even though interpretation of VO_2 measurements requires training, it remains the mainstay of the objective assessment of a heart failure patient's functional capacity.

In clinical practice, maximal VO_2, defined as the rise of VO_2 <1 mL/kg/minute for 30 seconds or more, despite an increase in workload, is rarely achieved *(37)*. The attainment of maximal VO_2 reflects the maximal cardiac output as well as the maximal extraction of peripheral oxygen extraction *(see* formula), and most patients stop exercise prior to achieving the true maximal VO_2. Thus, most VO_{2max} values reported are actually not maximal VO_2 values, but rather, peak

VO_2 values. There are several ways to sample the peak VO_2 values: by averaging the VO_2 values during the last 15, 30, or 60 seconds of exercise, take an average of the last eight breaths of exercise, or take the highest value recorded by the breath-by-breath analysis. In general, the 60-second average would yield the lowest VO_2 values, whereas the breath-by-breath measurement would yield the highest VO_2 value. In fact, Johnson et al. reported that the 60-second average (13.8 ± 4.2 mL/kg/minute) is 20% lower than the highest VO_2 value recorded by breath-by-breath measurement (17.3 ± 4.2 mL/kg/minute) (38). However, the other three intervals of peak VO_2 measurements yielded similar results (30-second average = 14.2 ± 3.7 mL/kg/minute; 15-second average = 14.5 ± 3.9 mL/kg/minute; eight-breath average = 14.7 ± 4.3 mL/kg/minute). Thus, as long as peak VO_2 values are reported based on a 15- to 30-second average or an average of eight breaths, the results should be consistent.

Weber and colleagues (39) at the University of Pennsylvania measured VO_2 and intracardiac hemodynamics in 62 patients with heart failure and defined four functional classes of exercise capacity (Table 7). He used the designation "classes A to D" to avoid confusion with the NYHA classification. He demonstrated that resting and exercise cardiac output and stroke volume decreased with advancing Weber class, thus validating this classification. Similar to the 6-minute walk test, VO_2 testing is associated with a "practice effect," with increases of VO_2 from the first to the second test (40), and subsequent values are reproducible over a period of 17 days to 22 months (40–42).

There are several other useful features of VO_2 testing. First of all, the VO_2 to heart rate relationship (known as O_2 pulse) is proportional to the stroke volume. Because the amount of oxygen bound to hemoglobin should remain relatively constant throughout exercise (assuming no significant arterial desaturation), the amount of oxygen carried per heartbeat should be a reflection of the amount of blood carried by each heartbeat, which is stroke volume. Weber and colleagues (39) also demonstrated that the O_2 pulse decreases with advancing Weber class, consistent with the observation that stroke volume response to exercise becomes progressively more limited from class A to D.

In addition, the measurement of carbon dioxide production (VCO_2) during exercise also yields useful clinical information. At rest, patients produce a certain amount of carbon dioxide based on their oxygen uptake. The respiratory exchange ratio (RER), or respiratory quotient (RQ) is the ratio of VCO_2/VO_2. This ratio ranges between 0.7–1.0 at rest, depending on the patient's predominant source of fuel (carbohydrate vs fat) (Table 8) (43). During the early phase of exercise, carbon dioxide

Table 7
Weber Classification of Functional Capacity
in Heart Failure Patients

Weber class	VO_2 (mL/kg/minute)
A	>20
B	16–20
C	10–15
D	<10

Used with permission from Weber et al. *(39)*.

Table 8
Relationship Between the Respiratory
Exchange Ratio (R; VCO_2/VO_2) and the
Types of Fuels Used in Caloric Production

	% Total caloric production	
R	CHO	Fats
0.70	0	100
0.75	14.6	84.4
0.80	33.4	66.6
0.85	50.7	49.3
0.90	67.5	32.5
1.00	100	0

Used with permission from Weber and
Janicki *(43)*.

increases proportionately with oxygen, but with the onset of anaerobic
metabolism, the excess lactate and other acids produced are buffered by
bicarbonate and are released as excess carbon dioxide. This is illustrated
by the following formula:

$$H^+ + HCO_3^- \leftrightarrow H_2O + CO_2$$

where H^+ is the proton of lactate or other acids, HCO_3^- is bicarbonate,
H_2O is water, and CO_2 is carbon dioxide. Thus, at AT, VCO_2 increases
abruptly compared to VO_2, and the plot of VCO_2 vs VO_2 reveals an abrupt
change in slope at AT (Fig. 4) *(44)*. This manner of AT detection is called
the V-slope method. This is the most sensitive method for AT detection
and is much simpler to utilize than the detection of AT by the measurement of lactate levels. Because the RER is less than 1.0 at rest, its rise over
1.0 is a specific, but a less sensitive indicator of the onset of anaerobic
metabolism. This "fixed value" method of detecting the AT consistently
overestimates true AT *(45)*. During the conduct of a stress test on heart

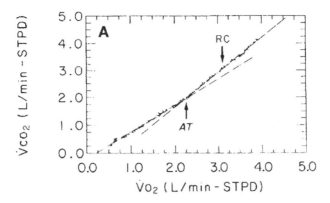

Fig. 4. Plots of VCO_2 vs VO_2 from 10 normal subjects for determination of the anaerobic threshold by the V-slope method (*see* text). The data are divided into two linear components that intersect at the anaerobic threshold (AT). This reflects the abrupt increase of VCO_2 in relation to VO_2 at the onset of AT. Reprinted with permission from Beaver et al. *(44)*.

failure patients, the achievement of AT by one of these methods is very important. If a patient stops exercise before the achievement of AT, it is either secondary to another cardiac limitation (angina, arrhythmias, blood pressure lability), a volitional discontinuation of exercise or because of pulmonary limitation to exercise (if the reduction in lung function limited exercise, the patient would not have a chance to reach AT).

The ventilatory characteristics of a patient are also useful in the assessment of a heart failure patient's functional impairment. The minute ventilation (VE; L/minute) is the product of respiratory rate and tidal volume and is the measurement of the amount of air moving through the lungs per minute. The maximal voluntary ventilation (MVV) is an estimate of the maximal lung capacity and is measured by 15 seconds of deep and rapid breathing *(46)*. Alternatively, the MVV can be estimated by multiplying the forced expiratory volume in one second (FEV_1) by 35 *(47)*. Under normal circumstances, the V_E/MVV ratio, or dyspnea index, rarely exceeds 50% even with heavy exercise, whereas patients with pulmonary disease have a dyspnea index higher than 50% *(48)*. Heart failure patients also demonstrate a VE/MVV of less than 50%, and Weber et al. *(39)* demonstrated that there was a significant difference ($p < 0.01$) in this index between class A/B patients (0.43–0.52) and class C/D patients (0.34–0.37). Thus, the assessment of this ventilatory characteristic can offer insight into the underlying etiology of dyspnea and perhaps the severity of heart failure.

The other useful ventilatory parameter is the ventilatory equivalent for CO_2 (V_E/VCO_2). This ratio indicates the amount of ventilation needed to release CO_2. V_E/VCO_2 is significantly higher in heart failure patients than in normals (46 vs 37), and the degree of elevation is correlated with the amount of physiologic dead space *(49)*. This may be a result of poor pulmonary perfusion with enhanced ventilation-perfusion mismatch at rest and with exercise. In addition, chronic elevations in pulmonary pressures secondary to left-ventricular failure may lead to pulmonary parenchymal abnormalities with resultant increased pulmonary dead space *(49)*. A recent study found V_E/VCO_2 to be a more specific indicator of heart failure in patients with poor exercise tolerance *(50)*. Heart failure patients had resting and peak exercise V_E/VCO_2 of 50 ± 9 and 43 ± 9, respectively, as opposed to 45 ± 9 and 36 ± 7 for cirrhotic patients. Thus, the noninvasive measurement of VO_2, VCO_2, and V_E reproducibly yields information about a patient's submaximal (AT) and maximal exercise capacity (VO_{2max}), as well as delineates the etiology of a patient's exercise intolerance (V_E/MVV, V_E/VCO_2).

Maximal and submaximal exercise testing can be performed using either a treadmill or bicycle. Walking is a more natural activity for patients than bicycle exercise, which tends to be more difficult for patients. VO_2 tends to be about 10–16% lower with bicycle testing in comparison with treadmill testing, because of the smaller muscle groups utilized for bicycle exercise *(51,52)*. There are many treadmill and bicycle testing protocols, but these can be separated into "staged" and "ramped" protocols. A staged protocol is one which employs a constant workload for a set amount of time (generally 2–3 minutes) and increases workload abruptly. A ramped protocol increases workload intensity gradually and yields "truer" results, which are much more closely related to the demands of the work compared to staged protocols *(52)*. The most common staged bicycle protocol begins either at 20 Watts of resistance, increasing by 20 W every 3 minutes *(53)*, or begins at 25 W of resistance, increasing by 25 W every 3 minutes *(28,49)*. Ramped bicycle exercise can vary from 10 W/minute *(54,55)* to 25 W/minute. However, it is difficult to have a true ramped bicycle protocol, because pedaling speed may decrease with increasing resistance, and workload varies with the speed of pedaling.

Treadmill exercise is the most common testing procedure. The most commonly utilized protocols are Bruce *(56)* (Table 9), modified Bruce *(56)* (Table 10), and Naughton/modified Naughton *(57)* (Table 11). The Bruce protocol is the most vigorous of these protocols and has the largest increase in workload with each stage. This protocol should be reserved for patients with no limitations in exercise. The modified Bruce protocol adds two "warm-up" stages to the Bruce protocol, beginning with no incline, then adds 5% incline to the second stage before begin-

Table 9
Bruce Protocol for Treadmill Testing

Stage	Speed (mph)	Incline (%)
1	1.7	10
2	2.5	12
3	3.4	14
4	4.2	16
5	5.0	18
6	5.5	20
7	6.0	22

Note. Each stage is 3 minutes. Used with permission from Bruce et al. (56).

Table 10
Modified Bruce Protocol for Treadmill Testing

Stage	Speed (mph)	Incline (%)
1	1.7	0
2	1.7	5
3	1.7	10
4	2.5	12
5	3.4	14
6	4.2	16
7	5.0	18
8	5.5	20
9	6.0	22

Note. Each stage is 3 minutes. Note that the only difference between this protocol and the Bruce protocol is the addition of two "warm-up" stages with lower inclines. Thus, stage 3 of the modified Bruce protocol is equivalent to stage 1 of the Bruce protocol, and so on. Used with permission from Bruce et al. (56).

ning the first stage of the Bruce protocol. Thus, stage 3 of the modified Bruce protocol is equivalent to stage 1 of the Bruce protocol, and so on. This protocol is slightly gentler and can be used in patients with mild exercise limitations. The Naughton protocol is the easiest of these protocols with 3-minute stages. This protocol tends to have inappropriately long exercise times (57), and the modified Naughton protocol (57), which utilizes 2-minute stages, is the most commonly utilized protocol for heart failure patients (58,59). However, this protocol would be too easy for the higher functioning patients (Class I and II), and peak exercise performance may be blunted from boredom. In fact, the American

Table 11
Naughton (3-Minute Stages) and Modified Naughton
(2-Minute Stages) Protocol for Treadmill Testing

Stage	Speed (mph)	Incline (%)
1	1.0	0
2	1.5	0
3	2.0	0
4	2.0	3.5
5	2.0	7.0
6	3.0	5
7	3.0	7.5
8	3.0	10
9	3.0	12.5
10	3.0	15

Used with permission from Patterson et al. *(57)*.

College of Cardiology (ACC) and American Heart Association (AHA) recommend choosing a testing protocol that allows 6–12 minutes of exercise *(60)*. This allows patients adequate time to reach anaerobic threshold, but is not too long as to induce boredom.

As a result, some investigators have advocated the routine use of ramped treadmill testing, especially because ramping allows a better response of VO_2 to workload *(52)*. The ramping Myers protocol *(52)* begins with a warm-up period of 2.0 mph for 1 minute, followed by an individualized increase in speed and grade to achieve a peak VO_2 in approximately 10 minutes. At the University of Pennsylvania, we utilize three levels of ramping treadmill exercise, to accommodate class I patients (high protocol), Class II–early III patients (moderate protocol) and advanced Class III to stable Class IV patients (low protocol). The programming of these protocols are illustrated in Tables 12 and 13 for the two most commonly utilized metabolic analyzer machines (Medical Graphics, Inc., Minneapolis, MN and SensorMedics, Yorba Linda, CA). All protocols begin at a treadmill speed of 1.5 mph, increasing to 2.0, 2.5, or 3.0 mph for the low, moderate, and high protocols, respectively. Thereafter, the treadmill increases by 0.5% at varying time intervals. After a treadmill elevation of 21 or 22% is achieved, treadmill speed is increased by 0.1 mph every 24, 18, or 12 seconds for the low, moderate, and high protocols, respectively. These three ramping protocols are chosen based on the physician's assessment of the patient's NYHA class.

Table 14 documents the VO_2 values from 400 exercise tests grouped into different exercise times using the three University of Pennsylvania

Table 12
University of Pennsylvania Ramping Treadmill Protocols for the Medical Graphic Breath-by-Breath Gas Analyzer System (Minneapolis, MN)

(For Medical Graphics Metabolic Cart)

Low ramping protocol: Ramp treadmill 2.0 mph, 7 METS in 12 minutes
    If the patient reaches final elevation of this protocol, manually increase speed 0.1 mph every 24 seconds until patient reaches maximum exercise capacity.
Moderate ramping protocol: Ramp treadmill 2.5 mph, 7 METS in 9 minutes
    If the patient reaches final elevation of this protocol, manually increase speed 0.1 mph every 18 seconds until patient reaches maximum exercise capacity.
High ramping protocol: Ramp treadmill 3.0 mph, 9 METS in 6 minutes
    If a patient reaches final elevation of this protocol, manually increase speed 0.1 mph every 12 seconds until patient reaches maximum exercise capacity.

Note. All protocols begin at a speed of 1.5 mph, increasing to 2.0 mph, 2.5 mph and 3.0 mph for the low, moderate and high protocols, respectively, before incline is added.

protocols. As evident from this table, these protocols yield significantly different VO_2 values after different exercise durations (4–8, 8–12, and 12–16 minutes). In addition, the three protocols yield significantly different VO_2 values within the same exercise duration (except for the low and moderate protocols at 12- to 16-minute exercise duration). Whereas the University of Pennsylvania treadmill ramping protocols are not as individualized as reported by Myers et al. *(52)*, the advantage is that only three protocols are utilized to suit the patient's exercise tolerance, yielding different VO_2 values. Even if the "wrong" protocol is chosen (too easy or too hard), these protocols still generate different results at short exercise times (if the protocol was too difficult for the patient), or if the exercise times are too long (if the protocol was too easy for the patient), with the exception of the low and moderate protocols yielding similar VO_2 values at the 12- to 16-minute exercise times. The disadvantage of these protocols is that the true Class IV patients will not be able to exercise 6–12 minutes, as recommended by the ACC/AHA guidelines *(60)*. However, it is arguable whether Class IV patients can exercise 6–12 minutes on any protocol. In fact, the ACC/AHA guidelines list uncontrolled symptomatic heart failure as a contraindication to exercise testing *(61)*.

Because exercise testing with breath-by-breath expired gas analysis involves a lot of procedures, it is important to have a worksheet with a checklist of procedures that allows the recording of events or complications during testing. The University of Pennsylvania cardiopulmonary

Table 13
University of Pennsylvania Ramping Treadmill Protocols

(For SensorMedics Metabolic Cart, Yorba Linda, CA)

Low ramping protocol

Stage	Speed (mph)	Grade (%)	Stage time (minutes)
1	1.5	0	1:00
2	2.0	0	2:30
3	2.0	3.5	2:30
4	2.0	7.0	2:00
5	2.0	10.5	2:00
6	2.0	14.0	2:00
7	2.0	17.5	2:00
8	2.0	21.0	2:00
9	2.5	21.0	2:00
10	3.0	21.0	2:00

If the patient reaches final elevation of this protocol, manually increase speed 0.1 mph every 24 seconds until patient reaches maximum exercise capacity.

Moderate ramping protocol

Stage	Speed (mph)	Grade (%)	Stage time (minutes)
1	1.5	0	1:30
2	2.5	0	1:30
3	2.5	2.5	3:00
4	2.5	7.0	3:00
5	2.5	11.5	3:00
6	2.5	16.5	3:00
7	2.5	21.0	3:00
8	3.4	21.0	3:00
9	4.2	21.0	3:00

If the patient reaches final elevation of this protocol, manually increase speed 0.1 mph every 18 seconds until patient reaches maximum exercise capacity.

High ramping protocol

Stage	Speed (mph)	Grade (%)	Stage time (minutes)
1	1.5	0	1:00
2	3.0	0	3:00
3	3.0	8.0	3:00
4	3.0	16.0	3:00
5	3.0	22.0	3:00
6	4.5	22.0	3:00
7	6.0	22.0	3:00
8	8.0	22.0	3:00
9	10.0	22.0	3:00

If the patient reaches final elevation of this protocol, manually increase speed 0.1 mph every 12 seconds until patient reaches maximum exercise capacity.

Note. All protocols begin at a speed of 1.5 mph, increasing to 2.0 mph, 2.5 mph and 3.0 mph for the low, moderate, and high protocols, respectively, before incline is added.

Table 14

Oxygen Consumption Values

	VO_2 at 4–8 min	VO_2 at 8–12 min	VO_2 at 12–16 min	p value 4–8 min vs 8–12 min	p value 4–8 min vs 12–16 min	p value 8–12 min vs 12–16 min
Low	11.3 ± 2.5	13.7 ± 2.9	18.4 ± 3.3	<0.001	<0.0001	<0.001
Moderate	13.0 ± 2.5	16.2 ± 3.5	18.7 ± 3.7	<0.0001	<0.0001	<0.001
High	18.6 ± 3.4	25.6 ± 4.9	33.7 ± 7.1	<0.0001	<0.0001	<0.0001
p value low vs mod	<0.001	<0.002	NS			
p value low vs high	<0.0001	<0.0001	<0.0001			
p value mod vs high	<0.0001	<0.0001	<0.0001			

Oxygen consumption (VO_2) values (mL/kg/minute) after three durations of exercise (4–8, 8–12, and 12–16 minutes) using the three University of Pennsylvania ramping treadmill exercise protocols (low, moderate, and high). The increase in VO_2 values is slowest for the low protocol and fastest for the high protocol. For patients exercising 8–12 minutes on each protocol, the individual values are consistent with Weber class C, B, and A functional status for the low, moderate, and high protocols, respectively. The VO_2 values for each duration of exercise (4–8, 8–12, and 12–16 minutes) are significantly different across the three protocols, except for the 12- to 16-minute duration between the low and moderate protocols. Within each protocol, different exercise times also yield significantly different VO_2 values. Unpublished data based on 400 exercise tests with expired gas analysis from the University of Pennsylvania.

exercise worksheet is illustrated in Appendix C. This worksheet is designed both as a checklist for testing procedures, as well as a source document for vital signs, symptoms, reason for test discontinuation, and physician/technician notes during exercise testing.

Because VO_2 measurement requires specialized training, practicing cardiologists often use treadmill exercise time to estimate the level of work achieved in metabolic equivalents (METs). One MET is the resting metabolic rate of an average 70-kg man, defined as a VO_2 of 3.5 mL/kg/minute *(60)*. Instead of calculating the actual resting metabolic demands in everyone, 3.5 mL/kg/minute is taken as an average of the resting metabolic rate of all patients for the purposes of standardization. A list of the METs associated with various daily activities is listed in Table 15 *(60)*. Unfortunately, this prediction is associated with wide confidence intervals *(62)* (Fig. 5). Thus, someone who exercised 10 minutes on the Bruce protocol can have a peak VO_2 between 25–47 mL/kg/minute! In addition, Roberts and colleagues *(63)* have demonstrated that normal subjects and patients with coronary artery disease exercising on the same protocol have significantly different peak VO_2 values, especially at higher workloads (Fig. 6), presumably owing to the lack of cardiac reserve in patients with cardiac disease. Bruce also documented this difference between healthy men and men with coronary disease (postmyocardial infarction and/or angina) *(56)*. Thus, the use of exercise time to estimate maximal exercise capacity is not accurate and should not be utilized.

PROGNOSTIC VALUE OF EXERCISE TESTING IN THE HEART FAILURE PATIENT

Even though the NYHA classification is subjective, its prognostic indications have been repeatedly demonstrated in large-scale heart failure studies. The angiotensin-converting enzyme (ACE) inhibitor studies illustrate this point. One of the first ACE inhibitor studies in heart failure was the Cooperative North Scandinavian Enalapril Survival Study (CONSENSUS) *(64)*. This study evaluated the efficacy of enalapril on the survival of patients with Class IV heart failure. The placebo group of this study had a 6-month mortality of 44% and a 1- year mortality of 52%. On the other hand, the Study of Left-Ventricular Dysfunction (SOLVD) treatment trial included predominantly patients with Class II and III heart failure patients (87%; only 2% were Class IV), and the 6-month mortality for the placebo group was 10% with 1-year mortality of 16% and a 3-year mortality of 35% *(65)*. The SOLVD Prevention trial included predominantly patients with Class I heart fail-

Table 15
METs Associated with Common Daily Activities

Activity	METs
Mild	
Billiards	2.4
Canoeing (leisurely)	2.5
Dancing, ballroom	2.9
Golf (with cart)	2.5
Horseback riding (walking)	2.3
Playing a musical instrument	1.8–2.5
Volleyball (noncompetitive)	2.9
Walking (2 mph)	2.5
Moderate	
Calisthenics (no weights)	4.0
Cycling (leisurely)	3.5
Golf (without cart)	4.9
Swimming (slowly)	4.5
Walking (3 mph)	3.3
Walking (4 mph)	4.5
Vigorous	
Chopping wood	4.9
Climbing hills (no load)	6.9
Climbing hills (5 kg load)	7.4
Cycling (moderate)	5.7
Dancing (aerobic or ballet)	6.0
Dancing (fast ballroom or square)	5.5
Jogging (10-minute mile)	10.0
Ice skating	5.5
Roller skating	6.5
Rope skipping	12.0
Skiing (water or downhill)	6.8
Squash	12.1
Surfing	6.0
Swimming	7.0
Tennis (doubles)	5.0
Walking (5 mph)	8.0
Activites of Daily Living	
Gardening (no lifting)	4.4
Household tasks, moderate effort	3.5
Lifting items continuously	4.0
Loading/unloading car	3.0
Lying quietly	1.0
Mopping	3.5
Mowing lawn (power mower)	4.5

Note. MET is a metabolic equivalent, and is the resting metabolic rate of an average 70-kg man, defined as a VO_2 of 3.5 mL/kg/minute. Used with permission from Fletcher GF et al. (60).

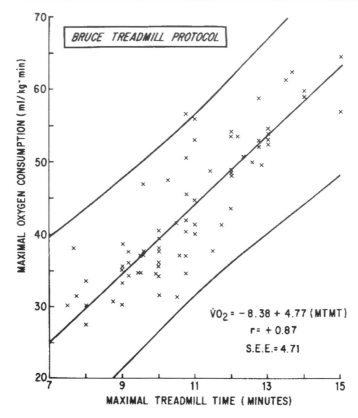

Fig. 5. Relationship between maximal treadmill time and peak VO_2 using the Bruce treadmill protocol in healthy pilots. Outer lines represent the 95% confidence intervals. Reprinted with permission from Froelicher et al. *(62)*.

ure (67%, with 33% Class II heart failure), and the mortality at a mean of 37 months of follow-up was only 16% *(66)*. The 1-year mortality in this study was less than 10%. Thus, the NYHA classification is useful in estimating outcomes in large populations of heart failure patients. However, it would be difficult to estimate an individual patient's mortality based on the NYHA classification, given the subjective nature of this system. The utility of this classification lies in the estimated outcomes of the asymptomatic and severely decompensated patients (Class I and IV), because it is very easy to differentiate these two patient populations. What is not clear is whether a patient's risk profile improves if his or her NYHA class decreases. The ACE inhibitor studies all had a positive impact on survival (except for the SOLVD prevention study), but it is not clear what the NYHA functional class of the patients were at the end of the studies *(64–67)*.

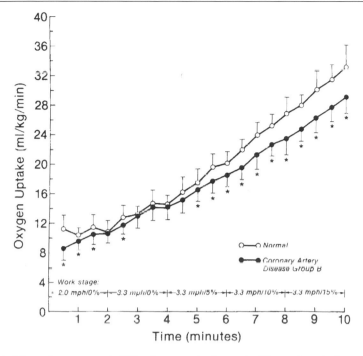

Fig. 6. Plot of mean peak VO$_2$ for matched treadmill workloads in normal subjects and patients with coronary artery disease. At higher workloads, VO$_2$ is significantly lower in patients with coronary artery disease. Reprinted with permission from Roberts et al. *(63)*.

The activity scales are not known to have prognostic indications, except as it may clarify a patient's NYHA functional class. The LIHFQ is also not known to have any prognostic implications, whereas the KCCQ scores were lower for patients who died or were rehospitalized for heart failure in the initial validation study *(23)*, but this needs to be confirmed in a larger study.

The 6-minute walk test is useful in estimating a patient's prognosis. In the SOLVD registry, 833 patients were stratified into four groups based on their walk test distance (Table 16) *(68)*. Level 1 patients walked less than 300 m, whereas level 2 patients walked between 300–374.9 m, level 3 patients walked between 375–449.9 m, and level 4 patients walked more than 450 m. There was a fair correlation between distance walked and the NYHA class: almost 75% of Class I patients were in levels 3 or 4, whereas around 80% of the Class III–IV patients were in levels 1 and 2. However, the Class II patients separated almost evenly into the four levels of distances walked, again highlighting the subjective nature of NYHA classification.

Table 16
Prognostic Significance of 6-Minute Corridor Walk Test

6MW distance	CHF readmissions	Mortality
<300 m	22.16%	10.23%
300–374.9 m	11.20%	7.88%
375–449.9 m	3.72%	4.19%
≥450 m	1.99%	2.99%

Relationship between 6-minute walk (6MW) distance and heart failure readmission rates and mortality in the SOLVD Registry, consisting of 833 patients followed for an average of 242 ± 82 days. Used with permission from Bittner et al. *(68)*.

As seen in Table 16, the 6-minute walk distance is inversely proportional to mortality ($p < 0.02$) *(68)*. The patients with the shortest walk distance (<300 m) had a 3.7-fold risk of dying compared to patients with the longest walk distance (≥450 m). Similarly, patients walking 300–374.9 m had a 2.78-fold increased mortality when compared to the group walking ≥450 m. In addition, admission for heart failure also increased with decreasing walk test distance. Thus, patients walking only <300 m had a 14-fold increased risk of heart failure admissions when compared to the highest functioning group, and patients walking 300–374.9 m had a 6.21-fold increase in heart failure admissions. Interestingly, the 6-minute walk distance also demonstrated prognostic significance for patients with preserved ejection fraction (>45%), with a 2.62-fold increase in the combined death/rehospitalization for heart failure for a 120 m difference in walk test distance *(68)*. Thus, the 6-minute walk test is not only an easy and inexpensive test to perform, it has significant prognostic implications.

Over the last 10–15 years, maximal exercise capacity as measured by VO_2 testing, has become the most important prognostic indicator in heart failure. Likoff et al. *(69)* examined 15 clinical variables in 201 patients with heart failure (60% with ischemic cardiomyopathy). Left-ventricular ejection fraction, ischemic etiology of heart failure and low peak VO_2 (less than 13 mL/kg/minute) were independent predictors of poor outcome. Cox proportional hazards revealed peak VO_2, S3 gallop, and ischemic cardiomyopathy as the best prognostic indicators. Patients with all three parameters have a 24% 6-month mortality, compared to 5% 6-month mortality in those patients without any of these three parameters. Based on this observation, Mancini et al. *(59)* utilized a peak VO2 of less than 14 mL/kg/minute as a criteria for heart transplant listing in 116 heart failure patients. Of the eight variables examined,

PEAK VO₂ (ml/kg/min)

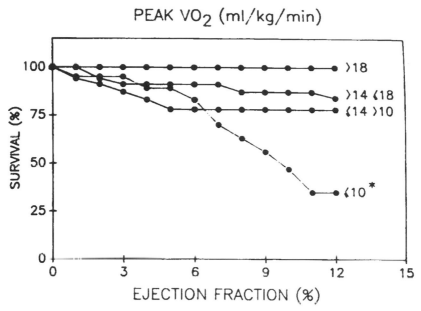

Fig. 7. One-year survival curves of heart failure patients with varying levels of exercise capacity (Maximal oxygen consumption >18 mL/kg/minute, >14 <18 mL/kg/minute, >10 <14 mL/kg/minute, and <10 kg/minute). Reprinted with permission from Mancini et al. (59).

peak VO_2 was the only significant predictor of death using multivariate analysis. Patients with peak VO_2 less than 10 mL/kg/minute had significantly worse survival compared to patients with peak VO_2 value greater than 14 mL/kg/minute (1 year survival about 30% as compared to greater than 80%) (Fig. 7). In fact, patients with peak VO_2 value greater than 14 mL/kg/minute had similar survival compared to patients posttransplant. Patients' whose peak VO2 value was between 10–14 mL/kg/minute had intermediate survival. A larger study from Italy recently confirmed that patients with VO_2 value less than 10 mL/kg/minute had a very poor outcome (70). Interestingly, patients with peak VO_2 value of less than 10 mL/kg/minute had a very poor prognosis, whether they reached AT or not.

To further evaluate the prognostic significance of moderate exercise intolerance, Kao and colleagues (71) evaluated VO_2 tests in 178 patients referred for cardiac transplantation. Patients were divided into three groups based on a VO_2 of <12 mL/kg/minute, 12–17 mL/kg/minute, and >17 mL/kg/minute. By chi square analysis, there was a significant difference in mortality between groups, but this was owing entirely to the difference in outcomes between the lowest and the highest VO_2 groups

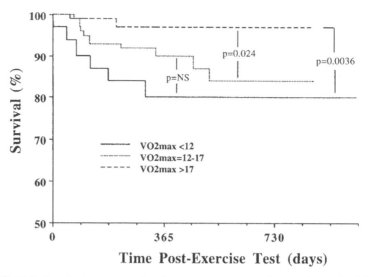

Fig. 8. Relation between maximal oxygen consumption and survival in all patients evaluated for transplant. By chi square analysis, there was an overall difference between groups ($p = 0.0162$; 2 degrees of freedom), but the only groups to differ were patients with maximal oxygen consumption <12 mL/kg/minute and those >17 mL/kg/minute. A p value of <0.0167 was considered significant because of Bonferroni correction. Reprinted with permission from Kao et al. *(71)*.

(Fig. 8). When the patients in the intermediate VO_2 group were further subdivided into tertiles (12–13.7 mL/kg/minute, 13.8–15.3 mL/kg/minute, and 15.4–17 mL/kg/minute), there was no difference in outcomes between tertiles. When patients are grouped according to the Weber classification, there was a significant decline in survival with decreasing VO_2 values (Fig. 9) *(72)*. A cardiac contraindication to exercise testing also identifies a high risk subgroup of patients. Opasich et al. *(70)* evaluated 653 patients for cardiac transplantation. Fifty-six of these patients could not complete exercise testing because of cardiac contraindications. These patients had a 77% likelihood of death/transplant during the 499-day follow-up period; 70% of these events occurred during the first 100 days of the study period. Finally, serial VO_2 testing has prognostic significance. When a group of patients listed for cardiac transplantation improved their VO_2 value to more than 12 mL/kg/minute, they had a 2-year 100% actuarial survival and a 2-year 85% transplant-free survival *(73)*. Thus, VO_2 testing is a useful prognostic indicator, especially with values less than 10 mL/kg/minute or greater than 14 mL/kg/minute.

However, using a fixed value of VO_2 to determine prognosis may bias unnecessarily against a younger cohort of patients, because a peak VO_2

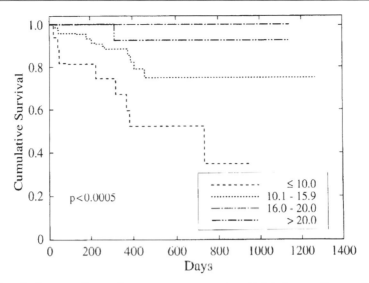

Fig. 9. Survival curves for peak oxygen consumption divided according to the Weber classification. There was a significant difference in survival between groups. Reprinted with permission from MacGowan et al. *(72).*

value of 14 mL/kg/minute represents severe exercise intolerance for younger patients. There are several formulas to estimate peak VO_2 for each gender and age group. The most frequently utilized formula by Wasserman *(74)* takes into account whether a patient is obese or not. The formulas for determining obesity are:

Males: Predicted wt = $(0.79 \times ht - 60.7)$

Females: Predicted wt = $(0.79 \times ht - 68.2)$

where wt is weight in kilograms and ht is height in centimeters. For patients whose weight is at or below the weight predicted above, the following equations predict peak VO_2 values:

Males: VO_2 peak (mL/minute) = Actual wt $\times$ $(56.36 - 0.413 \times age)$

Females: VO_2 peak (mL/minute) = Actual wt $\times$ $(44.37 - 0.413 \times age)$

For patients who are obese, the following equations predict peak VO_2 values:

Males: VO_2 peak (mL/minute) = Predicted wt $\times$ $(56.36 - 0.413 \times age)$

Females: VO_2 peak (mL/minute) = Predicted wt $\times$ $(44.37 - 0.413 \times age)$

Using Wasserman's formula, Stelken et al. *(75)* examined the use of the percent of predicted VO_2 as a prognostic factor in 181 patients evaluated for cardiac transplantation. The sensitivity and specificity of various "cut-off" points for percent predicted VO_2 are shown in Table 17. Using a threshold of 50% predicted peak VO_2 yields the best sensitivity/specificity. Table 18 illustrates the actuarial survival of patients stratified according to ≥50% of predicted peak VO_2. Patients with peak VO_2 <50% of predicted had a 1- and 2-year survival of 74 and 43%, as opposed to 98 and 90% for those whose VO_2 values are >50% of predicted. Multivariate analysis selected <50% predicted peak VO_2 as the most significant predictor of cardiac death. Receiver-operating characteristic curves indicated a significantly improved accuracy for the percent of predicted VO_2 as opposed to that for peak VO_2. Similarly, Osada et al. (76) found percent predicted VO_2 and peak exercise systolic blood pressure to be the most significant predictors of outcomes in 500 ambulatory heart failure patients referred for cardiac transplantation.

However, Aaronson and Mancini (77) examined the use of both actual weight-based peak VO_2 and percent of predicted VO_2 in 272 patients referred for cardiac transplantation. These authors used two different formulas for predicting peak VO2 values, and patients were stratified into <35% predicted VO_2, 35–50% predicted VO_2, and >50% predicted VO_2 groups. The lower two strata had similar survival, but both had significantly lower survival compared to the best functioning group. Similarly, patients were stratified into weight-based peak VO_2 values of <10 mL/kg/minute, 10–14 mL/kg/minute, and >14 mL/kg/minute. Similar to Mancini's study in 1991 (59), patients in the lower two VO_2 groups had similar survival, which were significantly lower than that of the highest VO_2 group. However, the use of the percent predicted peak VO_2 failed to improve the prognostic information provided by weight-based peak VO_2 values.

The prediction of peak VO_2 values is actually more complicated than that illustrated previously. The original Wasserman equations suggest that the "extra" weight of an obese patient is adipose tissue and does not contribute to exercise VO_2 values. However, these patients actually have to move more body mass during exercise owing to their obesity, and thus their peak VO_2 values should be higher than predicted by the formulas. In addition, patients with lower than predicted weight were assumed to have lower total-body adiposity as the reason for being underweight. However, thin patients have likely lost muscle mass (which contributes to peak VO_2 values), in addition to having a lower total-body fat. Therefore, Wasserman provided another set of equations in 1999 (78). The updated formulas for determining obesity are:

Table 17
Sensitivity and Specificity of Various Percent
Predicted VO_2 Cut-Off Points

	30%	40%	50%	60%
Sensitivity	11	55	86	93
Specificity	95	84	63	41

Reprinted with permission from Stelken et al. *(75)*.

Table 18
Actuarial Survival of Patients Stratified According
to Percent Predicted VO_2

	>50% Predicted VO_2	<50% Predicted VO_2
1-year survival	98%	74%
2-year survival	90%	43%

Note. Patients with peak VO_2 <50% of predicted have a significantly worse prognosis than those whose peak VO_2 values are >50% of predicted. Reprinted with permission from Stelken et al. *(75)*.

$$\text{Males: Predicted wt} = (0.79 \times ht) - 60.7$$
$$\text{Females: Predicted wt} = (0.65 \times ht) - 42.8$$

For patients whose weight equals that predicted by the above formulas, the following equations predict peak VO2 values with bicycle testing:

$$\text{Males: } VO_2 \text{ (mL/minute)} = \text{actual wt} \times (50.72 - 0.372 \times age)$$
$$\text{Females: } VO_2 \text{ (mL/minute)} = (\text{actual wt} + 43) \times (22.78 - 0.17 \times age)$$

For patients below their predicted body weight, the following equations predict peak VO_2 values with bicycle testing:

Males:
$$VO_2 \text{ (mL/minute)} = (\text{predicted wt} + \text{actual wt})/2 \times (50.72 - 0.372 \times age)$$
Females:
$$VO_2 \text{ (mL/minute)} = (\text{predicted wt} + \text{actual wt} + 86)/2 \times (22.78 - 0.17 \times age)$$

For the patients who are considered overweight or obese, the following equations are used to estimate predicted peak VO_2 values with bicycle testing. Thus:

$$\text{Males: } VO_2 \text{ (mL/minute)} = \text{predicted wt} \times (50.72 - 0.372 \times age) + 6 \times (\text{actual wt} - \text{predicted wt})$$

$$\text{Females: } VO_2 \text{ (mL/minute)} = (\text{predicted wt} + 43) \times (22.78 - 0.17 \times age) + 6 \times (\text{actual wt} - \text{predicted wt})$$

In all cases, when treadmill exercise is performed, the predictive formulas have to be multiplied by 1.11 to obtain the predicted peak VO_2 values.

Given the complexity of estimating a patient's predicted maximal VO_2, its use can be quite cumbersome. However, currently available metabolic carts often include predicted VO_2 values in the software, which makes this set of calculations much more accessible. Calculating percent predicted VO_2 may potentially be of prognostic value in the young patient whose measured VO_2 is greater than 14 mL/kg/minute, but whose predicted VO_2 is less than 50%. Similarly, percent predicted VO_2 analysis may also be of benefit in elderly patients with measured VO_2 of less than 14 mL/kg/minute, but whose percent predicted VO_2 is more than 50%. Further studies are needed to clarify the utility of percent predicted VO_2 in these situations. Finally, VO_2 analysis has been studied extensively only in patients who are transplant candidates; its predictive powers in a larger unselected heart failure population, who may be more functional, remains to be elucidated.

Although the prognostic studies of VO_2 testing may utilize bicycle testing (73), the majority are treadmill studies utilizing modified Naughton protocols (59,70–72,77). However, modified Bruce protocol has also been utilized (75), and the Bruce protocol yielded similar peak VO_2, percent predicted VO_2, and AT values as compared to the modified Naughton protocol (peak VO_2 Bruce 17.7 ± 3.8 mL/kg/minunt vs modified Naughton 18.0 ± 4.7 mL/kg/minute) in one study (79). Exercise time on the Bruce protocol was obviously shorter than that on the modified Naughton protocol, and Strzelczyk and colleagues recommend the routine use of the Bruce protocol to increase the efficiency of testing. However, most patients presenting for VO_2 testing will be considerably more limited than patients in this study and will likely do poorly with Bruce protocol exercise testing.

EXERCISE AS AN ENDPOINT IN EVALUATING HEART FAILURE THERAPY

Despite the tremendous utility of VO_2 testing in prognostication, its utility in monitoring the efficacy of drug therapy is much more limited. With the success of medical therapy for heart failure in the early 1980s, several investigators studied the impact of positive inotropic agents and vasodilators on exercise capacity in heart failure patients. Unfortunately, acute administration of dobutamine failed to improve exercise duration, despite an increase in cardiac output and reduction in pulmonary capillary wedge pressure (80). Similarly, acute administration of potent vasodilators, such as hydralazine (81), ACE inhibitors (82), nitrates (83), and prazosin (84) improved hemodynamics and femoral blood flow, but failed to increase exercise duration or peak VO_2.

As mentioned in the first section of this chapter, exercise capacity depends on the coordination between five organ systems—respiratory, hematologic, cardiac, vascular, and musculoskeletal. Acute improvements in intracardiac hemodynamics do not improve muscular conditioning, which will continue to limit exercise capacity. This point is well illustrated by Wilson and colleagues in a study of 64 heart failure patients undergoing transplant evaluation *(85)*. Patients underwent exercise testing with intracardiac hemodynamic measurements, as well as expired gas analysis. Surprisingly, there was absolutely no correlation between peak VO_2 and cardiac index or pulmonary capillary wedge pressures. Eighteen patients had a normal cardiac output response to exercise but had a peak VO_2 less than 14 mL/kg/minute, whereas seven patients had reduced cardiac reserve and elevated pulmonary capillary wedge pressures, but had peak VO_2 greater than 14 mL/kg/minute. This underscores the effects of deconditioning on exercise testing results and has limited the utility of exercise testing in large-scale clinical trials. In fact, there has often been a dissociation between the drug's effects on mortality and exercise capacity.

Perhaps the most dramatic examples of this are the oral inotrope studies. Several oral phosphodiesterase inhibitors were studied in the early 1990s, which were all associated with improved exercise duration and quality of life but increased mortality. Oral milrinone increased exercise duration by 17% *(86)*, but had a 28% increase in total mortality and a 34% increase in cardiovascular mortality over a 6-month period *(87)*. Similarly, another phosphodiesterase inhibitor, enoximone, significantly increased exercise time after four and eight weeks of treatment and improved a heart failure patient's ability to perform activities of daily living, with reduced dyspnea *(88)*, but increased mortality when compared to placebo *(89)*.

On the other hand, ACE inhibitors and β-blockers both improve mortality, but they do not have a consistent positive impact on exercise capacity. In V-HeFT-I, the hydralazine-isosorbide dinitrate combination therapy led to a 34% reduction in mortality *(90)*. In V-HeFT-II, enalapril was associated with a further 28% reduction in mortality in comparison to hydralazine-isosorbide dinitrate *(91)*. Interestingly, only the hydralazine-isosorbide dinitrate group improved their peak VO_2, but not the enalapril group. This improvement was seen as early as 13 weeks after medication initiation, and the effects persisted for 2 years. Similarly, a recent European study of various β-blockers (metoprolol, bisoprolol, sotalol, carvedilol, celiprolol) found no difference in NYHA class or peak VO_2 between the β-blocker group and no β-blocker group, but the β-blocker group had a significantly reduced rehospitalization and mortality rates *(92)*. This beneficial effect was especially evident in the Weber class D patients.

Carvedilol, a combined α and nonspecific β antagonist, has been associated with a significant 5–10% absolute increase in left ventricular ejection fraction with chronic use *(21,93–99)*. As a result, stroke volume increases in the carvedilol-treated patients compared to placebo *(94–96)*. However, resting cardiac index is unchanged *(94,95)*, owing to a 8–25 beat per minute reduction in resting heart rate *(94–97)*. The lack of improvement in resting cardiac index after carvedilol treatment may explain its neutral effect on maximal exercise capacity *(93–96,100)*. In addition, the effects of carvedilol on submaximal exercise performance is inconsistent, with modest improvement seen in some studies *(94,96)*, but no improvement seen in other studies *(21,22,93,100)*. Despite the lack of improvement in submaximal or maximal exercise capacity, the use of carvedilol is associated with a 23–73% reduction in mortality *(98,101,102)*, 38% reduction in heart failure admissions *(103)*, and a 24–38% reduction in the combined risk of heart failure hospitalization or death *(93,101,104)*.

As a result, submaximal and maximal exercise capacity cannot be used as a surrogate endpoint in large scale clinical studies of medications/devices for the treatment of heart failure *(105)*. Instead, clinical studies need to be designed to examine the effects of the treatment under study on heart failure morbidity and mortality, and exercise testing should be used to objectively document the effect of the proposed treatment on a patient's functional capacity.

SUMMARY

In summary, both central and peripheral factors are intimately involved in the performance of exercise. The heart failure state potentially impairs all of these factors, thus significantly limiting exercise capacity. There are subjective and objective measures of a heart failure patient's functional capacity. Although the subjective measures are inexpensive and easy to administer, they cannot reliably distinguish between those with intermediate levels of exercise impairment. Thus, it is useful to objectively document both submaximal and maximal exercise capacity. Both 6-minute walk test and maximal exercise testing with expired gas analysis are reproducible over time, and measurement of peak VO_2 has significant prognostic implications, especially in patients being evaluated for cardiac transplantation. Whereas the correlation between improved functional capacity and improved mortality is poor in large scale clinical studies, exercise testing can still be utilized to document a medication/device's effect on exercise capacity, because improvement in both submaximal and maximal exercise capacity can translate into improved endurance and increased ease with the performance of activities of daily living.

Appendix A:
The Kansas City Cardiomyopathy Questionnaire

The following questions refer to your **heart failure** and how it may affect your life. Please read and complete the following questions. There are no right or wrong answers. Please mark the answer that best applies to you.

1 **Heart failure** affects different people in different ways. Some feel shortness of breath while others feel fatigue. Please indicate how much you are limited by **heart failure** (shortness of breath or fatigue) in your ability to do the following activities over the past 2 weeks.

Place an **X** in one box on each line

Activity	Extremely Limited	Quite a bit Limited	Moderately Limited	Slightly Limited	Not at all Limited	Limited for other reasons or did not do the activity
Dressing yourself	❑	❑	❑	❑	❑	❑
Showering/Bathing	❑	❑	❑	❑	❑	❑
Walking 1 block on level ground	❑	❑	❑	❑	❑	❑
Doing yardwork, housework or carrying groceries	❑	❑	❑	❑	❑	❑
Climbing a flight of stairs without stopping	❑	❑	❑	❑	❑	❑
Hurrying or jogging (as if to catch a bus)	❑	❑	❑	❑	❑	❑

2. Compared with 2 weeks ago, have your symptoms of **heart failure** (shortness of breath, fatigue or ankle swelling) changed? My symptoms of **heart failure** have become ...

Much worse	Slightly worse	Not changed	Slightly better	Much better	I've had no symptoms over the last 2 weeks
❑	❑	❑	❑	❑	❑

3. Over the past 2 weeks, how many times did you have **swelling** in your feet, ankles or legs when you woke up in the morning?

Every morning	3 or more times a week, but not every day	1-2 times a week	Less than once a week	Never over the past 2 weeks
❑	❑	❑	❑	❑

4. Over the past 2 weeks, how much has swelling in your feet, ankles or legs bothered you? It has been ...

Extremely bothersome	Quite a bit bothersome	Moderately bothersome	Slightly bothersome	Not at all bothersome	I've had no swelling
❑	❑	❑	❑	❑	❑

5. Over the past 2 weeks, on average, how many times has **fatigue** limited your ability to do what you want?

All of the time	Several times per day	At least once a day	3 or more times per week but not every day	1-2 times per week	Less than once a week	Never over the past 2 weeks
❑	❑	❑	❑	❑	❑	❑

6. Over the past 2 weeks, how much has your **fatigue** bothered you? It has been ...

Extremely bothersome	Quite a bit bothersome	Moderately bothersome	Slightly bothersome	Not at all bothersome	I've had no fatigue
❑	❑	❑	❑	❑	❑

7. Over the past 2 weeks, on average, how many times has **shortness of breath** limited your ability to do what you wanted?

All of the time	Several times per day	At least once a day	3 or more times per week but not every day	1-2 times per week	Less than once a week	Never over the past 2 weeks
❑	❑	❑	❑	❑	❑	❑

8. Over the past 2 weeks, how much has your **shortness of breath** bothered you? It has been ...

Extremely bothersome	Quite a bit bothersome	Moderately bothersome	Slightly bothersome	Not at all bothersome	I've had no shortness of breath
❑	❑	❑	❑	❑	❑

9. Over the past 2 weeks, on average, how many times have you been forced to sleep sitting up in a chair or with at least 3 pillows to prop you up because of **shortness of breath**?

Every night	3 or more times a week, but not every day	1-2 times a week	Less than once a week	Never over the past 2 weeks
❑	❑	❑	❑	❑

10. **Heart failure** symptoms can worsen for a number of reasons. How sure are you that you know what to do, or whom to call, if your **heart failure** gets worse?

Not at all sure	Not very sure	Somewhat sure	Mostly sure	Completely sure
❑	❑	❑	❑	❑

11. How well do you understand what things you are able to do to keep your **heart failure** symptoms from getting worse? (for example, weighing yourself, eating a low salt diet, etc.)

Do not understand at all	Do not understand very well	Somewhat understand	Mostly understand	Completely understand
❑	❑	❑	❑	❑

12. Over the <u>past 2 weeks</u>, how much has your **heart failure** limited your enjoyment of life?

It has **extremely** limited my enjoyment of life	It has limited my enjoyment of life **quite a bit**	It has **moderately** limited my enjoyment of life	It has **slightly** limited my enjoyment of life	It has **not** **limited** my enjoyment of life at all
❑	❑	❑	❑	❑

13. If you had to spend the rest of your life with your **heart failure** the way it is <u>right now</u>, how would you feel about this?

Not at all satisfied	Mostly dissatisfied	Somewhat satisfied	Mostly satisfied	Completely satisfied
❑	❑	❑	❑	❑

14. Over the <u>past 2 weeks</u>, how often have you felt discouraged or down in the dumps because of your **heart failure**?

I felt that way **all of the time**	I felt that way **most of the time**	I **occasionally** felt that way	I **rarely** felt that way	I **never** felt that way
❑	❑	❑	❑	❑

15. How much does your **heart failure** affect your lifestyle? Please indicate how your **heart failure** may have limited your participation in the following activities over <u>the past 2 weeks</u>. Please place an **X** in one box on each line.

Activity	**Severely** limited	Limited **quite a bit**	Moderately limited	**Slightly** limited	**Did not** limit at all	Does not apply or did not do for other reasons
Hobbies, recreational activities	❑	❑	❑	❑	❑	❑
Working or doing household chores	❑	❑	❑	❑	❑	❑
Visiting family or friends out of your home	❑	❑	❑	❑	❑	❑
Intimate relationships with loved ones	❑	❑	❑	❑	❑	❑

Reprinted with permission from Green et al. *(23).*

Appendix B
University of Pennsylvania Heart Failure and Transplant Program 6-Minute Corridor Walk Test Worksheet

PATIENT NAME: _____   MRN: _____
DATE OF TEST: _____

Please check off each length of corridor completed and record the number of feet completed in the last lap (each ceiling tile represents 2 feet). Inform the patient at the end of 3 minutes and 5 minutes. Record vital signs prior to the start of test, immediately after the test, then 5 minutes after the test is completed.

Pretest:	HR:	_____	BP:	_____	SaO2:	_____
End of test:	HR:	_____	BP:	_____	SaO2:	_____
5 min. post:	HR:	_____	BP:	_____	SaO2:	_____

Lap 1 ____	Lap 2 ____	Lap 3 ____	Lap 4 ____
Lap 5 ____	Lap 6 ____	Lap 7 ____	Lap 8 ____
Lap 9 ____	Lap 10 ____	Lap 11 ____	Lap 12 ____
Lap 13 ____	Lap 14 ____	Lap 15 ____	Lap 16 ____
Lap 17 ____	Lap 18 ____	Lap 19 ____	Lap 20 ____
Lap 21 ____	Lap 22 ____	Lap 23 ____	Lap 24 ____
Lap 25 ____	Lap 26 ____	Lap 27 ____	Lap 28 ____
Lap 29 ____	Lap 30 ____	Lap 31 ____	Lap 32 ____
Lap 33 ____	Lap 34 ____	Lap 35 ____	Lap 36 ____

If the patient stops during the test, record the time stopped and time restarted below.

Time stopped:	_____	Time restarted:	_____	Reason:	_____
Time stopped:	_____	Time restarted:	_____	Reason:	_____
Time stopped:	_____	Time restarted:	_____	Reason:	_____

Symptoms at end of test: _____

CALCULATION OF 6 MINUTE WALK DISTANCE:

1. Each length of corridor is 60 feet.
2. Number of completed laps (A)   =
3. Number of feet in last lap (B)   = _____
4. Total distance: [(60 x A) + B] x 0.3048   = _____ meters

Signature of person completing test: _____

University of Pennsylvania 6-minute walk test worksheet, to facilitate the recording of laps completed, vitals, oxygen saturation, and any rest periods, if applicable. It also contains instructions for the conversion from feet to meters. Designed by Kao A, Division of Cardiology, Hospital of the University of Pennsylvania.

Appendix C
University of Pennyslvania Worksheet for Cardiopulmonary
Excercise Testing

Patient Name: _____   **Date:** _____

Height: _____   **Weight:** _____   **Sex:** _____   **Age:** _____

Which device was used? ❑ MASK :   ❑ SMALL   ❑ MEDIUM   ❑ LARGE   ❑ GEL SEAL

❑ MOUTHPIECE / NOSECLIP

Which flow meter was used?   #_____   **Was elastic net used?**   ❑ YES   ❑ NO

Which protocol was used?   ❑ LOW RAMP   ❑ MODERATE RAMP   ❑ HIGH RAMP
❑ OTHER: _____

Baseline EKG: _____	**Baseline BP:** _____
Peak EKG: _____	**Peak BP:** _____
Recovery EKG: _____	**Recovery BP:** _____

Total rest time: _____ MINUTES ____ SECONDS   **MVV:** _____ Good effort? ❑ YES   ❑ NO

Total exercise time: _____ MINUTES ____ SECONDS   **Peak BORG:** _____

Total recovery time: _____ MINUTES ____ SECONDS   **Was an RQ of 1.1 reached?**   ❑ YES   ❑ NO

Reason for termination:

Patient complaint (Rank in order):   Technician terminated:

❑	____	DYSPNEA
❑	____	LEG FATIGUE
❑	____	GENERAL FATIGUE
❑	____	CHEST DISCOMFORT
❑	____	DRY MOUTH
❑	____	LIGHTHEADEDNESS
❑	____	LACK OF MOTIVATION
❑	____	SYNCOPE / NEAR SYNCOPE
❑	____	OTHER (Specify): _____

❑   ARRHYTHMIA (Specify): _____
❑   ECG CHANGES (Specify): _____
❑   ICD DISCHARGE
❑   HYPOTENSION
❑   HYPERTENSION
❑   LOSS OF BALANCE / INABILITY TO COORDINATE
❑   DANGEROUS SITUATION (i.e. loose clothing, loose shoelace)
❑   ORTHOPEDIC LIMITATIONS (Specify): _____
❑   OTHER (Specify): _____

Technician:

Supervising MD:

Notes:

Worksheet for cardiopulmonary excercise testing at the University of Pennsylvania, documenting patient demographics, testing protocol and equipment, vitals, reason for termination, and provides space for physician or technician notes for documentation. This worksheet also serves as a checklist for testing procedures. Designed by DeRosa, R, and Kao, A, University of Pennsylvania.

REFERENCES

1. Lehninger AL. Principles of Biochemistry. Worth Publishers, Inc., New York, New York: 1982, p. 498.
2. Lehninger AL. Principles of Biochemistry. Worth Publishers, Inc., New York, New York: 1982. p. 428.
3. Sullivan MJ, Knight JD, Higginbotham MB, Cobb FR. Relation between central and peripheral hemodynamics during exercise in patients with chronic heart failure: muscle blood flow is reduced with maintenance of arterial perfusion pressure. Circulation 1989;80:769–781.

4. White M, Yanowitz F, Gilbert EM, et al. Role of beta-adrenergic receptor downregulation in the peak exercise response in patients with heart failure due to idiopathic dilated cardiomyopathy. Am J Cardiol 1995;76:1271–1276.

5. Katz SD. The role of endothelium-derived vasoactive substances in the pathophysiology of exercise intolerance in patients with congestive heart failure. Prog Cardiovasc Dis 1995;38:23–50.

6. Mancini DM, Coyle E, Coggan A, et al. Contribution of intrinsic skeletal muscle changes to 31P NMR Skeletal muscle metabolic abnormalities in patients with chronic heart failure. Circulation 1989;80:1338–1346.

7. MacDougall JD, Edler GCB, et al. Effects of strength training and immobilization on human muscle fibres. Eur J Appl Physiol Occ Physiol 1980;43:25–34.

8. Lindboe CF, Presthus J. Effects of denervation, immobilization and cachexia on fibre size in the anterior tibial muscle of the rat. Acta Neuropathol 1985;66:42–51.

9. Mancini DM, Walter G, Reichek N, et al. Contribution of skeletal muscle atrophy to exercise intolerance and altered muscle metabolism in heart failure. Circulation 1992;85:1364–1373.

10. Wilson JR, Fink L, Maris J, et al. Evaluation of energy metabolism in skeletal muscle of patients with heart failure with gated phosphorus-31 nuclear magnetic resonance. Circulation 1985;71:57–62.

11. Massie B, Conway M, Yonge R, et al. 31P Nuclear magnetic resonance evidence of abnormal skeletal muscle metabolism in patients with congestive heart failure. Am J Cardiol 1987;60:309–315.

12. Massie B, Conway M, Yonge R, et al. Skeletal muscle metabolism in patients with congestive heart failure: relation to clinical severity and blood flow. Circulation 1987;76:1009–1019.

13. The Criteria Committee of the New York Heart Association, Inc. Diseases of the Heart and Blood Vessels; Nomenclature and Criteria for Diagnosis. Little, Brown, Co.; Boston, MA: 1964, pp. 112,113.

14. Smith RF, Johnson G, Ziesche S, et al. Functional capacity in heart failure: comparison of methods for assessment and their relation to other indexes of heart failure. Circulation 1993;87:V188–V193.

15. Goldman L, Hashimoto B, Cook EF, Loscalzo A. Comparative reproducibility and validity of systems for assessing cardiovascular functional class: advantages of a new specific activity scale. Circulation 1981;64:1227–1234.

16. Hlatky MA, Boineau RE, Higginbotham MB, et al. A brief, self-administered questionnaire to determine functional capacity (The Duke Activity Status Index). Am J Cardiol 1989;64:651–654.

17. Rector T, Kubo S, Cohn J. Patient's self-assessment of their congestive heart failure. Part 2: content, reliability and validity of a new measure, the Minnesota Living with Heart Failure questionnaire. Heart Failure 1987;3:198–209.

18. Rector TS, Cohn JN. Assessment of patient outcome with the Minnesota Living with Heart Failure questionnaire: reliability and validity during a randomized, double-blind, placebo controlled trial of pimobendan. Am Heart J 1992;124:1017–1025.

19. Kubo SH, Gollub S, Bourge R, et al. Beneficial effects of pimobendan on exercise tolerance and quality of life in patients with heart failure: results of a multicenter trial. Circulation 1992;85:942–949.

20. Rector TS, Kubo SH, Cohn JN. Validity of the Minnesota Living with Heart Failure questionnaire as a measure of therapeutic response: effects of enalapril and placebo. Am J Cardiol 1993;71:1106,1107.

21. Colucci WS, Packer M, Bristow MR, et al. Carvedilol inhibits clinical progression in patients with mild symptoms of heart failure. Circulation 1996;94:2800–2806.

22. Packer M, Colucci WS, Sackner-Bernstein JD, et al. Double-blind, placebo-controlled carvedilol in patients with moderate to severe heart failure: the PRECISE

trial. Prospective randomized evaluation of carvedilol on symptoms and exercise. Circulation 1996;94:2793–2799.

23. Green CP, Porter CB, Bresnahan DR, Spertus JA. Development and evaluation of the Kansas City Cardiomyopathy questionnaire: a new health status measure for heart failure. J Am Coll Cardiol 2000;35:1245–1255.

24. McGavin CR, Gupta SP, McHardy GJ. Twelve minute walking test for assessing disability in chronic bronchitis. Br Med J 1976;1:822,823.

25. Lipkin DP, Scriven AJ, Crake T, Poole-Wilson PA. Six Minute walking test for assessing exercise capacity in chronic heart failure. Br Med J 1986;292:653–655.

26. Guyatt GH, Pugsley S, Sullivan MJ, et al. Effect of encouragement on walking test performance. Thorax 1984;39:818–822.

27. Riley M, McParland J, Stanford CF, Nicholls DP. Oxygen consumption during corridor walk testing in chronic cardiac failure. Eur Heart J 1992;13:789–793.

28. Simonton CA, Higginbotham MB, Cobb FR. The ventilatory threshold: quantitative analysis of reproducibility and relation to arterial lactate concentration in normal subjects and in patients with chronic congestive heart failure. Am J Cardiol 1988;62:100–107.

29. Wasserman K, Beaver WL, Whipp BJ. Gas exchange theory and the lactic acidosis (anaerobic) threshold. Circulation 1990;81:II14–II30.

30. Katz SD, Berkowitz R, LeJemtel TH. Anaerobic threshold detection in patients with congestive heart failure. Am J Cardiol 1992;69:1565–1569.

31. Weber KT, Janicki JS. Lactate production during maximal and submaximal exercise in patients with chronic heart failure. J Am Coll Cardiol 1985;6:717–724.

32. Fick A. Über die Messung des Blutquantums in den Herzventrikeln. Sitz der Physik. Med. Ges. Wurzburg 1870, p. 16.

33. Braunwald E. Heart Disease: A Textbook of Cardiovascular Medicine. W. B. Saunders Co., Philadelphia, PA: 1988, pp. 251,252.

34. Harrison TR, Pilcher C. Studies in congestive heart failure. II. The respiratory exchange during and after exercise. J Clin Invest 1930;8:291–315.

35. Wasserman K. Measures of functional capacity in patients with heart failure. Circulation 1990;81:II1–II4.

36. Beaver WL, Wasserman K, Whipp BJ. On-line computer analysis and breath-to-breath graphical display of exercise function tests. J Appl Physiol 1973;34:128–132.

37. Weber KT, Janicki JS. Cardiopulmonary Exercise Testing: Physiologic Principles and Clinical Applications. W. B. Saunders Co., Philadelphia, PA: 1986, p. 152.

38. Johnson JS, Carlson JJ, VanderLaan RL, Langholz DE. Effects of sampling interval on peak oxygen consumption in patients evaluated for heart transplantation. Chest 1998;113:816–819.

39. Weber KT, Kinasewitz GT, Janicki JS, Fishman AP. Oxygen utilization and ventilation during exercise in patients with chronic cardiac failure. Circulation 1982;65:1213–1223.

40. Elborn JS, Stanford CF, Nicholls DP. Reproducibility of cardiopulmonary parameters during exercise in patients with chronic cardiac failure. The need for a preliminary test. Eur Heart J 1990;11:75–81.

41. Nordehaug JE, Danielsen R, Stangeland L, et al. Respiratory gas exchange during treadmill exercise testing: reproducibility and comparison of different exercise protocols. Scand J Clin Lab Invest 1991;51:655–658.

42. Janicki JS, Gupta S, Ferris ST, McElroy PA. Long-term reproducibility of respiratory gas exchange measurements during exercise in patients with stable cardiac failure. Chest 1990;97:12–17.

43. Weber KT, Janicki JS. Cardiopulmonary Exercise Testing: Physiologic Principles and Clinical Applications. W. B. Saunders Co., Philadelphia, PA: 1986, p. 21.

44. Beaver WL, Wasserman K, Whipp BJ. A New method for detecting anaerobic threshold by gas exchange. J Appl Physiol 1986;60:2020–2027.
45. Dickstein K, Barvik S, Aarsland T, et al. A comparison of methodologies in detection of the anaerobic threshold. Circulation 1990;81:II38–II46.
46. Weber KT, Janicki JS. Cardiopulmonary Exercise Testing: Physiologic Principles and Clinical Applications. W. B. Saunders Co., Philadelphia, PA: 1986, p. 78.
47. Weber KT, Janicki JS. Cardiopulmonary Exercise Testing: Physiologic Principles and Clinical Applications. W. B. Saunders Co., Philadelphia, PA: 1986, p. 81.
48. Weber KT, Janicki JS. Cardiopulmonary Exercise Testing: Physiologic Principles and Clinical Applications. W. B. Saunders Co., Philadelphia, PA: 1986, p. 297.
49. Sullivan MJ, Higginbotham MB, Cobb FR. Increased exercise ventilation in patients with chronic heart failure: intact ventilatory control despite hemodynamic and pulmonary abnormalities. Circulation 1988;77:552–559.
50. MacGowan GA, Panzak G, Murali S. Exercise-related ventilatory abnormalities are more specific for functional impairment in chronic heart failure than reduction in peak exercise oxygen consumption. J Heart Lung Transplant 2001;20:1167–1173.
51. Page E, Cohen-Solal A, Jondeau G, et al. Comparison of treadmill and bicycle exercise in patients with chronic heart failure. Chest 1994;106:1002–1006.
52. Myers J, Buchanan N, Walsh D, et al. Comparison of the ramp versus standard exercise protocols. J Am Coll Cardiol 1991;17:1334–1342.
53. Wilson JR, Fink LI, Ferraro N, et al. Use of maximal bicycle exercise testing with respiratory gas analysis to assess exercise performance in patients with congestive heart failure secondary to coronary artery disease or to idiopathic dilated cardiomyopathy. Am J Cardiol 1986;58:601–606
54. Hansen JE. Exercise instruments, schemes, and protocols for evaluating the dyspneic patient. Am Rev Respir Dis 1984;129;5525–5527.
55. Cohen-Solal A, Zannad F, Guèret P, et al. Multicenter determination of the oxygen uptake and the ventilatory threshold. Eur Heart J 1991;12:1055–1063.
56. Bruce RA, Kusumi F, Hosmer D. Maximal oxygen uptake and nomographic assessment of functional aerobic impairment in cardiovascular disease. Am Heart J 1973;85:546–562.
57. Patterson JA, Naughton J, Pietras RJ, Gunnar RM. Treadmill exercise in assessment of the functional capacity of patients with cardiac disease. Am J Cardiol 1972;30:757–762.
58. Liang C, Stewart DK, LeJemtel TH, et al. Characteristics of peak aerobic capacity in symptomatic and asymptomatic subjects with left ventricular dysfunction. Am J Cardiol 1992;69:1207–1211.
59. Mancini DM, Eisen H, Kussmaul W, et al. Value of peak exercise oxygen consumption for optimal timing of cardiac transplantation in ambulatory patients with heart failure. Circulation 1991;83:778–786.
60. Fletcher GF, Balady GJ, Amsterdam EA, et al. Exercise standards for testing and training: a statement for healthcare professionals from the American Heart Association. Circulation 2001;104:1694–1740.
61. Gibbons RJ, Balady GJ, Beasley JW, et al. ACC/AHA guidelines for exercise testing: a report of the American College of Cardiology/American Heart Association Task Force on practice guidelines (committee on exercise testing). J Am Coll Cardiol 1997;30:260–315.
62. Froelicher VF, Thompson AJ, Noguera I, et al. Prediction of maximal oxygen consumption: comparison of the Bruce and Balke treadmill protocols. Chest 1975;68:331–336.

63. Roberts JM, Sullivan M, Froelicher VF, et al. Predicting oxygen uptake from treadmill testing in normal subjects and coronary artery disease patients. Am Heart J 1984;108:1454–1460.

64. The CONSENSUS Trial Study Group. Effects of enalapril on mortality in severe congestive heart failure: results of the Cooperative North Scandinavian Enalapril Survival Study (CONSENSUS). N Engl J Med 1987;316:1429–1435.

65. The SOLVD Investigators. Effect of enalapril on survival in patients with reduced left ventricular ejection fractions and congestive heart failure. N Engl J Med 1991;325:293–302.

66. The SOLVD Investigators. Effect of enalapril on mortality and the development of heart failure in asymptomatic patients with reduced left ventricular ejection fractions. N Engl J Med 1992;327:685–691.

67. Garg R, Yusuf S, for the Collaborative Group on ACE Inhibitor Trials. Overview of randomized trials of angiotensin-converting enzyme inhibitors on mortality and morbidity in patients with heart failure. JAMA 1995;273:1450–1456.

68. Bittner V, Weiner DH, Yusuf S, et al. Prediction of mortality and morbidity with a 6-minute walk test in patients with left ventricular dysfunction. JAMA 1993;270:1702–1707.

69. Likoff MJ, Chandler SL, Kay HR. Clinical determinants of mortality in chronic congestive heart failure secondary to idiopathic dilated or to ischemic cardiomyopathy. Am J Cardiol 1987;59:634–638.

70. Opasich C, Pinna GD, Bobbio M, et al. Peak exercise oxygen consumption in chronic heart failure: toward efficient use in the individual patient. J Am Coll Cardiol 1998;31:766–775.

71. Kao W, Winkel EM, Johnson MR, et al. Role of maximal oxygen consumption in establishment of heart transplant candidacy for heart failure patients with intermediate exercise tolerance. Am J Cardiol 1997;79:1124–1127.

72. MacGowan GA, Janosko K, Cecchetti A, Murali S. Exercise-related ventilatory abnormalities and survival in congestive heart failure. Am J Cardiol 1997;79:1264–1266.

73. Stevenson LW, Steimle AE, Fonarow G, et al. Improvement in exercise capacity of candidates awaiting heart transplantation. J Am Coll Cardiol 1995;25:163–170.

74. Wasserman K, Hansen JE, Sue DY, Whipp BJ. Principles of Exercise Testing and Interpretation. Lea & Febiger, Philadelphia, PA: 1987, p. 73.

75. Stelken AM, Younis LT, Jennison SH, et al. Prognostic value of cardiopulmonary exercise testing using percent achieved of predicted peak oxygen uptake for patients with ischemic and dilated cardiomyopathy. J Am Coll Cardiol 1996;27:345–352.

76. Osada N, Chaitman BR, Miller LW, et al. Cardiopulmonary exercise testing identifies low risk patients with heart failure and severely impaired exercise capacity considered for heart transplantation. J Am Coll Cardiol 1998;31:577–582.

77. Aaronson KD, Mancini DM. Is percentage of predicted maximal exercise oxygen consumption a better predictor of survival than peak exercise oxygen consumption for patients with severe heart failure? J Heart Lung Transplant 1995;14:981–989.

78. Wasserman K, Hansen JE, Sue DY, et al. Principles of Exercise Testing and Interpretation, Including Pathophysiology and Clinical Applications. Lippincott Williams & Wilkins, Philadelphia, PA: 1999, p. 148.

79. Strzelczyk TA, Cusick DA, Pfeifer PB, et al. Value of the Bruce protocol to determine peak exercise oxygen consumption in patients evaluated for cardiac transplantation. Am Heart J 2001;142:466–475.

80. Wilson JR, Martin JL, Ferraro N. Impaired skeletal muscle nutritive flow during exercise in patients with congestive heart failure: role of cardiac pump dysfunction as determined by the effect of dobutamine. Am J Cardiol 1984;53:1308–1315.
81. Wilson JR, Martin JL, Ferraro N, Weber KT. Effect of hydralazine on perfusion and metabolism in the leg during upright bicycle exercise in patients with heart failure. Circulation 1983;68:425–432.
82. Kugler J, Maskin C, Frishman WH, et al. Regional and systemic metabolic effects of angiotensin-converting enzyme inhibition during exercise in patients with severe heart failure. Circulation 1982;66:1256–1261.
83. Franciosa JA, Goldsmith SR, Cohn JN. Contrasting immediate and long-term effects of isosorbide dinitrate on exercise capacity in congestive heart failure. Am J Med 1980;69:559–566.
84. Wilson JR, Ferraro N, Wiener DH. Effect of the sympathetic nervous system on limb circulation and metabolism during exercise in patients with heart failure. Circulation 1985;72:72–81.
85. Wilson JR, Rayos G, Yeoh T, Gothard P. Dissociation between peak exercise oxygen consumption and hemodynamic dysfunction in potential heart transplant candidates. J Am Coll Cardiol 1995;26:429–435.
86. Colucci WS, Sonnenblick EH, Adams KF, et al. Efficacy of phosphodiesterase inhibition with milrinone in combination with converting enzyme inhibitors in patients with heart failure. J Am Coll Cardiol 1993;22:113A–118A.
87. Packer M, Carver JR, Rodeheffer RJ, et al. Effects of oral milrinone on mortality in severe chronic heart failure. N Engl J Med 1991;325:1468–1475.
88. Narahara KA, Western Enoximone Study Group. Oral enoximone therapy in chronic heart failure: a placebo-controlled randomized trial. Am Heart J 1991;121:1471–1479.
89. Uretsky BF, Jessup M, Konstam MA, et al. Multicenter trial of oral enoximone in patients with moderate to moderately severe congestive heart failure: lack of benefit compared with placebo. Circulation 1990;82:774–780.
90. Cohn JN, Archibald DG, Ziesche S, et al. Effect of vasodilator therapy on mortality in chronic congestive heart failure: results of a Veterans Administration cooperative study. N Engl J Med 1986;314:1547–1552.
91. Cohn JN, Johnson G, Ziesche S, et al. A comparison of enalapril with hydralazine-isosorbide dinitrate in the treatment of chronic congestive heart failure. N Engl J Med 1991;325:303–310.
92. Zugck C, Haunstetter A, Krüger C, et al. Impact of beta-blocker treatment on the prognostic value of currently used risk predictors in congestive heart failure. J Am Coll Cardiol 2002;39:1615–1622.
93. Australia/New Zealand Heart Failure Research Collaborative Group. Randomised, placebo-controlled trial of carvedilol in patients with congestive heart failure due to ischaemic heart disease. Lancet 1997;349:375–380.
94. Krum H, Sackner-Bernstein JD, Goldsmith RL, et al. Double-blind, placebo-controlled study of the long-term efficacy of carvedilol in patients with severe chronic heart failure. Circulation 1995;92:1499–1506.
95. Olsen SL, Gilbert EM, Renlund DG, et al. Carvedilol improves left ventricular function and symptoms in chronic heart failure: a double-blind randomized study. J Am Coll Cardiol 1995;25:1225–1231.
96. Metra M, Nardi M, Giubbini R, Dei Cas L. Effects of short- and long-term carvedilol administration on rest and exercise hemodynamic variables, exercise capacity and clinical conditions in patients with idiopathic dilated cardiomyopathy. J Am Coll Cardiol 1994;24:1678–1687.

97. Doughty RN, Whalley GA, Gamble G, et al. Left ventricular remodeling with carvedilol in patients with congestive heart failure due to ischemic heart disease. J Am Coll Cardiol 1997;29:1060–1066.

98. Bristow MR, Gilbert EM, Abraham WT, et al. Carvedilol produces dose-related improvements in left ventricular function and survival in subjects with chronic heart failure. Circulation 1996;94:2807–2816.

99. Quaife RA, Gilbert EM, Christian PE, et al. Effects of carvedilol on systolic and diastolic left ventricular performance in idiopathic dilated cardiomyopathy or ischemic cardiomyopathy. Am J Cardiol 1996;78:779–784.

100. Australia/New Zealand Heart Failure Research Collaborative Group. Effects of carvedilol, a vasodilator-β-blocker, in patients with congestive heart failure due to ischemic heart disease. Circulation 1995;92:212–218.

101. Packer M, Bristow MR, Cohn JN, et al. The effect of carvedilol on morbidity and mortality in patients with chronic heart failure. N Engl J Med 1996;334:1349–1355.

102. The CAPRICORN Investigators. Effects of carvedilol on outcome after myocardial infarction in patients with left-ventricular dysfunction: the CAPRICORN randomised trial. Lancet 2001;357:1385–1390.

103. Fowler MB, Vera-Llonch M, Oster G, et al. Influence of carvedilol on hospitalizations in heart failure: incidence, resource utilization and costs. J Am Coll Cardiol 2001;37:1692–1699.

104. Packer M, Coats AJS, Fowler MB, et al. Effect of carvedilol on survival in severe chronic heart failure. N Engl J Med 2001;344:1651–1658.

105. Anand IS, Florea VG, Fisher L. Surrogate end points in heart failure. J Am Coll Cardiol 2002;39:1414–1421.

12 Understanding the Syndrome of Heart Failure

Mariell L. Jessup MD, FCC, FAHA

INTRODUCTION

The definition of heart failure is a clinical syndrome resulting from a structural or functional cardiac disorder that impairs the ability of the ventricle to fill with or eject blood commensurate with the needs of the body. This syndrome, which is a constellation of signs and symptoms, is primarily manifested by dyspnea, fatigue, fluid retention, and a decreased exercise tolerance. Heart failure may result from disorders of the pericardium, the myocardium, the endocardium or valvular structures, the great vessels of the heart, or from rhythm disturbances. However, from a clinical standpoint, we tend to think about heart failure in terms of myocardial dysfunction. This may be because many valvular or pericardial disorders and arrhythmias are easily amenable to either very effective surgery or other definitive treatments, which go a long way towards correcting the symptoms of heart failure. We are left, then,

From: *Contemporary Cardiology: Heart Failure:*
A Clinician's Guide to Ambulatory Diagnosis and Treatment
Edited by: M. L. Jessup and E. Loh © Humana Press Inc., Totowa, NJ

with patients who have myocardial dysfunction that ultimately accounts for their symptoms of congestion or fatigue.

In the United States, the most common cause of heart failure is coronary artery disease *(1,2)*, causing an ischemic cardiomyopathy (*see* Chapter 9). However, the pathophysiologic mechanisms that cause a patient's symptoms to worsen over time and cause cardiac function to deteriorate usually develop irrespective of the underlying etiology of the cardiomyopathy. From a practical standpoint, it is useful to divide up patients with heart failure into those with primarily systolic dysfunction and those with diastolic dysfunction. For the clinician, this usually means assessing the patient's left-ventricular ejection fraction (LVEF) by a variety of techniques during the initial evaluation *(3–7)* (*see* Chapters 7 and 8). Thus, if a patient has a low LVEF, usually less than 40–45%, their condition is called systolic heart failure. If a patient has symptoms consistent with heart failure but has a preserved or normal LVEF, they are labeled as diastolic heart failure or diastolic dysfunction. Patients with systolic heart failure typically have a low LVEF, a dilated left-ventricular cavity, and a reduced cardiac output because of diminished contractility of the myocardium. In contrast, patients with diastolic heart failure have a normal LVEF, normal contractility, but impaired filling of the heart secondary to a variety of pathophysiologic abnormalities (*see* Chapter 20).

Most of the clinical trials that have contributed to our improved management of the patient with heart failure have focused on the patient with systolic dysfunction. Nevertheless, the neurohormonal and inflammatory cytokine activation that is commonly described seems to occur in all forms of heart failure. Thus, any discussion of heart failure almost always stems from research with dilated cardiomyopathic models, either animal or human studies, but is most likely applicable to patients with diastolic heart failure as well.

HEART FAILURE IS A PROGRESSIVE DISORDER

Heart failure begins with an initial injury to the myocardium. This may be as obvious as a transmural myocardial infarction with large tissue loss or as seemingly innocuous as mild systemic hypertension. Ultimately, the loss of myocyte viability or the altered structure of the cardiac wall results in a decrease in cardiac output, as ventricular function becomes increasingly impaired. Underperfusion of a variety of vascular receptors and organs results in the activation of several neurohormonal pathways, the most clearly elucidated of which is the renin-angiotensin-aldosterone (RAA) system and the sympathetic nervous pathway *(8)*. These and other systems induce inappropriate expansion of the intravascular and extravascular volumes, causing the congestion and sodium retention that is the hallmark of the disease. In addition, the pathophysiologic pathways induce cytokine release, myocyte hypertrophy and collagen formation, and trigger myocyte apoptosis *(9)*. These increasingly understood mechanisms account for the subsequent further deterioration of ventricular function. Thus, heart failure is a progressive disorder, often initiated by myocyte destruction or alteration that occurred years before the onset of clinical symptoms.

Drugs that inhibit the RAA and the adrenergic nervous systems have slowed the relentless progression of heart failure. In select populations, primarily middle-aged white men with systolic dysfunction secondary to ischemic cardiomyopathy, angiotensin-converting enzyme (ACE) inhibitors and β-blockers have substantially reduced both morbidity and mortality *(10–12)*. However, the impact of heart failure on public health in the United States cannot be overstated, and mortality for all patients with heart failure remains unacceptably high *(13–21)*. Unfortunately, progression of myocardial dysfunction is often asymptomatic and becomes apparent only when a patient is hospitalized, or when testing reveals a deterioration in the LVEF. Moreover, utilization of effective pharmacological and other management strategies for heart failure continues to be less than optimal in this country. All too often, physicians treat patients only if their symptoms worsen and use signs and symptoms as a stimulus to add additional therapy, most of which has been shown to be effective even in the absence of a worsening clinical picture.

Most investigators agree that earlier recognition of the syndrome or better identification of patients at risk for heart failure, may be our best hope for the future reduction of heart failure's death toll. This is very analogous to the concerted efforts to screen for and detect cancer at the earliest stages of the malignancy, before the disease can defy therapy. It was for this reason that the committee charged with revising the American College of Cardiology/American Heart Association (ACC/AHA) Guidelines for the Evaluation and Management of Heart Failure *(22)* decided to take the bold step of developing a new classification for patients with heart failure. For years, clinicians have used the New York Heart Association's (NYHA) functional assessment as a short-hand for discussion about patients' limitations. *(23,24)*. However, depending on an individual patient's therapy, more or less diuretic, or more or less activity, the symptoms that the patient reports are subjectively interpreted by the clinician to determine the appropriate NYHA class. A patient could move back and forth among the NYHA classes, theoretically even in the space of a few days, whereas the underlying state of the myocardial function remains unchanged, e.g., a 60-year-old male might be admitted with acute heart failure from a remote myocardial infarction. His LVEF is documented as low, and he responds immediately to the addition of digitalis, diuretics, and ACE inhibitors to his regimen. He is discharged much improved and with minimal symptoms. One week following his discharge, his primary physician sees him in the office and determines his NYHA status as Class I and does not further adjust his medications because of his stable clinical picture. The opportunity to add β-blockers is missed, and this man will undoubtedly have additional hospital admission because of the disease progression.

The ACC/AHA guidelines propose the following stages of heart failure that serve as the foundation on which subsequent discussions of therapy are built (22). Stage A represents those patients who are at high risk for developing heart failure. These include patients with hypertension and/or diabetes mellitus, coronary artery disease, or all three diseases. Included in this group are patients with a family history of dilated cardiomyopathy, as the genetic basis of this disease is becoming more clearly elucidated. Patients who have been exposed to toxic chemotherapeutic agents are also in this group. Perhaps intensive intervention in Stage A patients will prevent their subsequent development of heart failure symptoms. Stage B are those patients who have been found to have left-ventricular systolic dysfunction in the absence of symptoms of heart failure. Usually these patients are discovered coincidentally, often during screening for other problems, such as a preoperative medical clearance. A typical example is a young man who is to undergo orthopedic surgery and found to have a left-bundle branch block (LBBB) pattern on his electrocardiogram (ECG). Subsequent evaluation reveals a dilated cardiomyopathy, which has not yet caused symptoms of breathlessness or fluid retention. Other groups of patients who might develop asymptomatic left-ventricular systolic dysfunction are those with longstanding hypertension or left-ventricular hypertrophy (LVH), an old myocardial infarction, or chronic valvular disease. For instance, some women with chronic mitral valve prolapse and progressive mitral regurgitation can ultimately develop left-ventricular dilatation and systolic failure, despite minimal change in their exercise tolerance. There is already some data that have shown a beneficial effect of both β-blockers and ACE inhibitors when given to patients at this stage of their cardiac dysfunction (25,26). Stage C are all those patients with current or prior symptoms of heart failure, including those patients who are currently asymptomatic because they have been given appropriate therapy. Stage D are those patients with advanced or refractory symptoms of heart failure. Despite all appropriate therapy, these patients have undergone

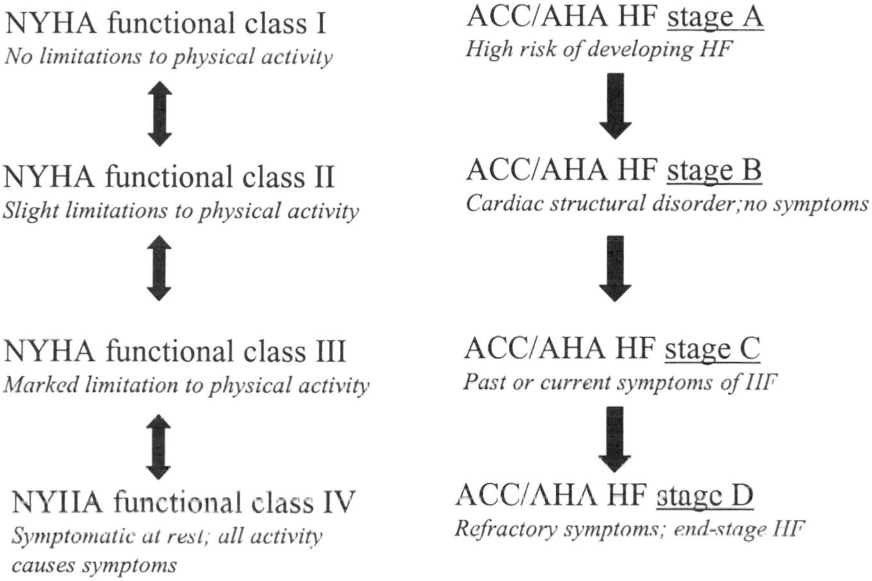

NYHA functional class I
No limitations to physical activity

⇕

NYHA functional class II
Slight limitations to physical activity

⇕

NYHA functional class III
Marked limitation to physical activity

⇕

NYIIA functional class IV
Symptomatic at rest; all activity causes symptoms

ACC/AHA HF stage A
High risk of developing HF

⬇

ACC/AHA HF stage B
Cardiac structural disorder;no symptoms

⬇

ACC/AHA HF stage C
Past or current symptoms of HF

⬇

ACC/AHA HF stage D
Refractory symptoms; end-stage HF

Fig. 1. NYHA functional class contrasted to the ACC/AHA stages of heart failure.

multiple hospitalizations or are under consideration for cardiac transplantation or awaiting a donor organ, or are terminal and require hospice. One advantage of this classification is that patients can't move backwards from a higher class to a lower class, as one might with the NYHA functional classification (*see* Fig. 1). Moreover, assignment of a particular stage depends less on the patients' reporting an accurate description of their symptoms and more on the recognition of therapy.

PROGNOSIS AND CLINICAL IMPLICATIONS OF THE ACC/AHA STAGES OF HEART FAILURE

Stage A (High Risk of Developing Heart Failure)

A recent finding from the Framingham Heart Study concludes that 9 out of 10 middle-aged and older adults are likely to develop hypertension over their remaining lifetime *(27)*. Approximately 50 million Americans have hypertension, yet only one-fourth of patients with hypertension have their blood pressure adequately controlled *(28)*. The impact of hypertension on the subsequent development of cardiovascular disease is enormous; even "high-normal" blood pressure in patients is associated with a risk-factor-adjusted hazard ratio for heart disease of 2.5 in women and 1.6 in men *(29)*. And, for the purposes of this discussion, effective treatment of hypertension has been shown to reduce the subsequent development of heart failure by nearly 50% (21,30–34). Thus, a patient with uncontrolled or poorly controlled hypertension is generally at high risk for developing heart disease and, more specifically, heart failure and is a Stage A patient.

At least 10.3 million Americans carry a diagnosis of diabetes mellitus (35). A large body of epidemiological and pathological data document that diabetes is an independent risk factor for cardiovascular disease in both men and women. More importantly, patients with diabetes are unusually prone to congestive heart failure (CHF). Unfortunately, as opposed to the evidence with hypertension, data are not yet available to suggest that control of hyperglycemia will prevent or reduce the development of heart failure. However, the co-existence of hypertension and type 2 diabetes mellitus renders a diabetic patient about twice as likely to experience cardiovascular events as a nondiabetic patient (36). In addition, in patients with left-ventricular dysfunction from another etiology, the presence of diabetes increases the risk of morbidity and mortality (37).

Thus, the convergence of risk factors in an elderly patient makes the risk of the development of heart failure significantly higher than in a population without such risk factors. As can be seen in Fig. 2, patients may develop heart failure either by the primary path of a dilated cardiomyopathy or by the initial manifestations of coronary artery disease with subsequent progression to an ischemic cardiomyopathy.

There are several other risk factors that should be taken into consideration in the determination of the Stage A patient, one who is at high risk for developing heart failure. Inheritable predilections for the development of cardiomyopathy may function via a variety of pathophysiologic processes. Certainly, a strong family history of premature coronary artery disease may make a patient more likely to develop significant occlusive coronary obstruction, often leading to an ischemic cardiomyopathy. But, a large number of patients in the United States with dilated or congestive cardiomyopathy have no obvious coronary artery obstruction, no apparent toxin ingestion (e.g., alcohol or exposure to antineoplastic agents), and no infiltrative process of the myocardium (e.g., sarcoidosis, hemachromatosis or amyloid). The diagnosis of idiopathic-dilated cardiomyopathy remains. Over the past several years, there has been increased recognition that many of these "idiopathic" dilated cardiomyopathies are familial, and a number of centers are actively focusing on the identification of the genetic irregularities responsible for the abnormal phenotypes (38).

The most common mode of inheritance of familial-dilated cardiomyopathy is autosomal-dominant. However, not all members of a family

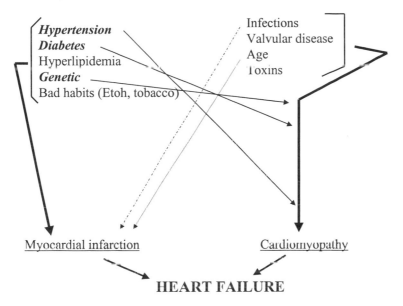

Fig. 2. Risk factors for the development of heart failure.

may present with the same clinical syndrome, a phenomenon called incomplete penetrance. This is presumably related to the presence of other modifying genes and the influence of environmental stressors, e.g., it could be that some forms of familial cardiomyopathy are not evident unless a patient drinks excessive alcohol or becomes pregnant. The genetic abnormalities may result in defects of the myocytes themselves, so that force generation is less effective. Or, the aberrant genes may code for an abnormal extracellular matrix that binds the myocytes, promoting ventricular dilatation. These and many other issues will undoubtedly be resolved over the next decade or so of intensive investigation. The challenge to clinicians will be to recognize the patient with incipient heart failure and apply measures that will forestall the clinical manifestations of the disease.

Stage B (Asymptomatic Patient with Left-Ventricular Systolic Dysfunction)

Patients in stage B heart failure, who have had a documentation of a low LVEF, but are apparently asymptomatic, are discovered in many ways. However, the clinician must often discern whether the patient is truly without symptoms. Frequently, patients have unconsciously decreased their activity so that they don't experience breathlessness. Another manner in which Stage B patients may declare their cardiac dysfunction is with a life-threatening arrhythmia. All too often, a patient is resuscitated from sudden cardiac death and subsequently found to have severe left-ventricular systolic dysfunction. Therefore, though it is true that the patient was asymptomatic with respect to heart failure symptoms, the disease process was already causing havoc.

We have learned the most about patients in Stage B heart failure from the large, multicenter trials performed to investigate the utility of ACE inhibitors and/or β-blockers. Many of the earliest β-blocker trials were enrolling patients following a myocardial infarction, and an important subgroup in some of those studies was patients with a reduced ejection fraction *(25,39–41)*. Not all of these patients had symptoms of heart failure, so today they would be classified as Stage B patients. It was the Study of Left-Ventricular Dysfunction (SOLVD) trials, however, that really focused on what is now called the Stage B patient *(26)*. More than 4000 patients with LVEF below 35% who were not being treated for heart failure were randomized to placebo or the ACE-inhibitor enalapril. Although overall mortality was not significantly reduced, the rate of progression to symptomatic heart failure or to the need for hospitalization was meaningfully and significantly decreased with enalapril. One might speculate that this population, without symptoms of heart failure despite a low LVEF, had a predicted low-mortality rate irrespective of treatment regimens. Yet, the 1-year mortality rate of the group who received placebo was calculated at 5.1% for a population with a mean age of 59 years! This study was the first of several that lent considerable credibility to the concept that the relentless progression of heart failure could be halted.

What are the clinical implications of these large trials? First, we need to actively look for the patient at risk for developing symptomatic heart failure and screen for the presence of left-ventricular systolic dysfunction. When a low LVEF is fortuitously discovered, guideline recommendations now suggest the addition of both ACE inhibitor and a β-blocker to the medical regimen, despite the absence of symptoms *(10,22,42,43)*.

Stage C (Patient with Past or Present Symptoms of Heart Failure)

Most of the advances that have been made in the treatment of heart failure have been made in patients with Stage C heart failure. That is, patients with significant symptoms of breathlessness and fatigue, and patients who had a low LVEF, were the principle subjects of the majority of the large randomized trials that serve as our evidence-based recommendations about heart failure. We have learned a great deal about the prognosis of this population, recognizing that most of these trials studied a very select subset of the heart failure population at large. One-year mortality for symptomatic heart failure has ranged from 52% in elderly patients with severe symptoms and multiple comorbid conditions *(44)*, to 12.5% in the large DIG trial that entered much less sick patients *(45)*. The SOLVD treatment trial studied patients not using an ACE inhibitor and documented a 1-year mortality of 15.5%, an unexpectedly low rate at the time *(46)*.

The statistics have to be considered as representative of the age, concomitant medical conditions of the patients entered into the trials, and the associated medical therapy used as baseline. At the end of the last century, not all patients with heart failure could expect such a relatively good outcome from the lethal disease that was heart failure. A report from Scotland studied 66,547 consecutive patients with first-time admission to hospital for heart failure *(17)* This group was elderly, evenly distributed in gender, and had a 1-year mortality of 44.5%. This actually represented a modest improvement in comparison to the previous 10-year data. This result partly reflects the age of the general population that experiences heart failure in contrast to the younger age of patients suitable for randomized trials. Older patients do less well and have a much higher incidence of comorbidities.

On a positive note, however, appropriate therapy still has the potential to decrease mortality and morbidity in a meaningful manner, despite age, comorbid conditions and advanced symptoms of heart failure. The RALES trial studied NYHA Class III and IV patients, most of who were already on adequate doses of diuretics, digitalis, ACE inhibitors, and even β-blockers in some. Overall mortality was reduced 30%, an outcome that astonished most investigators *(47)*. The addition of β-blockers to a patient already on average doses of ACE-inhibitor has the potential to decrease mortality another 30–35% *(48)*. Thus, judicious application of medical therapies can have an important impact on an individual's quality and duration of life, even in cases of advance heart failure.

Stage D (Patient with Refractory Symptoms of Heart Failure)

Few guidelines exist to help us manage the patient who has failed medical and/or surgical therapy and has recurrent symptoms of heart failure. The multiple hospitalizations and the increasing desperation of the patient, their family, and the medical personnel are likely familiar to anyone who has cared for these patients. The FIRST trial enrolled such patients in attempting to investigate the role of epoprostenol in the management of end-stage heart failure *(49)*. The observed mortality rate of these patients was in excess of 40% over a period of a few months.

Indeed, unless the patient is a candidate for heart transplantation, there is little to offer that can realistically be expected to substantially reduce morbidity or mortality. These grim facts account for the enthusiasm for mechanical assist devices, which have been studied in patients considered ineligible for transplant *(50)*. In the REMATCH trial, mortality in the group of patients who did not receive a left-ventricular assist device (LVAD) was 80% over a 2-year period. LVAD therapy, in many forms of devices, may offer some hope in the future to patients with debilitating symptoms and no hope for a transplant.

SUMMARY

The steps to the development of symptomatic heart failure are increasingly recognized. Impediments to the progression of the seemingly relentless syndrome are similarly being developed. Our role as clinicians is clear in this very real battle with life and death. We need to recognize the patient at risk for the heart failure syndrome and prescribe conclusive, evidenced-based therapy so that risk is reduced. Failing that, we need to apply therapy to the patient with early manifestations of the disease so that more morbid symptoms can be avoided. In some respects, this story is all about hope, and the impact that our management can make in the future.

REFERENCES

1. Soto JR, Beller GA. Clinical benefit of noninvasive viability studies of patients with severe ischemic left ventricular dysfunction. Clin Cardiol 2001;24:428–434.
2. Gheorghiade M, Bonow RO. Chronic heart failure in the United States: a manifestation of coronary artery disease. Circulation 1998;97:282–289.
3. Albin G, Rahko P. Comparison of echocardiographic quantitation of left-ventricular ejection fraction to radionuclide angiography in patients with regional wall motion abnormalities. Am J Cardiol 1990;65:1031,1032.
4. Eagle K, Quertermous T, Singer D, et al. Left-ventricular ejection fraction: physician estimates compared with gated blood pool scan measurements. Arch Intern Med 1988;148:882–885.
5. Gadsboll N, Hoilund-Carlsen P, Neilsen G, et al. Interobserver agreement and accuracy of bedside estimation of right and left-ventricular ejection fraction in acute myocardial infarction. Am J Cardiol 1989;63:1301–1307.
6. Mattleman S, Hakki A, Iskandrian A, et al. Reliability of bedside evaluation in determining left-ventricular function:correlation with left-ventricular ejection fraction determined by radionuclide ventriculography. J Am Coll Cardiol 1983;1:417–420.
7. Philbin E, Garg R, Danisa K, et al. The relationship between cardiothoracic ratio and left ventricular ejection fraction in congestive heart failure. Digitalis Investigation Group. Arch Intern Med 1998;158:501.
8. Schrier RW, Abraham WT. Hormones and hemodynamics in heart failure. N Engl J Med 1999;341:577–585.

9. Williams R. Apoptosis and heart failure. N Engl J Med 1999;341:759,760.
10. Gomberg-Maitland M, Baran DA, Fuster V. Treatment of congestive heart failure: guidelines for the primary care physician and the heart failure specialist. Arch Intern Med 2001;161:342–352.
11. Konstam MA. Progress in heart failure Management? Lessons from the real world. Circulation 2000;102:1076–108.
12. Rodgers JE, Patterson JH. The role of the renin-angiotensin-aldosterone system in the management of heart failure. Pharmacotherapy 2000;20:368S–378S.
13. Aronow WS, Ahn C, Kronzon I. Prognosis of congestive heart failure in elderly patients with normal versus abnormal left ventricular systolic function associated with coronary artery disease. Am J Cardiol 1990;66:1257–1259.
14. Kupari M, Lindroos M, Iivanainen AM, et al. Congestive heart failure in old age: prevalence, mechanisms and 4-year prognosis in the Helsinki Ageing Study. J Intern Med 1997;241:387–394.
15. Jaagosild P, Dawson NV, Thomas C, et al. Outcomes of acute exacerbation of severe congestive heart failure: quality of life, resource use, and survival. SUPPORT Investigators. The Study to Understand Prognosis and Preferences for Outcomes and Risks of Treatments. Arch Intern Med 1998;158:1081–1089.
16. Vasan RS, Larson MG, Benjamin EJ, et al. Congestive heart failure in subjects with normal versus reduced left ventricular ejection fraction: prevalence and mortality in a population-based cohort. J Am Coll Cardiol 1999;33:1948–1955.
17. MacIntyre K, Capewell S, Stewart S, et al. Evidence of improving prognosis in heart failure: trends in case fatality in 66 547 patients hospitalized between 1986 and 1995. Circulation 2000;102:1126–1131.
18. McMurray JJ, Stewart S. Epidemiology, aetiology and prognosis of heart failure. Heart 2000;83:596–6002.
19. Adams KF, Jr. New epidemiologic perspectives concerning mild-to-moderate heart failure. Am J Med 2001;110.6S–13S.
20. Eichhorn EJ. Prognosis determination in heart failure. Am J Med 2001;110:14S–36S.
21. Lloyd-Jones DM. The risk of congestive heart failure: sobering lessons from the Framingham Heart Study. Curr Cardiol Rep 2001;3:184–190.
22. Hunt SA, Baker DW, Chin MH, et al. ACC/AHA guidelines for the evaluation and management of chronic heart failure in the adult: executive summary. A report of the American College of Cardiology/American Heart Association Task Force on Practice Guidelines (Committee to revise the 1995 Guidelines for the Evaluation and Management of Heart Failure). J Am Coll Cardiol 2001;38:2101–2113.
23. Gibelin P. An evaluation of symptom classification systems used for the assessment of patients with heart failure in France. Eur J Heart Fail 2001;3:739–746.
24. Mezzani A, Corra U, Baroffio C, et al. Habitual activities and peak aerobic capacity in patients with asymptomatic and symptomatic left ventricular dysfunction. Chest 2000;117:1291–1299.
25. Vantrimpont P, Rouleau JL, Wun C, et al. Additive beneficial effects of beta-blockers to angiotensin-converting enzyne inhibitors in the Survival and Ventricular Enlargement (SAVE) Study) SAVE Investigators. J Am Coll Cardiol 1997;29:229–236.
26. The SOLVD Investigators. Effect of enalapril on mortality and the development of heart failure in asymptomatic patients with reduced left ventricular ejection fraction. N Engl J Med 1992;327:685–691.
27. Vasan RS, Beiser A, Seshadri S, et al. Residual lifetime risk for developing hypertension in middle-aged women and men. The Framingham Heart Study. J Am Med Assoc 2002;287:1003–1010.

28. Hyman DJ, Pavlik VN. Characteristics of patients with uncontrolled hypertension in the United States. N Engl J Med 2001;345:479–486.
29. Vasan RS, Larson MG, Leip EP, et al. Impact of high-normal blood pressure on the risk of cardiovascular disease. N Engl J Med 2001;345:1291–1297.
30. Joint National Committee. The sixth report of the Joint National Committee on detection,evaluation,and treatment of high blood pressure(JNC IV). Arch Intern Med 1997;157:2413–2446.
31. Furberg CD, Psaty BM, Pahor M, et al. Clinical implications of recent findings from the Antihypertensive and Lipid-Lowering Treatment to Prevent Heart Attack trial (ALLHAT) and other studies of hypertension. Ann Intern Med 2001;135:1074–108.
32. Kaplan NM. Management of hypertensive patients with multiple cardiovascular risk factors. Am J Hyperten 2001;14:221S–224S.
33. Kostis JB, Davis BR, Cutler J, et al. Prevention of heart failure by antihypertensive drug treatment in older persons with isolated systolic hypertension. SHEP Cooperative Research Group. J Am Med Assoc 1997;278:212–216.
34. Levy D, Larson MG, Vasan RS, et al. The progression from hypertension to congestive heart failure. JAMA 1996;275:1557–1562.
35. Grundy SM, Benjamin IJ, Burke GL, et al. Diabetes and cardiovascular disease: a statement for healthcare professionals from the American Heart Association. Circulation 1999;100:1134–1146.
36. Deedwania P. Hypertension and diabetes: new therapeutic options. Arch Intern Med 2000;160:1585–1594.
37. Dries DL, Sweitzer NK, Drazner MH, et al. Prognostic impact of diabetes mellitus in patients with heart failure according to the etiology of left ventricular systolic dysfunction. J Am Coll Cardiol 2001;38:421–428.
38. Schonberger J, Seidman CE. Many roads lead to a broken heart: the genetics of dilated cardiomyopathy. Am J Human Genet 2001;69:249–260.
39. Aronow WS. Postinfarction use of beta-blockers in elderly patients. Drugs Aging 1997;11:424–432.
40. Chen J, Marciniak TA, Radford MJ, et al. Beta-blocker therapy for secondary prevention of myocardial infarction in elderly diabetic patients. J Am Coll Cardiol 1999;34:1388–1394.
41. Lee S, Spencer A. Beta-blockers to reduce mortality in patients with systolic dysfunction: a meta-analysis. J Family Prac 2001;50:499–504.
42. Heart Failure Society of America. HFSA Guidelines for management of patients with heart failure caused by left ventricular systolic dysfunction pharmacological approaches. J Cardiac Fail 1999;5:357–382.
43. Packer M, Cohn JN, Abraham WT, et al. Consensus recommendations for the management of chronic heart failure. Am J Cardiol 1999;83:1A–38A.
44. The CONSENSUS Trial Study Group. Effects of enalapril on mortality in severe congestive heart failure. Results of the Cooperative North Scandinavian Enalapril Survival Study (CONSENSUS). N Engl J Med 1987;316:1429–1435.
45. The Digitalis Investigators Group. The effect of digoxin on mortality and morbidity in patients with heart failure. N Engl J Med 1997;336:525–533.
46. The SOLVD Investigators. Effect of enalapril on survival in patients with reduced left ventricular ejection fractions and congestive heart failure. N Engl J Med 1991;325:293–302.
47. Pitt B, Zannad F, Remme W, et al. The effect of spironolactone on morbidity and mortality in patients with severe heart failure. N Engl J Med 1999;341:709–717.

48. Lechat P, Packer M, Chalon S, et al. Clinical ef
chronic heart failure: a meta-analysis of double
ized trials. Circulation 1998;98:1184–1191.
49. Califf RM, Adams KF, McKenna WJ, et al.
epoprostenol therapy for severe congestive he
Randomized Survival Trial (FIRST). Am Hear
50. Rose EA, Gelijns AC, Moskowitz AJ, et al. Loi
assistance for end-stage heart failure. N Engl J

13 Education and Management of the Whole Patient

Kathleen M. McCauley PhD, RN, CS, FAAN

CONTENTS

INTRODUCTION

Given the magnitude of heart failure as a public health problem, with 5 million affected patients and its recognition as the most costly cardiovascular illness in the United States, efforts are needed to enable patients to live optimally with the disease, avoiding costly and preventable recurrent hospitalizations *(1)*. Nearly 50% of rehospitalizations are preventable *(2,3)*. An analysis of International Classification of Diseases-9th Revision (ICD-9) codes associated with heart failure admissions identified 16 codes that are modifiable through improved patient self-care. These include volume depletion or overload, hyper and hypopotassemia, edema, orthopnea, dyspnea, and poisoning by agents such as cardiac glycosides *(4)*. Factors prompting readmission include inadequate discharge planning, and patient behaviors such as failure to adhere to diet

From: *Contemporary Cardiology: Heart Failure:*
A Clinician's Guide to Ambulatory Diagnosis and Treatment
Edited by: M. L. Jessup and E. Loh © Humana Press Inc., Totowa, NJ

restrictions, take medications appropriately, and report symptoms promptly *(3,5–7)*. Nonadherence is greatest in patients who lack motivation and strong social-support systems *(5)*. In a study of more than 7000 patients with newly prescribed digoxin, only 10% had filled enough prescriptions to ensure daily dosing *(8)*. Other authors in this volume describe the significant advances in therapies that promise both to prolong life and increase its quality. However, these therapies will be largely unsuccessful if patients fail to take the medications as prescribed and engage in lifestyles that hinder wellness.

In 1997, the American Heart Association (AHA) published an expert panel report, "The Multilevel Compliance Challenge: Recommendations for a Call to Action," charging health care professionals with incorporating strategies into clinical practice to enhance patients' compliance with treatment regimens and lifestyle modifications *(9)*. The findings of the expert panel indicated that improved patient adherence is dependent on actions by the patient, the provider, and the organization. This framework provides the organizational structure for this chapter. Strategies to improve adherence are discussed, as well as management programs that have been shown to decrease rehospitalizations and health service utilization.

THE PATIENT: STRENGTHENING THE PATIENT'S ROLE IN SELF-MANAGEMENT

The prevalence of heart failure has increased as more effective treatment of its predisposing causes, primarily coronary artery disease and hypertension, has occurred. A detailed analysis by Funk and colleagues *(10)* of multiple population studies has shown that the aging of our population is the primary driving force behind the increased incidence of heart failure. This presents challenges for patients, clinicians, and family support systems as they try to manage not only the manifestations of heart failure but also multiple comorbid conditions and the normal effects of aging. An analysis of the characteristics of heart failure patients referred for home health care revealed that the majority had major functional limitations in the areas of endurance (95%), dyspnea (87.5%), and ambulation (67.5%). Whereas the majority was oriented to time and place, more than half experienced agitation, confusion, or depression, and the availability of a caregiver decreased as the age of patient increased. Despite receiving the full services of the home care agency, only half of subjects were considered recovered or improved at the time of termination of services *(11)*.

A disease management program limited to management of heart failure alone may miss the significant contribution of other existing diseases to the patients' symptoms and complexity of the treatment regimen. Treatment and adherence challenges increase for patients, such as those with both heart failure and diabetes, who need to manage complex medication regimens, as well as more restrictive diets. In a qualitative study of factors predisposing elders with heart failure to rehospitalization, poor health behaviors such as smoking, substance abuse, and a history of nonadherence were much more common in those experiencing rehospitalization *(5)*. Factors identified as causes of nonadherence include lack of patient understanding of expected behaviors, patient forgetfulness, lack of acceptance of the benefits of treatment, and financial barriers to adherence *(12)*.

Identification of the underlying causes of nonadherence is critical to improving patient behaviors. For example, if a patient is hospitalized with an exacerbation of heart failure resulting from medication nonadherence, a targeted strategy to modify patients' behavior must be rooted in knowing exactly what caused the problem. Failure to take medications as prescribed may be because of knowledge deficit, lack of reminder systems, financial burden, patient biases, or significant depression. Lifestyle interference by diuretics, cost, and lack of transportation to the physician's office and pharmacy are the most commonly sited reasons why patients failed to take medications or renew prescriptions *(5)*.

Simplifying the treatment regimen by once per day dosing when possible and eliminating unnecessary polypharmacy, as well as diminishing the use of agents with burdensome side effects can improve adherence. Helping patients differentiate between side effects of medication vs symptoms of the disease is critical to ongoing adherence. Some patients may benefit from a proactive discussion of potential side effects to prevent overreaction when they occur *(13)*. Ongoing efforts to educate and motivate patients are needed, as adherence is likely to decrease with longer duration of treatment. Developing the habit of adherence to therapies takes time, and patients can be helped to understand that repetition will make the lifestyle change less of an effort over time *(14)*.

However, accurate assessment of adherence is challenging. Use of indirect methods such as patient interview, prescriptions filled, pill counts, patient tendency to make and keep appointments, and monitoring of patient progress toward achieving treatment goals have some inherent weaknesses *(9,14)*. Patients may overrepresent their adherence in an effort to please their provider, "dump" pills to avoid detection, or become extremely compliant shortly before an office visit to improve objective parameters. Use of compliance devices such as microprocessor-enhanced pill bottles that record data related to time and frequency of dosing may uncover problems with medication usage. These devices enable the provider to assess not only the number of times the bottle is opened as a measure of medication adherence, but also the time of day so that dosing according to prescribed frequency can be determined *(14)*.

Educating patients with a goal of increasing their knowledge is essential, but it must be combined with efforts to help them address the other real barriers *(9,12,15)*. Conversations with patients and caregivers to uncover and address actual barriers to adherence, coupled with written or other forms of education (videotapes, audiotapes, accurate Internet resources, etc.) are helpful in correcting knowledge deficits and motivating patients. Many patients will benefit from the use of devices such as special medication containers, calendar reminder systems, and tailoring of medication dosing to other activities such as meals. Given the importance of distinguishing between patients who fail to fully use a recommended treatment vs those for whom the therapy is not working, minimizing nonadherence is critically important.

Efforts to enable patients to live with a chronic illness such as heart failure extend beyond strategies to improve adherence. Self-management enables patients to become partners with their providers in recognizing symptoms, taking appropriate action, and thereby preventing deterioration and unnecessary rehospitalizations. Riegel and colleagues *(16)* conceptualized self management as involving four stages: the recognition that a sign or symptom is related to the illness; evaluation of the change in their condition; implementation of a treatment strategy; and evaluation of the treatment's effectiveness. This process requires patients to understand their illness well enough so that they can identify the subtle symptoms that predict future deterioration. They must differentiate between symptoms that are to be managed or reported vs those that can be safely ignored. The action taken in response to key symptoms should be one that has been negotiated with the provider as part of the overall treatment plan. This may involve specific actions such as taking an additional dosage of a diuretic for weight gain or generalized strategies to manage fatigue by clustering activities and more frequent rest periods. Inherent in the success of this self-management strategy is the patient's ability to recognize symptoms when they occur, evaluate the effectiveness of the negotiated treatment and to know when and how to access the provider.

Riegel and colleagues *(16)* have developed a clinical tool for measuring patient's self-management of heart failure. Adequate face and content validity have been demonstrated, as well as internal consistency for most of the subscales, so that its use in clinical practice is supported. The investigators recommend additional testing prior to use of the tool for research purposes. In the process of validating this instrument, the investigators learned that patients attach more importance to the severity of the symptom than to its significance as a predictor. The symptom of shortness of breath was particularly problematic for patients in that they failed to understand the link between the symptom and treatment actions. This finding was supported by another study where dyspnea was evident for 3 days prior to hospital admission in 91% of elderly hospitalized with heart failure. Symptom severity failed to prompt action for 37% of patients who experienced acute dyspnea for 12 hours prior to admission. The study design failed to identify whether the delays were caused by patient misinterpretation of the significance of symptoms and lack of notification of health care providers; by efforts of the patient and provider to manage the symptom without admission; or by patient's unsuccessful early efforts to access the health care system (11). Efforts to prevent the next admission should begin with a careful analysis of the exact cause of the current admission. Educational and management strategies should be identified to enhance patient, caregiver, and provider effectiveness in treating early deterioration in function.

THE PROVIDER: BUILDING A PARTNERSHIP TO IMPROVE PATIENT OUTCOMES

Recent efforts to synthesize current knowledge in heart failure have resulted in consensus guidelines (18–21) describing evidenced-based treatment strategies. There are also data that suggest that multidisciplinary provider models incorporating coordinated inpatient care, transitional care from hospital to home, specialized home interventions, and/or specialized heart failure clinics can improve outcomes. The organizational strategy that seems to be most effective is program management by an advanced practice nurse or specially trained heart failure nurse working in close collaboration with physicians who are committed to implementing evidence-based practice. Key features include optimization of medication regimens, patient education and interventions to improve adherence, and ready access to health care providers for symptomatic patients. These features have been incorporated into in-patient disease management programs (22), specialty heart failure clinics (23–27), and home visit programs (26,28–34), and/or telemonitoring systems (24,30,34). Outcomes include reduced length of stay (26,33–35), reduced hospital days (22), lower readmission rates (22–26,28–32,34–36), cost savings (24,29,31,36), improved functional status (23,24,28,30), improved dietary adherence (30), improved overall compliance (6), improved quality of life (23,29), achievement of target medication dosages *(23,30)*, and lower mortality *(32,33,35)*. Common intervention strategies include frequent patient access to a nurse or other knowledgeable provider to identify general health status and educational needs via telemonitoring, home visits, and educational mailings. Education of primary care physicians has also been found to be helpful *(34)*.

The transition from hospital to home is recognized as a particularly vulnerable time for elderly patients. They are at risk for incomplete understanding of how to implement changes in their treatment program. Temporary or permanent decrease in functional status or inadequate social support may contribute to problems with filling new prescriptions and obtaining and preparing food. In randomized clinical trials (RCTs) designed specifically to address this transition for elders with a variety of cardiac medical, surgical and other conditions, Naylor and colleagues found that advanced practice nurse (APN) coordination of discharge planning and a 2-week home telephone follow-up *(37)* and, in a later study, a 1-month home care component *(38)* resulted in fewer readmissions, fewer total days of rehospitalization, and significant cost savings. Heart failure patients reverted back to a pattern of frequent readmissions after the end of the intervention. This group of investigators has recently submitted for publication data from an RCT designed to test a longer (3-month) home care intervention implemented by APNs with specialized expertise in management of heart failure. The APN visited the patient within 24 hours of discharge because of evidence in earlier studies that patients arrive home with prescriptions that conflict with verbal or written discharge instructions and with social supports that are inadequate to support adherence to dietary and activity recommendations. A particularly vulnerable time for deterioration and readmission is 7–10 days postdischarge. Unstable co-existing conditions and poor general health behaviors require attention as the patient learns to incorporate new treatment regimens and adopt healthier behaviors. The APN's actively participated in reviewing food available in the home and in helping patients shop for food in order to help them see, in concrete terms, dietary changes that needed to be made.

Consultation with specialists such as pharmacists and dieticians may be particularly helpful in improving management and adherence with medication and diet therapy. A clinical pharmacist who provided therapeutic recommendations to physicians, as well as education and follow-up of patients, resulted in significantly lower all-cause mortality and fewer heart failure events in comparison with a control group receiving usual care. Intervention patients achieved a higher dose of angiotensin-converting enzyme (ACE) inhibitor agents and this may have contributed to the difference in outcomes *(39)*.

Nurses in all settings are actively involved in educating patients about heart failure. A recent study of patients' perceived learning needs about heart failure as compared to nurses' perceptions of priorities for patient education revealed that patients and nurses agreed that knowledge of medications and signs and symptoms of heart failure were highly important. Patients differed from nurses in that patients placed less importance on knowledge of their diet (ranked eighth by patients) but more importance on learning about their prognosis *(40)*. A similar study by Frattini and colleagues *(41)* confirmed the lack of patient emphasis on diet education. They recommend that discussing diet within the context of salt and fluid management may increase its importance to patients. Patients may be reluctant to accept personal accountability for symptom control through diet and expect that medications will accommodate an occasional indiscretion. To the extent that these findings can be generalized, providers should consider the fact that factors such as long-standing food preferences may influence how receptive patients are to dietary recommendations.

HEALTH CARE ORGANIZATIONS: SYSTEMS TO PROMOTE OPTIMUM CARE

Increased efforts to shorten length of stay present challenges to providers in their efforts to educate patients and families about strategies to manage the specific causes of the admission and the transition to home. To the extent that patient care is fragmented and in-patient care is disconnected from ambulatory care, the transition between acute exacerbations of illness and ongoing management will continue to be problematic. Specialized heart failure management programs address both the causes of rehospitalization and the ongoing treatment and management needs of patients with chronic illnesses. Evidence of the cost effectiveness of these programs is becoming increasingly apparent. Reimbursement of programs with demonstrated effectiveness is needed.

In July 2000, the Health Care Financing Administration (HCFA) published a call for demonstration projects to test established models of coordinated care to improve the quality of care to Medicare Part A and B beneficiaries *(42)*. Case management and disease management programs in both urban and rural settings were invited to apply with the goal of identifying new models of care that ultimately could be developed into established and funded models of care delivery. Programs that focused on managing care for beneficiaries with chronic conditions that produce high costs to the Medicare program were favored. Heart failure was named specifically as a targeted diagnosis. At least eight programs were proposed to be funded using experimental designs with the formal program evaluation to be designed and analyzed by HCFA. Costs of actual care and some administrative costs were covered. These have the potential to become mainstream programs with long-standing governmental support through Medicare.

Telehealth

As more sophisticated telecommunication and portable patient-monitoring technologies are developed, clinicians can gain current and accurate information about patients' status, and patients can receive management advice and education without having to travel to the provider's office. In an RCT of 497 male Veteran Administration patients with a variety of chronic diseases, substitution of more frequent telephone calls for office visits resulted in fewer scheduled or unscheduled clinic visits, fewer hospital admissions, shorter hospital stays, fewer intensive care unit days, and reduced cost of care over the 2-year follow-up period. Their medication use lessened, and physical function improved. Providers included internists, nurse practitioners, and physician assistants who used a standard form to record patient concerns about symptoms. Patient–provider continuity was assured. The intervention was most effective for the subgroup of patients reporting fair or poor overall health. This subgroup, known to have greater utilization of medical services, had significant improvement in physical activity and incurred significantly less health care service costs. The beneficial effect on mortality approached significance. The investigators attributed the improved clinical outcomes to the more frequent monitoring that the telephone calls provided *(43)*.

Technologies now exist to gather physical assessment, hemodynamic and electrocardiographic (ECG) data and transmit them electronically. Video conferencing can be used to provide distance consultation to identify patients who may benefit most from specialist care or to provide management consultation to primary providers *(44)*.

A pilot study evaluating the ease of use and accuracy of a transtelephonic stethoscope found that patients easily learned how to use the device, and there was agreement on the interpretation of the heart and lung sounds by a nurse in the home and a nurse at the receiving unit *(45)*. Transtelephonic ECG monitoring has long been available. New devices now exist that can transmit not only ECG data but also blood pressure, temperature, and pulse oximetry findings. Systems with video links can aid in assessment of wounds and other physical findings such as edema. Computerized ECG systems can be used to download 12-lead or single-lead data with interpretation to physician offices, home care nursing agencies, or 24-hour service centers. Hemodynamic data via impedance cardiography can assist the clinician in identifying low-cardiac output states, volume status problems, and in evaluating patient responses to pharmacological management. For patients who are candidates for home infusion of inotropic agents, accurate clinical data enhance management of patients who are too ill for frequent office visits. Accurate assessment of volume status, appropriate diuresis, and maximization of vasodilator therapy can prevent unnecessary hospitalization, particularly for patients with advanced heart failure *(46)*.

Improved adherence to daily weights was seen in patients who used a daily telephone reporting system to record their weight and answer a series of heart failure symptom questions using a touch-tone phone. Responses were monitored and triaged by a nurse. Increased weight was associated with symptoms of congestion. Overall adherence to daily reporting was 86% *(47)*. Similar adherence (89.5%) was seen with the use of a computerized phone system, the CHF Tel-Assurance™ program that enabled an APN to track clinical variances including patient failure to call daily, changes in patient symptoms, and weight changes warranting intervention. Patients reported high satisfaction with the device. Telemonitoring was part of a comprehensive in-patient and out-patient heart failure disease management program that resulted in favorable comparisons with nationally reported benchmarking data on the parameters of length of stay and readmissions *(48)*.

Use of a telemonitoring system that measured weight and recorded symptoms resulted in fewer emergency room visits and single rehospitalization events for 30 patients with severe heart failure. The DayLink monitor transmitted the patient's weight and responses to questions assessing symptoms of shortness of breath, edema, fatigue, and patient adherence to medications. A nurse monitored the data and contacted the physician for significant weight changes and symptoms. The study was limited by a nonrandomized comparison group that included patients who refused to use the device. Cost data were not provided. Further analyses of this device are underway *(49)*.

The Internet as a Tool for Patient Education

For patients who want to assume an active role in their health care, accurate information about the illness, treatment options, and personal behavior is critical. The internet is increasingly becoming an important source of health care information. As the number of senior citizens grows, it is expected that many more of them will use the internet to obtain that information. A recent study designed to teach seniors to conduct internet health information searches revealed that at a 90-day post-training follow-up session, 66% continued to use the internet, and 47% were using it to access health information. Of those who had obtained internet health information, two-thirds had discussed their findings with their physician. The information and physician discussion was associated with greater treatment satisfaction for more than half of subjects *(50)*.

Patient-focused internet websites have been developed by major cardiology associations such as the AHA's Living with Heart Failure site that features information specifically for caregivers, opportunities for patients to share their experiences, as well as links to learn about heart failure management. Some programs, such as CorSolutions, provide information and tracking programs for body mass index, weight, exercise progress, blood sugar, and blood pressure. Patients can participate in discussion groups and post questions that are answered by health professionals. A cardiologist-monitored site, Cardiology Community, supports patient chats and allows patients to register for live chats with physicians. Several sites, such as the San Diego Cardiac Center and the Sharp Foundation Heart Failure Online, have options for Spanish-speaking patients. A brief review of these sites revealed accurate and supportive information that focused on patient ownership of their illness and ongoing communication with their physicians. Sites differed in the reading level of the information provided as well as the degree of sophistication. Several included animated graphics. Many sites provided a link for patients to provide feedback about their perceptions of the site. However, an internet search will reveal multiple sites that are unmonitored by clinicians and hold the risk of providing patients with inaccurate or misleading information. Patients should be encouraged to use sites under the direct supervision of professional associations or other groups where the quality of information is assured.

SUMMARY

Effective management of heart failure requires a partnership between the patient, providers, and the patient's caregivers. Given current knowledge about the underlying disease process and the resulting advances in therapies, patients must be helped to incorporate these therapies and a healthier lifestyle into their daily behaviors. Care strategies that support patients in the transition from hospital to home and educate them about how to be effective partners in care hold promise for improving patient outcomes and quality of life. Technologies including internet-based educational and monitoring programs and in-home electronic monitoring systems can support the patient–provider relationship and their joint efforts to manage heart failure.

REFERENCES

1. O'Connell JB. The economic burden of heart failure. Clin.Cardiol. 2000;23:III-6–III-10.
2. Rich M. Heart failure disease management: A critical review. J Cardiac Fail 1999;5:64–75.
3. Vinson J, Rich M, Sperry J, et al. Early readmission of elderly patients with congestive heart failure. J Am Geriatr Soc 1990;38:1290–1295.
4. Thomas V, Riegel B. A computerized method of identifying potentially preventable heart failure admissions. J Nurs Care Qual 1999;13:1–10.
5. Happ MB, Naylor M, Roe-Prior P. Factors contributing to rehospitalization in elderly patients with heart failure. Journal of Cardiovascular Nursing 1997;11:75–84.
6. Rich M, Bray DB, Beckham V, et al. Effect of a multidisciplinary intervention on medication compliance in elderly patients with congestive heart failure. Am J Med 1996;101:270–276.
7. Ghalli J, Kadikia S, Cooper R, et al. Precipitating factors leading to decompensation of heart failure: Traits among urban blacks. Arch Intern Med 1988;148:2013–2016.
8. Monane M, Bohn R, Gurwitz I, et al. Noncompliance with congestive heart failure therapy in the elderly. Arch Intern Med 1994;154:433–437.
9. Houstin Miller N, Hill M, Kottke T, et al. A multilevel compliance challenge: Recommendations for a call to action. Circulation 1997;95:1085–1090.
10. Funk M, Milner K, Krumholz,H. Epidemiology of heart failure. In Moser D, Riegel B, eds. Improving Outcomes in Heart Failure, An Interdisciplinary Approach. Aspen Publisher, Gaithersburg, MD: 2001, pp. 3–17.
11. Anderson MA, Pena RA, Helms L. Home care utilization by congestive heart failure patients: a pilot study. Public Health Nursing 1998;15:146–162.
12. Dracup K, Baker D, Dunbar S, et al. Management of heart failure II. Counseling, education and lifestyle modification. JAMA 1994;272:1442–1446
13. Lassleben M, Cullen M, Wilson A. Compliance by collaboration: effectively addressing problems of treatment adherence. Australian Family Phys 1999;28:850–853.
14. Bond W, Hussar D. Detection methods and strategies for improving medication compliance. Am J Hosp Pharm 1991;48:1978–1988.
15. Padgett D, Mumford E, Hynes M, et al. Meta-analysis of the effects of educational and psychosocial intervention on management of diabetes mellitus. J Clin Epidemiol 1988;41.1007–1030.
16. Riegel B, Carlson B, Glaser D. Development and testing of a clinical tool measuring self-management of heart failure. Heart Lung 2000;29:4–12.
17. Friedman M. Older adults' symptoms and their duration before hospitalization for heart failure. Heart Lung 1997;26:169–176.
18. Konstam M, Dracup K, Baker D, et al. Heart Failure: Evaluation and Care of Patients with Left-Ventricular Systolic Dysfunction; Clinical Practice Guideline No. 11. Agency for Health Care Policy and Research, US Department of Health and Human Services, Public Health Service; June 1994. Publication 94-0612.
19. Packer M, Cohn J. on behalf of the Steering Committee and Membership of the Advisory Council to Improve Outcomes Nationwide in Heart Failure. Consensus recommendations for the management of chronic heart failure. Am J Cardiol 1999;83:2A–38A.
20. American College of Cardiology/American Heart Association Task Force on Practice Guidelines. Guidelines for the evaluation and management of heart failure. Circulation 1995;92:2764–2784.

21. Adams K. on behalf of the committee, Heart Failure Society of America (HFSA). HFSA guidelines for the management of patients with heart failure due to left ventricular systolic dysfunction - pharmacological approaches. Congestive Heart Failure 2000;6:11–39.

22. Riegel B, Thomason T, Carlson B, et al. Implementation of a multidisciplinary disease management program for heart failure patients. Congestive Heart Failure 1999;5:164–170.

23. Smith L, Fabbri S, Pai R, et al. Symptomatic improvement and reduced hospitalization for patients attending a cardiomyopathy clinic. Clin Cardiol 1997;20 949–954.

24. Fonarow G, Stevenson L, Walden J, et al. Impact of a comprehensive heart failure management program on hospital readmission and functional status in patients with advanced heart failure. J Am Coll Cardiol 1997;30:725–732.

25. Hanumanthu S, Butler J, Chomsky D, et al. Effects of a heart failure program on hospitalization frequency and exercise tolerance. Circulation 1997;96:2842–2848.

26. Chapman D, Torpy J. Development of a heart failure center: A medical center and cardiology practice join forces to improve care and reduce costs. Am J Managed Care 1997;3:431–437.

27. Lasater M. The effect of a nurse-managed CHF clinic on patient readmission and length of stay. Home Healthcare Nurse 1996;14:351–356.

28. Kornowski R, Zeeli D, Averbuch M, et al. Intensive home-care surveillance prevents hospitalization and improves morbidity rates among elderly patients with severe congestive heart failure. Amer Heart J 1995;129:762–766.

29. Rich M, Beckman V, Wittenberg C, et al. A multidisciplinary intervention to prevent readmission of elderly patients with congestive heart failure. N Engl J Med 1995;333:1190–1195.

30. West J, Miller N, Parker K, Set al. A comprehensive management system for heart failure improves clinical outcomes and reduces medical resources. Am J Cardiol 1997;79:58–63.

31. Stewart S, Pearson S, Horowitz J. Effects of a home-based intervention among patients with congestive heart failure discharged from acute hospital care. Arch Intern Med 1998;158:1067–1072.

32. Stewart S, Pearson S, Luke C, et al. Effects of a home-based intervention on unplanned readmissions and out of hospital deaths. J Am Geriatric Soc 1998;46:174–180.

33. Stewart S, Vandenbroek A, Pearson ., et al. Prolonged beneficial effects of a home-based intervention on unplanned readmissions and mortality among patients with congestive heart failure. Arch Intern Med 1999;159:257–261.

34. Roglieri J, Futterman R, McDonough K, et al. Disease management interventions to improve outcomes in congestive heart failure. Am J Managed Care 1997;3:1831–1839.

35. Dahl J, Penque S. The effects of an advanced practice nurse – directed heart failure program. Nurse Practitioner 2000;25:61–77.

36. Rauh RA, Schwabauer N, Enger E, et al. A community hospital-based congestive heart failure program: impact on length of stay, admission and readmission rates, and cost. Am J Managed Care 1999;5:37–43.

37. Naylor M, Brooten D, Jones R, et al. Comprehensive discharge planning for the hospitalized elderly. Ann Intern Med 1994;120:999–1006.

38. Naylor M, Brooten D, Campbell R, et al. Comprehensive discharge planning and home follow-up of hospitalized elders. JAMA 1999;281:613–620.

39. Gattis W, Hasselblad V, Whelan D, et al. Reduction in heart failure events by the addition of a clinical pharmacist to the heart failure management team: results of the pharmacist in heart failure assessment recommendation and monitoring (PHARM) study. Arch Intern Med 1999;159:1939–1945.

40. Wehby D, Brenner P. Perceived learning needs of patients with heart failure. Heart Lung 1999;28:31–40.
41. Frattini E, Lindsay P, Kerr E, et al. Learning needs of congestive heart failure patients. Prog Cardio Nursing 1998;13:11–16, 33.
42. Department of Health and Human Services, Health Care Financing Administration. Medicare program: sSolicitation for proposals for Medicare Coordinated Care Demonstration. Federal Register 2000;65:46,466–46,473.
43. Wasson J, Gaudette C, Whaley F, et al. Telephone care as a substitute for routine clinic follow-up. JAMA 1992;267:1788–1793.
44. Peters L, Peters D. Teleheath Part II, a total system approach. ASHA 1998;20:31–33.
45. Carroll T. Remote symptom monitoring: home management of heart failure patients using transtelephonic stethoscope – a pilot study. Nurs Admin Q 2000;25:148–153.
46. Frantz A, Lynn C. Cardiac technology in the home. Home Health Care Manage Prac 1999;11:9–16.
47. Williams R, Keller L, Sprang M, et al. Telemanagement of congestive heart failure: Results of daily weight and symptom tracking. Abstract. J Am Coll Cardiol 1997;Feb. 247A.
48. Knox D, Mischke L. Implementing a congestive heart failure disease management program to decrease length of stay and cost. J Cardio Nursing 1999;14:55–74.
49. Cordisco M, Benjaminovitz A, Hammond K, et al. Use of telemonitoring to decrease the rate of hospitalization in patients with severe congestive heart failure. Am J Cardiol 1999;84:860–862.
50. Leaffer T, Gonda B. The Internet: an undcrutilized tool in patient education. Comp Nursing 2000;18:47–52.

14 Pharmacologic Therapy for Symptomatic Congestive Heart Failure

Evan Loh, MD, FACC, FAHA

CONTENTS

INTRODUCTION

Treatment for symptomatic congestive heart failure (CHF) is aimed at two goals: improvement in symptoms and prolongation of survival. Improvement in symptoms can be achieved by a variety of drugs, including diuretics, digitalis, angiotensin-converting enzyme (ACE) inhibitors, angiotensin receptor blockers, and β-blockers *(1)*. Reductions in mortality have been documented in CHF patients treated with ACE inhibitors, β–blockers, and spironolactone *(1)*. The recommendations for therapy in this chapter are aligned with the American College of Cardiology/American Heart Association (ACC/AHA) task force recommendations published in 2001 *(1)*. As a theme throughout this chap-

From: *Contemporary Cardiology: Heart Failure:*
A Clinician's Guide to Ambulatory Diagnosis and Treatment
Edited by: M. L. Jessup and E. Loh © Humana Press Inc., Totowa, NJ

ter, it remains important to remember and to consider all potential side effects of these pharmacologic interventions because of the combinatorial therapy approach that is now advocated given the positive survival and symptom benefits of these therapies. Furthermore, the hemodynamic abnormalities seen in patients with CHF will affect vital organ function (i.e., liver and kidney) that will alter metabolic and elimination rates for these agents (*see* Table 1).

DIURETICS

Although there are no mortality data to support their use, diuretics are vital to control the excessive fluid retention that is classically seen in patients with heart failure. The fluid retention is secondary to compensatory neurohormonal activation characterized by elevations in angiotensin II, aldosterone, and antidiuretic hormone. This represents an attempt by the kidneys to restore effective plasma volume in the setting of perceived relative hypovolemia secondary to renal hypoperfusion secondary to reduced cardiac output. The reduced cardiac output and reduced tissue perfusion can be manifest clinically as an otherwise unexplained rise in BUN. The most common signs of volume overload and retention are pulmonary and peripheral edema. This is often accompanied clinically by dyspnea. These symptoms can usually be controlled by the judicious use of diuretics.

Loop diuretics, such as furosemide, remain the mainstay of diuretic therapy for volume control in patients with CHF. When administered to patients with pulmonary edema, intravenous furosemide can induce transient venodilation similar to morphine secondary to increased production of prostaglandins from the kidney. These venodilation effects precede the onset of the diuretic effects of the diuretic. The net effect is a fall in cardiac filling pressures and decreased pulmonary congestion *(2)*. Parodoxically, there can also be an acute increase in increase in afterload from lasix therapy, presumed secondary to an increase in plasma renin and norepinephrine levels *(3)*. This can lead to a reduction in cardiac output and a rise in pulmonary wedge pressure with possible worsening of dyspnea. These changes are usually reversed quickly but may need the addition of morphine, oxygen, and the subsequent diuretic effect of the loop diuretic.

Thiazide-type diuretics are generally less effective and carry a risk of inducing or worsening the hyponatremia and hypokalemia that is commonly seen in CHF. A potassium-sparing diuretic (such as amiloride or spironolactone) has traditionally been added for control of the plasma potassium concentration, whereas a thiazide diuretic can be added to a

Table 1
Pharmacologic Therapy of Heart Failure

Drug class	Drug name	AHA/ACC class (1)	Dose range	Side effects
Diuretics	Lasix	C–D	20–200 mg QD	Hypokalemia
	Spironolactone	C–D	25–50 mg QD	Renal insufficiency
				Ototoxicity
				Hyperkalemia
				Gynecomastia
ACE inhibitors (including asymptomatic LV dysfunction)	Captopril	B–D	6.25–50 mg TID	Hypotension
	Enalapril	B–D	2.5–20 mg BID	Cough
	Fosinopril	B–D	5–40 mg QD	Renal insufficiency
	Lisinopril	B–D	2.5–40 mg QD	Hyperkalemia
	Quinapril	B–D	10–40 mg QD	Dysgeusia (metallic taste)
	Ramipril	B–D	1.25–10 mg QD	
Direct vasodilators (if ACE inhibitor intolerant)	Losartan	C–D	25–100 mg QD/BID	Hypotension
	Irbesartan	C–D	150–300 mg QD	Renal insufficiency
	Valsartan	C–D	80–320 mg QD	
Inotropes	Digoxin	C–D	0.125–0.375 mg QD	Visual
				GI (nausea, vomiting)
				Conduction disturbances
				Increase VEA
β-blockers (including post-MI LV dysfunction)	Carvedilol	B–D	3.125–50 mg QD	Hypotension
	Metoprolol-XL	B–D	12.5–200 mg QD	Bradycardia
	Bisoprolol	B–D	1.25–10 mg QD	Heart block
				Worsening CHF

loop diuretic in refractory patients to block sodium reabsorption at a different site in the kidney and amplify the action of the loop diuretic.

It is important to remember that the major side effect of these agents is hypokalemia. Hypokalemia will result in an increased susceptibility for ventricular arrhythmias and possibility sudden cardiac death. In an analysis from the Study of Left-Ventricular Dysfunction (SOLVD) trial, diuretic use, in comparison to no diuretic use at baseline, was associated with a higher incidence of overall morality, cardiovascular deaths (11.4 vs 4.6% per year), and arrhythmic or sudden cardiac death *(4)*. The risk for arrhythmic death associated with the use of nonpotassium-sparing diuretics was significantly elevated (relative risk 1.33) after controlling for disease severity, comorbid illnesses, and concomitant medications including ACE inhibitors. Other complications of diuretic therapy include hypovolemia, hypotension, and worsening azotemia. These side effects are all exacerbated by the underlying reduced cardiac output in patients with heart failure.

In contrast to the concern with regards to increased mortality secondary to hypokalemia with the standard nonpotassium-sparing diuretic therapy, recent data suggest improved survival in CHF patients treated with spironolactone, a potassium-sparing diuretic. In the Randomized Aldactone Evaluation Study (RALES) trial *(5)*, 1663 patients with New York Heart Association (NYHA) Class III to IV CHF who were receiving an ACE inhibitor and a loop diuretic, with or without digoxin, were randomized to placebo or spironolactone (25–50 mg daily—a nondiuretic dose of spironolactone). After an average follow-up of 24 months, the study was discontinued because of a 30% reduction in overall mortality with spironolactone (35 vs 46% for placebo), including a 36% reduction in death from heart failure ($p < 0.001$), a 29% reduction in sudden death ($p = 0.02$), and a 35% reduction in hospitalization for heart failure. The benefit of spironolactone was evident in both ischemic and nonischemic cardiomyopathy patients. The most common side effects seen in this trial were hyperkalemia and gynecomastia.

ACE INHIBITORS

ACE inhibitors have emerged as standard therapy in the treatment of CHF. These agents work by inhibiting angiotensin converting enzyme, which is the privotal enzyme responsible for the conversion of angiotensin I to angiotensin II, one of the most potent vasoconstrictors produced by the body.

Prospective, randomized trials have demonstrated a significant reduction in morbidity and mortality in patients with left-ventricular

dysfunction (LVEF < 40%) with and without symptomatic heart failure
(6–10). The improvement in outcome is clinically associated with
diminished progression of left-ventricular remodeling secondary to
antagonism of the deleterious effects of increased angiotensin II production.

The Cooperative North Scandinavian Enalapril Survival Study
(CONSENSUS) study group evaluated 253 patients with advanced
NYHA III or IV CHF who were already treated with diuretics, digitalis,
and other vasodilating agents (mostly nitrates [6]) who were then randomized to therapy with enalapril or placebo. The administration of
enalapril reduced the 6-month mortality by 40%, from 44 to 26%, and
the 12-month mortality by 31%, from 52 to 36% ($p = 0.003$). This
benefit was sustained for at least 4 years (11). Similarly, the SOLVD
trial evaluated 2569 patients with symptomatic NYHA Class II to III
heart failure (7) treated with enalapril or placebo. When compared to
placebo, enalapril resulted in a 16% risk reduction in mortality ($p =
0.0036$) vs placebo. The Vasodilator Heart Failure Trial (VHeFT) II
study randomized 806 men with NYHA Class II and III heart failure
symptoms to either isosorbide dinitrate/hydralazine or enalapril (8).
After 2 years, the mortality rate was 25% in the former group vs only
18% with enalapril ($p = 0.016$).

Benefit in Asymptomatic Left-Ventricular Dysfunction

ACE inhibitors are also beneficial for patients with asymptomatic
left-ventricular dysfunction. This was demonstrated in a study by the
SOLVD investigators, which included 4228 patients with asymptomatic left-ventricular dysfunction with an LVEF below 35% (mean LVEF
28% [9]). The combined incidence of symptomatic heart disease or
cardiovascular death was reduced 29% by enalapril (29.8 vs 38.6% for
placebo) at a mean follow-up of just over 3 years.

The Survival and Ventricular Enlargement (SAVE) trial evaluated
2231 asymptomatic patients with LVEF ≤ 40% were randomized to
treatment with either captopril (12.5 mg TID increasing to a final target
dose of 50 mg TID) or placebo starting 3–16 days after myocardial
infarction (mean of 11 days post-infarction [10]). Captopril therapy was
associated with a 37% reduction in the incidence of severe heart failure,
a 22% reduction in hospitalization for heart failure, and a 19% fall in
mortality (20 vs 25% for placebo) at a mean follow-up of 42 months.

Two meta-analyses have analyzed the randomized trials with ACE
inhibitors (12,13). One meta-analysis demonstrated that ACE inhibition
had the following benefits in comparison to placebo in patients with
CHF (13): (1) A lower total mortality (23 vs 26.8% for placebo, odds

ratio 0.80). Most of the mortality benefit was a result of fewer deaths from progressive heart failure *(12)*; (2) A lower rate of readmission for heart failure (13.7 vs 18.9%) and a lower mortality combined with hospitalization (30.7 vs 36.9%, odds ratio 0.74); *(3)* A lower incidence of myocardial infarction (8.9 vs 11%). These data provide the evidence that supports the use of ACE inhibitors as standard therapy for patient with asymptomatic and symptomatic CHF.

The side effect profile of ACE inhibitors include hypotension, worsening azotemia, hyperkalemia, cough, and angioedema. The hemodynamic and azotemia/hyperkalemia consequences can be avoided by initiation of therapy in patients who are not hypovolemic from excessive diuresis or relatively "hypovolemic" from reduced cardiac output. The cough from ACE inhibitors is characterized by a dry, hacking cough, most commonly seen at night. The cough is most likely secondary to the relative increases in bradykinin secondary to inhibition of neutral endopeptidases and is managed most effectively by cessation of therapy with ACE inhibitors. The angioedema from ACE inhibitors is rare but can be life-threatening, thereby mandating cessation of therapy with ACE inhibitors.

Angiotensin Receptor Blockers (ARB)

The angiotensin II receptor blockers (e.g., losartan, valsartan, irbesartan, and candesartan) act by competitively inhibiting the binding of angiotensin II to the AT1 receptor. Increases in bradykinin, because of the inhibition of neutral endopeptidase by ACE inhibitors, is important in the cough side effect seen with agents. Because ARB agents do not affect kinin metabolism, they do not appear to induce cough. Therefore, these agents may be of particular benefit in patients who are intolerant of ACE inhibitors. However, there remains no data to suggest that these ARB agents provide the same beneficial survival effects observed with the ACE inhibitors. The ELITE II *(14)* and the ValHeft *(15)* trials have been the largest to date to examine ACE inhibitors vs ARB effects on survival.

The Evaluation of Losartan in the Elderly (ELITE) II trial randomized symptomatic, CHF patients ($n = 3152$; age > 65 years) to losartan (50 mg daily) or captopril (50 mg TID). No difference in mortality between either treatment group was observed. Further, there was no difference in the incidence of progressive heart failure or the number of hospital admissions for heart failure. The discontinuation rate for an adverse event was significantly lower with losartan (9.7 vs 14.7%). The Val-HeFT trial randomized patients in Class II or III heart failure ($n = 5010$) to valsartan (40 up to 160 mg BID) or placebo *(15)*. After a 2-year follow-up, valsartan had no effect on all-cause mortality (19.7 vs 19.4% for placebo); it did reduce the combined endpoint of mortality and morbidity (29 vs 32%), largely because of a reduction in hospitalizations for heart failure. In this trial, 36% of patients were receiving a β-blocker in addition to an ACE inhibitor (15). There was a trend toward an increase in mortality with the addition of valsartan compared to placebo, whereas those not receiving a β-blocker had a significant improvement in outcome with valsartan.

DIGOXIN

Digitalis has been used for more than 200 years to treat patients with CHF. By inhibiting the Na-K-ATPase pump in myocardial cells, an increase in intracellular calcium concentration (16) is observed which results in enhanced myocyte contractile performance. Another theoretically beneficial effect of digoxin is through its effects on the withdrawal of sympathetic tone. The recommendation for its use in CHF patients comes from clinical evidence that it improves cardiac function, symptoms and exercise capacity. There is no survival advantage to its use. Finally, it remains unclear if digitalis has a role in patients with asymptomatic left-ventricular dysfunction.

In the last decade, a number of trials have demonstrated that digoxin improves clinical symptoms and quality of life. One trial compared the effects of the initiation of therapy with digoxin, captopril, vs placebo (17). Both treatment regimens were effective. Compared to placebo, digoxin led to an increase in LVEF of 4.4%, reduced need for increased diuretic use, and reduced hospitalizations for heart failure.

The Digoxin Investigators' Group (DIG) trial (21) randomized almost 6800 patients with symptomatic CHF to digoxin or placebo. For entry into the study, patients had to have an LVEF less than or equal to 45% and normal sinus rhythm. Most patients (84%) had NYHA Class II/III heart failure symptoms and ischemic heart disease (70%); 94% were treated with an ACE inhibitor.

After 3 years, there was no difference in survival between the digoxin and placebo groups. However, digoxin therapy was associated with a trend toward a lower mortality from worsening CHF (11.6 vs 13.2% for placebo, $p = 0.06$); this benefit was counter-balanced by an apparent increase in non-CHF cardiac deaths, which included death from arrhythmia (15 vs 13%, $p = 0.04$). However, in contrast to all other oral inotropes, digoxin did not demonstrate an *increase* in mortality rates. Digoxin was also associated with a decrease in hospitalization rates, primarily because of a decrease in hospitalization for CHF (26.8 vs

34.7%, $p < 0.001$). There was also a significant reduction in the combined secondary endpoints of death from heart failure and hospitalization for CHF.

Effects of Digoxin Withdrawal

Two important trials (RADIANCE and PROVED) examined the effects of digoxin withdrawal on exercise capacity and worsening of heart failure symptoms in stable heart failure patients *(18,19)*. These studies randomized patients to continuation of digoxin therapy vs placebo. Patients withdrawn from digoxin demonstrated worsened maximal exercise capacity, increased incidence of treatment failures, and lower ejection fractions after 12 weeks of follow-up. Based on these data, predictors of clinical deterioration after digoxin withdrawal include cardiothoracic ratio ≥ 0.57, absence of ACE inhibitor therapy, and reduced LVEF *(20)*.

Optimal Dose

Despite the hemodynamic, exercise, clinical and neurohormonal evidence suggesting that digoxin should be used in patients with CHF, there are few data to guide dosing in patients. Digoxin also possesses a very narrow toxic to therapeutic ratio. Most studies suggest that levels above 0.6 ng/mL and below 1.2 ng/mL should be the dosing goal for patients with symptomatic heart failure. Above these ranges, the toxicity of digitalis increases rapidly. It is also important to remember that there is little to no data to support the concept that dosing within these "therapeutic" levels is associated with any clinically meaningful changes in exercise tolerance or reduction in symptoms. Further caution can be gleened from the mortality data in the DIG trial with regards to serum levels of digoxin. Mortality was reduced in patients with a serum digoxin concentration less than 1.0 ng/mL but increased in those with a serum digoxin above 1.5 ng/mL.

The side effects of digoxin include arrhythmias (both ventricular and supraventricular), conduction system, visual, and gastrointestinal. The development of side effects is not predictable based on the serum levels of digoxin and can be idiosyncratic on a patient-to-patient basis. It is important to note that digoxin is clear primarily via renal excretion and therefore, extra care needs to be taken when patients have clinical renal insufficiency.

Digoxin is the only agent that can induce arrhythmias that are associated with increased automaticity as well as increased atrioventricular (AV) block. In patients with atrial fibrillation, a typical side effect is regularization of the ventricular response. In other patients, there can be increased ventricular ectopy or frank ventricular tachycardia. There can also be increased AV block with complete heart block or severely reduced ventricular conduction response across the AV node. Other symptoms of digoxin toxicity can include yellow-green halos, as well as profound nausea and vomiting. In patients with mild symptoms of digoxin toxicity, simply withholding digoxin therapy usually allows the abnormalities to resolve. In patients with life-threatening complications, there is a Fab antibody fragment commercially available that will bind all circulating digoxin and remove its toxic effects immediately. Once this Fab fragment is administered, digoxin levels are not accurately determined by the standard assay because the Fab fragment crossreacts in the assay.

INOTROPIC AGENTS

Several other oral inotropic drugs have been studied in patients with symptomatic heart failure. These agents include phosphodiesterase inhibitors (such as milrinone, vesnarinone, and enoximone), β receptor agonists (such as xamoterol), and dopamine agonists (such as ibopamine). These agents have all been shown to increase patient mortality and therefore have never been approved for use in patients with CHF.

β-BLOCKERS

CHF is associated with activation of the sympathetic nervous system and renin-angiotensin system. These responses are intended to increase blood pressure and perfusion to vital organ systems via increased cardiac output (via β-receptor stimulation of myocyte contractility). However, the increased afterload work of the heart in the setting of increased peripheral vasoconstriction increases cardiac work and contributes to the progressive ventricular dilation typically observed over the course of the natural history of patients with left-ventricular dysfunction. Furthermore, direct myocyte injury has also been demonstrated as a result of chronic exposure to increased levels of norepinephrine and angiotensin II.

These observations provide the rationale for β-receptor antagonism therapy for patients with symptomatic CHF. Early studies involving a small number of patients suggested that therapy with a β-blocker might improve patient outcome in heart failure (22,23). Subsequently, several major trials have demonstrated an improvement in survival with a number of β–blockers (e.g., metoprolol, carvedilol, and bisoprolol) in selected heart failure patients.

Metoprolol Trials

The efficacy of metoprolol has been evaluated in a number of randomized trials, including Metoprolol in Dilated Cardiomyopathy

(MDC) *(24)* and Metoprolol Randomized Intervention Trial-Heart Failure (MERIT-HF) *(25)*.

METOPROLOL IN DILATED CARDIOMYOPATHY TRIAL

The MDC trial randomly assigned 383 patients to placebo or metoprolol (beginning at a dose of 10 mg and increasing slowly to a maximum of 150 mg/day) *(24)*. Eligible patients had to have idiopathic dilated cardiomyopathy, symptomatic heart failure, LVEF less than 40%, and a systolic blood pressure over 90 mm Hg. Potential participants were excluded if they had significant coronary disease, active myocarditis, other life-threatening disease, or they deteriorated after a test dose of 5 mg of metoprolol BID for 2 to 7 days.

Of the patients who entered the study, despite the lack of survival improvement, the following benefits were noted in the metoprolol group when compared to therapy with placebo at 12 to 18 months:

- A reduced likelihood of progressing to cardiac transplantation (1 vs 10%).
- A greater increase in LVEF (12 vs 6%) and exercise tolerance.
- An improvement in quality of life.

MERIT-HF TRIAL

In contrast to the MDC trial, a mortality benefit with metoprolol (Toprol XL) was demonstrated in the much larger MERIT-HF trial *(25,26)*. In this study, 3991 patients with Class II to IV heart failure and an LVEF ≤40% were randomized to extended-release metoprolol or placebo. The mean dose was 159 mg/day, with 64% of patients achieving the target dose; the discontinuation rate for patients taking active drug was 14% at 1 year. This study demonstrated that for patients treated with Toprol XL: (1) A decrease in all-cause mortality at 12 months (7.2 vs 11% for placebo, $p = 0.006$); (2) a reduction in the combined end point of death or need for cardiac transplantation (7.5 vs 10.3%, $p < 0.001$); (3) A decrease in the incidence of hospitalization for cardiovascular causes (20 vs 25%, $p < 0.001$) or for heart failure (10 vs 15%, $p < 0.001$); and (4) improved NYHA functional class and quality of life.

CARVEDILOL TRIALS

Four individual carvedilol trials, including PRECISE, the US Carvedilol Heart Failure Study, and MOCHA, were initially designed to evaluate improvements in submaximal exercise tolerance; mortality (which was not a prospectively designated primary endpoint) was also measured to assess safety and potential benefit *(27–30)*. The results were combined to form a double-blind controlled study of nearly 1100 patients with mild, moderate, and severe heart failure *(30)*. Patients were maintained on digoxin, diuretics, and ACE inhibitors and then randomly assigned to treatment with carvedilol or placebo, following a 2-week open-label tolerability phase with carvedilol.

These studies were stopped early as a result of a significant improvement in survival in patients treated with carvedilol. The benefit was due primarily to reductions in death from progressive heart failure (0.7 vs 3.3%) and sudden cardiac death (1.7 vs 3.8%). The benefit was independent of age, sex, heart failure etiology, LVEF, exercise tolerance, systolic blood pressure, or heart rate. There was also a reduction in the need for hospitalization (14.1 vs 19.6%, $p = 0.036$) and a 38% increase in event-free survival, i.e., need for hospitalization or death (15.8 vs 24.6%, $p = 0.001$). The most common adverse reaction was worsening heart failure, which was less frequent with carvedilol than with placebo (1.6 vs 2.3%).

BISOPROLOL TRIALS

After demonstration that bisoprolol had both hemodynamic benefits and a trend to improved survival in 557 patients in CIBIS I *(31)*, the efficacy of bisoprolol was studied in the larger CIBIS II trial *(32)*. CIBIS II randomly assigned 2647 patients with Class III/IV heart failure and an LVEF less than 35% to bisoprolol vs placebo; the patients also received standard therapy with diuretics and ACE inhibitors. After an average follow-up of 1.4 years, the trial was stopped early when the following benefits were observed in the bucindolol group: (1) A significant reduction in total all-cause mortality (11.8 vs 17.3%), primarily because of a reduction in SCD (3.6 vs 6.3%, $p < 0.001$) and (2) a 15% reduction in all-cause hospitalizations admissions and a 30% reduction in admissions for heart failure ($p < 0.0001$).

META-ANALYSIS OF TRIALS

A number of meta-analyses have confirmed the benefits of beta blockade *(33–35)*. The most recent meta-analysis consisted of 21 trials involving 5849 patients who were treated for median of 6 months: β-blockers reduced overall mortality, cardiovascular mortality, heart failure death, and sudden death by 39, 39, 34, and 30%, respectively *(35)*. The decrease in overall mortality was the same in those with ischemic and nonischemic heart disease, and, as noted above, was greater with vasodilating agents. An earlier meta-analysis confirmed the equivalent efficacy in ischemic and nonischemic cardiomyopathies *(33)*. To date, there are no comparative data to give firm guidance as to which β-blocker may be superior. Accordingly, at this time, recommendations for β-blocker use in heart failure consider the beneficial effects of these agents as a class effect.

NITRATES

Organic nitrates have a beneficial effect on hemodynamics, myocardial ischemia, the magnitude of mitral regurgitation, endothelial function, cardiac remodeling, and exercise capacity. However, no study has evaluated the effects of long-term treatment with nitrates alone in patients with symptomatic heart failure. The VHeFT I trial compared the combination of hydralazine (300 mg/day) and isosorbide dinitrate (160 mg/day) to placebo *(36,37)*. Three-year mortality was reduced by 22%. This combination is difficult for patients to adhere to given the QID administration regimen for isordil and accordingly has not been considered the standard of care, especially given the ACE inhibitor data cited above.

Nitrates may have beneficial effects when used in combination with ACE inhibitors. In one study, the effect of high-dose transdermal nitroglycerin was evaluated in 29 patients with Class II/III heart failure who were on background ACE inhibitor therapy *(38)*. Compared to placebo, nitroglycerin significantly improved exercise time over a 3-month period of time, decreased left-ventricular end-systolic and end-diastolic dimensions, and increased left-ventricular fractional shortening. However, no beneficial effects on heart failure symptoms, quality of life, or the need for additional diuretics or hospitalization.

DIRECT-ACTING VASODILATORS

A meta-analysis of several studies has not demonstrated any benefit from direct vasodilators *(39)*. As an example, therapy with the α-blocker prazosin constituted one arm of the V-HeFT I trial; no difference in survival was observed compared with the placebo group *(37,38)*. The negative inotropic effects of calcium-channel blockers and their undesirable activation of the renin-angiotensin and sympathetic nervous systems remain a major concern in patients with CHF *(40)*. In several studies, the degree of clinical deterioration was greater in patients treated with nifedipine or diltiazem than in those receiving placebo or isosorbide dinitrate *(41,42)*. In addition, short-acting calcium-channel blockers may increase coronary mortality. Long-acting dihydropyridines, such as amlodipine or felopidine, have also been studied in patients with heart failure but have not been demonstrated to improve the outcome in patients with heart failure (PRAISE or VHeFT III trials *[43,44]*). Because these agents were not associated with an increase in mortality, amlodipine and felodipine appear to be safe and well tolerated and can be used, especially if treatment with a calcium-channel blocker is necessary, such as for angina or hypertension.

RECOMMENDATIONS

Diuretics

Loop diuretics should be the diuretic of choice in patients with symptomatic CHF and associated volume overload. Spironolactone also has a role in patients with advanced heart failure. Patients already receiving maximal therapy with an ACE inhibitor, digoxin, and loop diuretic, who remain symptomatic (NYHA Class III or IV) or who have a large-loop diuretic requirement with a plasma potassium concentration below 4.0 meq/L should considered the addition of spironolactone.

Digoxin

Digoxin has been demonstrated to be safe and to decrease the morbidity associated with heart failure. Despite its narrow toxic to therapeutic ratio, it should be used in all patients with symptomatic CHF. Dose ranges for this agent should be aimed at achieving the therapeutic ranges below 1.0ng/ml. It should not be forgotten that digoxin excretion is mainly via the kidneys, and that dose adjustments must be made in the setting of renal insufficiency.

ACE Inhibitors

All patients with symptomatic left-ventricular dysfunction or an LVEF below 40% should be placed on an ACE inhibitor. Beginning therapy with low doses (2.5 mg of enalapril BID or 6.25 mg of captopril TID) will reduce the likelihood of hypotension and azotemia (26,27) and then gradually increased to maintenance doses of 20 mg BID of enalapril, 20 mg/day of lisinopril, 50 mg TID of captopril, or 5 mg BID of quinapril are reached. It remains uncertain if lower doses provide the same magnitude of clinical improvements in survival. If an ACE inhibitor is not tolerated, or significant renal dysfunction occurs, therapy with hydralazine and isosorbide dinitrate (40 mg TID or QID) or mononitrate (40–120 mg/day) is appropriate. Hydralazine should be started at 25 mg TID and titrated upward to 100 mg TID. It remains unclear if the angiotensin receptor blockers will demonstrate improved survival similar to what has been observed with the ACE inhibitors.

β-Blockers

Initial and target doses for β-blocker therapy are 3.125 mg BID and 25 to 50 mg BID (the higher dose being used in subjects over 85 kg) for carvedilol, 6.25 mg BID and 50–75 mg BID for metoprolol or 12.5 or 25 mg daily and titrated up to 200 mg/day for therapy with extended-release metoprolol, and 1.25 mg QD and 5–10 mg QD for bisoprolol. Dose-increment intervals should not be earlier than at 2-week intervals. Even lower starting doses should be given to patients with recent decompensation of a systolic pressure below 85 mm Hg. Every effort should be made to achieve the target dose because the improvement appears to be dose-dependent.

REFERENCES

1. ACC/AHA guidelines for the evaluation and management of chronic heart failure in the adult: Executive summary. J Am Coll Cardiol 2001;38:2101.
2. Dikshit, K, Vyden, JK, Forrester, JS, et al. Renal and extrarenal hemodynamic effects of furosemide in congestive heart failure after acute myocardial infarction. N Engl J Med 1973;288:1087.
3. Francis, GS, Siegel, RM, Goldsmith, SR, et al. Acute vasoconstrictor response to intravenous furosemide in chronic congestive heart failure. Activation of the neurohumoral axis. Ann Intern Med 1985;103:1.
4. Cooper, HA, Dries, DL, Davis, CE, et al. Diuretics and risk of arrhythmic death in patients with left ventricular dysfunction (In Process Citation). Circulation 1999;100:1311.
5. Pitt, B, Zannad, F, Remme, WJ, et al., for the Randomized Aldactone Evaluation Study Investigators. The Effect of spironolactone on morbidity and mortality in patients with severe heart failure. N Engl J Med 1999;341:709.
6. The CONSENSUS Trial Study Group. Effects of enalapril on mortality in severe congestive heart failure: Results of the Cooperative North Scandinavia Enalapril Survival Study (CONSENSUS). N Engl J Med 1987;316:1429.
7. The SOLVD Investigators. Effect of enalapril on survival in patients with reduced left ventricular ejection fractions and congestive heart failure. N Engl J Med 1991;325:293.
8. Cohn, JN, Johnson, G, Ziesche, S, et al. A comparison of enalapril with hydralazine-isosorbide dinitrate in the treatment of chronic congestive heart failure. N Engl J Med 1991;325:303.
9. The SOLVD Investigators. Effect of enalapril on mortality and the development of heart failure in asymptomatic patients with reduced left ventricular ejection fractions. N Engl J Med 1992;327:685.
10. Pfeffer, MA, Braunwald, E, Moyé, LA, et al. Effect of captopril on mortality and morbidity in patients with left ventricular dysfunction after myocardial infarction. Results of the Survival and Ventricular Enlargement trial. The SAVE Investigators. N Engl J Med 1992;327:669.
11. Swedberg, K, Kjekshus, J, Snapinn, S for the CONSENSUS Investigators. Long-term survival in severe heart failure in patients treated with enalapril. Ten year follow-up of CONSENSUS I. Eur Heart J 1999;20:136.
12. Garg, R, Yusuf, S, for the Collaborative Group on ACE Inhibition Trials. Overview of randomized trials of angiotensin-converting enzyme inhibitors in patients with heart failure. JAMA 1995;273:1450.
13. Flather, MD, Yusuf, S, Kober, L, et al. Long-term ACE-inhibitor therapy in patients with heart failure or left-ventricular dysfunction: a systematic overview of data from

individual patients. ACE-Inhibitor Myocardial Infarction Collaborative Group. Lancet 2000;355:1575.

14. Pitt, B, Poole-Wilson, PA, Segal, R, et al. Effect of losartan compared with captopril on mortality in patients with symptomatic heart failure: randomised trial—the Losartan Heart Failure Survival Study ELITE II. Lancet 2000;355:1582.

15. Cohn JN, Tognani G and the Valsartan Heart Failure Trial Investigators. A randomized trial of the angiotensin receptor blocker valsartan in chronic heart failure. N Engl J Med 2001;345:1667.

16. Smith, TW. Digitalis: Mechanisms of action and clinical use. N Engl J Med 1988;318:358.

17. The Captopril-Digoxin Multicenter Research Group. Comparative effects of therapy with captopril and digoxin in patients with mild to moderate heart failure. JAMA 1988;259:539.

18. Packer, M, Gheorghiade, M, Young, JB, et al. Withdrawal of digoxin from patients with chronic heart failure treated with angiotensin-converting-enzyme inhibitors. N Engl J Med 1993;329:1

19. Uretsky, BF, Young, JB, Shahidi, FE, et al. Randomized study assessing the effect of digoxin withdrawal in patients with mild to moderate chronic congestive heart failure: results of the PROVED trial. J Am Coll Cardiol 1993;22:955.

20. Adams, KF, Gheorghiade, M, Uretsky, BF, et al. Clinical predictors of worsening of heart failure during withdrawal from digoxin therapy. Am Heart J 1998;135:389.

21. The Digitalis Investigation Group. The effect of digoxin on mortality and morbidity in patients with heart failure. N Engl J Med 1997;336:525.

22. Swedberg, K, Waagstein, F, Hjalmarson, A, Wallentin, I. Prolongation of survival in congestive cardiomyopathy by beta receptor blockade. Lancet 1979;1:1374.

23. Anderson, JL, Lutz, JR, Gilbert, EM, et al. A randomized trial of low-dose beta-blockade therapy for idiopathic dilated cardiomyopathy. Am J Cardiol 1985;55:471.

24. Waagstein, F, Bristow, MR, Swedberg, K, et al. Beneficial effects of metoprolol in idiopathic dilated cardiomyopathy. Lancet 1993;342:1441.

25. MERIT-HF Study Group. Effect of metoprolol CR/XL in chronic heart failure: Metoprolol CR/XL Randomised Intervention Trial in Congestive Heart Failure (MERIT-HF). Lancet 1999;353:2001.

26. Hjalmarson, A, Goldstein, S, Fagerberg, B, et al. Effects of controlled-release metoprolol on total mortality, hospitalizations, and well-being in patients with heart failure: the Metoprolol CR/XL Randomized Intervention Trial in congestive heart failure (MERIT-HF). MERIT-HF Study Group. JAMA 2000;283:1295.

27. Packer, M, Colucci, WS, Sackner-Bernstein, JD, et al. Double-blind, placebo-controlled study of the effects of carvedilol in patients with moderate to severe heart failure. The PRECISE Trial. Prospective Randomized Evaluation of Carvedilol on Symptoms and Exercise. Circulation 1996;94:2793.

28. Colucci, WS, Packer, M, Bristow, MR, et al. Carvedilol inhibits clinical progression in patients with mild symptoms of heart failure. US Carvedilol Heart Failure Study Group. Circulation 1996;94:2800.

29. Bristow, MR, Gilbert, EM, Abraham, WT, et al. Carvedilol produces dose-related improvements in left ventricular function and survival in subjects with chronic heart failure. MOCHA Investigators. Circulation 1996;94:2807.

30. Packer, M, Bristow, MR, Cohn, JN, et al for the US Carvedilol Heart Failure Study Group. The effect of carvedilol on morbidity and mortality in patients with chronic heart failure. N Engl J Med 1996;334:1349.

31. Lechat, P, Escolano, S, Golmard, JL, et al. Prognostic value of bisoprolol-induced hemodynamic effects in heart failure during the Cardiac Insufficiency Bisoprolol study (CIBIS). Circulation 1997;96:2197.

32. CIBIS-II Investigators and Committees. The Cardiac Insufficiency Bisoprolol Study II (CIBIS-II): A randomised trial. Lancet 1999;353:9.
33. Heidenreich, PA, Lee, TT, Massie, BM. Effect of beta-blockade on mortality in patients with heart failure: A meta-analysis of randomized clinical trials. J Am Coll Cardiol 1997;30:27.
34. Lechat, P, Packer, M, Chalon, S, et al. Clinical effects of beta-adrenergic blockade in chronic heart failure: a meta-analysis of double-blind, placebo-controlled, randomized trials. Circulation 1998;98:1184.
35. Bonet, S, Agusti, A, Arnau, JM, et al. Beta-adrenergic blocking agents in heart failure: benefits of vasodilating and non-vasodilating agents according to patients' characteristics: a meta-analysis of clinical trials. Arch Intern Med 2000;160:621.
36. Cohn, JN, Archibald, DG, Francis, GS, et al. Veterans Administration Cooperative Study on Vasodilator Therapy of Heart Failure: Influence of pre-randomization variables on the reduction of mortality by treatment with hydralazine and isosorbide dinitrate. Circulation 1987;75:IV49.
37. Cohn, JN, Archibald, DG, Ziesche, S, et al. Effect of vasodilator therapy on mortality in chronic congestive heart failure: Results of a Veterans Administration Cooperative Study. N Engl J Med 1986;314:1547.
38. Elkayam, U, Johnson, JV, Shotan, A, et al. Double-blind, placebo-controlled study to evaluate the effect of organic nitrates in patients with chronic heart failure treated with angiotensin-converting enzyme inhibition. Circulation 1999;99:2652.
39. Furberg, CD, Yusuf, S. Effect of drug therapy on survival in chronic congestive heart failure. Am J Cardiol 1988;62:41A
40. Packer, M. Treatment of chronic heart failure. Lancet 1992;340:92.
41. Elkayam, U, Amin, J, Mehra, A, et al. A prospective, randomized, double-blind, crossover study to compare the efficacy and safety of chronic nifedipine therapy with that of isosorbide dinitrate and their combination in the treatment of chronic congestive heart failure. Circulation 1990;82:1954.
42. Goldstein, RE, Boccuzzi, SJ, Cruess, D, Nattel, S. Diltiazem increases late-onset congestive heart failure in postinfarction patients with early reduction in ejection fraction. The Adverse Experience Committee; and the Multicenter Diltiazem Postinfarction Research Group. Circulation 1991;83:52.
43. Packer, M, O'Connor, CM, Ghali, JK, et al. Effect of amlodipine on morbidity and mortality in severe chronic heart failure. N Engl J Med 1996;335:1107.
44. Cohen, JN, Ziesche, S, Smith, R, et al., for the Vasodilator-Heart Failure Trial (V-HeFT) Study Group. Effect of the calcium antagonist felodipine as supplementary vasodilator therapy in patients with chronic heart failure treated with enalapril. V-HeFT III. Circulation 1997;96:856.

15 Evaluation and Treatment of Arrhythmias in Heart Failure

David J. Callans, MD

OVERVIEW: SHOULD ALL ARRHYTHMIAS BE TREATED?

Arrhythmias contribute substantially to morbidity and mortality in patients with symptomatic heart failure. Atrial fibrillation is a frequent cause and effect of heart failure exacerbation (1,2). As discussed below, the onset of atrial fibrillation is an independent negative prognostic sign in advanced heart failure (3,4). Approximately 300,000 people in the United States die suddenly each year, presumably largely a result of ventricular arrhythmias; the majority have pre-existing ventricular dysfunction (5). It has been estimated that 50% of deaths in patients with symptomatic heart failure are sudden, presumably arrhythmic (6,7). Furthermore, the relative contribution of sudden death to total mortality seems to be highest in patients with more preserved functional class. Against this highly emotionally charged back drop, the desire to find

From: *Contemporary Cardiology: Heart Failure:*
A Clinician's Guide to Ambulatory Diagnosis and Treatment
Edited by: M. L. Jessup and E. Loh © Humana Press Inc., Totowa, NJ

effective treatment for all patients with congestive heart failure (CHF) is certainly understandable.

What are then the barriers to treating all arrhythmias in the setting of CHF, or even further, using antiarrhythmic agents as part of a primary prevention strategy in all patients? First, on closer inspection, there are substantial difficulties in better defining our preconceptions about sudden cardiac death. Despite significant improvements in classification (8), the cause of sudden death in patients with structural heart disease may be impossible to determine, even in patients with implanted defibrillators (9). Although "unexpected death without warning" (of prior worsening of heart failure symptoms) or "death within 1 hour of symptom onset" is generally considered caused by ventricular tachycardia or fibrillation, many other mechanisms can cause sudden unexpected death. Although sometimes criticized because of the highly selected nature of the patients involved (transplant-listed, undergoing-inpatient heart failure therapy), Luu and collegues reported that more than 50% of sudden deaths in monitored patients were a result of bradyarrhythmias and/or electromechanical dissociation (10). In addition, a recently published autopsy substudy of the Assessment of Treatment with Lisinopril and Survival (ATLAS) trial demonstrated that the majority of sudden deaths in patients with ischemic cardiomyopathy were associated with acute coronary thrombosis (11). This was true despite the absence of preceding angina and the firm perception of the treating physicians that the presumed cause of death was arrhythmic. Thus, even if perfect empiric therapy for ventricular arrhythmias existed, the actual impact this therapy would have on sudden death in heart failure is difficult to determine.

A second barrier to generalized antiarrhythmic treatment of heart failure patients has been difficulties in risk stratification. The rationale behind this is that even if perfect therapy does not exist, antiarrhythmic treatment may benefit a subpopulation of those patients at the highest risk of arrhythmic death. Variables that are helpful in determining risk of ventricular arrhythmias post-myocardial infarction (MI) are either controversial or not useful in patients with heart failure, even those with "pure" ischemic etiologies. Rational treatment algorithms have been constructed for patients who are obviously at high risk (resuscitated cardiac arrest, syncope, NSVT in the setting of prior myocardial infarction; see below), but the real difficulty exists in defining primary prevention strategies in the majority of patients. Etiology of heart failure (i.e., ischemic vs idiopathic) does not seem to be a consistent factor in determining risk of sudden death (12–14), or a defining characteristic of response to preventative interventions. With the exception of the combination of nonsustained ventricular tachycardia and depressed LVEF in patients with prior myocardial infarction, noninvasive or invasive testing has not been helpful in determining risk of sudden death in patients with heart failure without a history of sustained arrhythmias. More recently, it was demonstrated that patients with decreased LVEF (<30) in the setting of prior MI were at sufficiently high risk to benefit from prophylactic implantable defibrillators *(14a)*. Although screening factors such as advanced New York Heart Association (NYHA) symptom class, QRS duration, low ejection fraction, frequent ventricular ectopy, positive signal-averaged electrocardiogram, and reduced heart rate variability are powerful predictors of mortality, they do not specifically distinguish the likelihood of death from progressive heart and sudden death in patients without prior MI *(6,7,13–16)*.

One possible explanation for the difficulty in predicting risk of arrhythmic death is the number of variables that upset homeostasis in the heart failure syndrome. Starting from a background of advanced ventricular dysfunction that provides the substrate for ventricular arrhythmias (fibrosis either from infarct scar or myocyte loss in idiopathic-dilated cardiomyopathy), the onset of symptomatic heart failure brings to bear a multiplicity of interacting situations that may provide "triggers" to induce specific arrhythmia episodes. Even in patients with a relatively "pure" and well-understood arrhythmia substrate of healed MI, the development of heart failure introduces new and less well-appreciated risks. Neurohormonal activation, differential regional responses to injury (e.g., hypertrophy with resultant increases in wall stress) ischemia, progressive ventricular dilatation all interact with each other and with the structural arrhythmia substrate. Susceptibility to electrolyte abnormalities and drug side effects also increases in this setting, further adding to risk.

The final, and perhaps most important barrier to empiric and widespread specific antiarrhythmic therapy, has been the realization of the great potential for harm. The PVC hypothesis, that prevention of frequent ectopy would prevent sudden cardiac death, although logically sound, provided disastrous results when field-tested in the Cardiac Arrhythmia Suppression Trial (CAST). The use of flecainide and encainide in patients with depressed left-ventricular function post-myocardial infarction, lead to a increased risk of death or cardiac arrest (RR: 2.64, $p = 0.0001$) in the treatment group, despite marked suppression of PVCs *(17)*. Although the analysis was not randomized or controlled, a substudy of antiarrhythmic drug use in the Stroke Prevention in Atrial Fibrillation Trial (SPAF) demonstrated a 4.7-fold risk of total mortality (3.7-fold increase in arrhythmic death) in patients with heart failure treated with Class I antiarrhythmic drugs, predominately for atrial fibrillation *(18)*. Antiarrhythmic drugs did not confer a survival disadvantage in patients without heart failure. A meta-analysis suggested that Type 1 agents (Na+ channel blockers) are detrimental in the primary prevention of the post-infarct patient *(19)*. The negative effects of antiarrhythmic drugs are not limited to those that block the sodium channel. The Survival With Oral d-Sotalol (SWORD) study, which used d-sotolol (a relatively pure Class III agent) in patients with depressed ejection fraction post-MI, was terminated prematurely because of increased mortality in the treatment arm (5.0 vs 3.1%, $p = 0.006$) *(20)*. In summary, although somewhat counterintuitive, most attempts at targeted antiarrhythmic drug therapy in the setting of advanced structural heart disease have led to worsened rather than improved outcome. Although it is generally considered that the excess mortality is a result of proarrhythmia, the negative inotropic effects caused by the majority of antiarrhythmic agents may also contribute. In fact, in a review of the general improvement in prognosis of patients listed for transplantation comparing pre- and post-1990, Stevenson et al. *(21)* focus the modern avoidance of harmful antiarrhythmic agents as one of the more important factors *(21)*.

The exception to the otherwise uniformly negative effect of antiarrhythmic agents in primary prevention is amiodarone, which has in general, been demonstrated to have a neutral to mildly positive effect on survival. Amiodarone is almost difficult to consider as a pure antiarrhythmic agent, as in addition to effects on the cardiac sodium and potassium channel, it also has potent β blockade, calcium-channel blockade, and anti-ischemic effects *(22)*. Amiodarone therapy was shown to improve survival and freedom from cardiac arrest and sustained ventricular arrhythmias in comparison to placebo and "individualized" conventional antiarrhythmic drug therapy in post-MI patients in the Basel Antiarrhythmic Study of Infarct Survival (BASIS) *(23)*.

Two trials have evaluated amiodarone therapy as primary prevention in the setting of symptomatic CHF independent of etiology. The Grupo de Estudio de la Sobrevida en la Insuficiencia Cardiaca en Argentina (GESICA) compared amiodarone to placebo in patients with Class II–IV heart failure and demonstrated reductions in total and sudden death mortality of 28 and 27%, respectively, at 2 years *(24)*. This study is often criticized as nonrepresentative, given the relatively high proportion of patients with Chagastic cardiomyopathy (who may respond especially well to amiodarone) and the relatively low incidence (<40%) of ischemic cardiomyopathy. The Survival Trial of Antiarrhythmic Treatment–Congestive Heart Failure (CHF-STAT) trial tested whether amiodarone therapy reduced mortality in patients with congestive heart failure, EF ≤40% and > 10 PVC/hour. The majority of patients in this trial had NYHA Class II symptoms (55%) and ischemic heart disease (70%). After a median follow-up of 45 months in 674 patients, no difference in mortality was observed between the two treatment groups ($p = 0.6$) (25).

Two further trials, European Myocardial Infarction Amiodarone Trial (EMIAT) and Canadian Myocardial Infarction Amiodarone Trial (CAMIAT) examined the effect of treatment with amiodarone in patients with depressed left-ventricular function following MI (26,27). In EMIAT, 1486 patients with prior MI and EF ≤ 40% were randomized to either amiodarone (200 mg/day) or placebo. After a median follow-up of 21 months, no difference in mortality was observed between the two groups. In CAMIAT, 1202 patients with prior MI and frequent ventricular ectopy (>10 PVC/hour or 1 run of VT) were randomized to either amiodarone (200 mg/day) or placebo. The primary endpoint was an outcome cluster of arrhythmic death and resuscitated VF. After a mean follow-up of 1.79 years, the amiodarone group was associated with a lower outcome cluster than placebo (0.6 vs 3.3%, $p = 0.016$). Patients in the amiodarone group treated with β-blockers had an even more favorable outcome.

In summary, multicenter, placebo-controlled trials of amiodarone in patients with congestive heart failure demonstrate that amiodarone therapy is at least safe and at most mildly effective in improving total mortality; this effect is assumed but not proven to be secondary to effects on sudden cardiac death. Most trials were performed prior to widespread therapy with modern heart failure therapy; however, the CAMIAT trial suggests that concomitant amiodarone and β-blocker therapy may exert an additive protective effect.

Although attempts at *specific* antiarrhythmic therapy (with the exception of amiodarone) have resulted in increased mortality, other current therapies for CHF also may have significant effects on risk of sudden death.

β-blocker therapy was initially studied in patients post-MI and were found to improve survival, related in part to the reduction of sudden cardiac death (28,29). More recently, large-scale multicenter trials have demonstrated that the benefit of β-blocker therapy extends beyond those patients with ischemic cardiomyopathy. In the Metoprolol CR/XL Randomised Intervention Trial in Congestive Heart Failure (MERIT-HF) trial, patients with heart failure (NYHA Class II–IV; ischemic cardiomyopathy in 65%) and decreased ejection fraction (≤ 40%) were randomized to long-acting metoprolol or placebo. After a mean follow-up of 1 year, metoprolol therapy reduced all-cause mortality, sudden death, and death from worsening heart failure; the relative risk of sudden death was 0.59 ($p = 0.0002$) in the metoprolol-treated group *(30)*. Similar beneficial effects were demonstrated using carvedilol in The US Carvedilol Heart Failure Study Group *(31)*. Carvedilol was associated with a significant reduction in overall mortality compared with placebo (3.2 vs 7.8%, $p < 0.001$) and a reduction in sudden death (1.7 vs 3.8%). The Carvedilol Prospective Randomized Cumulative Survival Trial (COPERNICUS) suggested that the benefit of carvedilol therapy to extends to patients with NYHA Class IV symptoms *(32)*. In contrast, the β-Blocker Survival Trial (BEST), which used bucindolol hydrochloride in patients with NYHA Classes III and IV, was terminated early because of increased mortality *(33)*.

An overview of β-blocker mortality trials in CHF demonstrates compelling evidence of a mortality benefit of these agents in patients with heart failure; and in particular a significant reduction in sudden death *(34)*. The reduction in sudden death in these trials is substantially greater than in trials using other drugs including angiotensin-converting enzyme (ACE) inhibitors. Some investigators further hypothesize that lipophilic β-blockers (e.g., propranolol, metoprolol, carvedilol) may have a more protective effect than hydrophilic β-blockers *(35)*.

The data on the role of ACE inhibition specifically for the prevention of sudden death in infarct survivors is somewhat less compelling. The first Cooperative North Scandinavian Enalapril Survival Study (CONSENSUS I) evaluated the effect of enalopril vs placebo in patients with NYHA Class IV heart failure. Although enalopril therapy resulted in 40% reduction in total mortality, the effect was almost entirely because of prevention of deaths as a result of progressive heart failure rather than sudden cardiac death *(36)*. Similar results were observed in the Study of Left-Ventricular Dysfunction (SOLVD) trial in patients with Class II–IV heart failure *(37)*. However, the second second Vasodilator-Heart Failure Trial (VHeFT II) demonstrated that the reduction in total mortality conferred by enalopril in comparison to hydralazine plus isosorbide dinitrate was attributable mostly to a reduction in sudden death *(38)*. Subsequently, two large-scale multicenter trials have suggested that ACE inhibitor therapy specifically reduces risk of sudden cardiac death in patients with heart failure following myocardial infarction. Trandolapril (TRACE) and ramipril (AIRE) therapy compared with placebo-reduced sudden-death mortality by approximately 30% *(39–41)*. This benefit did not appear to extend to patients without symptomatic heart failure following MI in the Survival and Ventricular Enlargement Trial (SAVE) study *(42)*.

A post-hoc analysis of Evaluation of Losartan in the Elderly (ELITE) study initially raised the hope that angiotensin II receptor antagonists would provide further reduction in total and sudden-death mortality compared to ACE inhibition *(43)*. However, the definitive trial of this hypothesis, the ELITE II study, which compared losartan and captopril, demonstrated no difference (yearly mortality 11.7 vs 10.4% in losartan vs captopril treated patients, $p = 0.16$) Losartan was better tolerated than captopril, however *(44)*. These findings support the conclusion that ACE inhibitors should be initially used for patients with heart failure, and angiotensin II receptor blockers reserved for those who do not tolerate ACE inhibitors.

In the Randomized Aldactone Evaluation Study (RALES), sprinolactone had a 30% reduction in total mortality with reduction in both sudden and progressive heart failure death in patients with severe heart failure (NYHA Class III–IV symptoms, ejection factor < 35%) who were already treated with ACE inhibitors, loop diuretics, and digitalis *(45)*.

In summary, primary prevention for the prevention of sudden death in the majority of patients with symptomatic heart failure should focus on contemporary therapy with agents demonstrated to significantly reduce total mortality, such as β-blockers, ACE inhibitors, and spirono-lactone. Aggressive lipid management and coronary revascularization when appropriate and avoidance of other are known arrhythmia triggers (electrolyte abnormalities, medication side effects) are also important factors. General usage of antiarrhythmic drugs, with the possible exception of amiodarone, is contraindicated. As discussed here, in patients with symptomatic arrhythmias, the choice of antiarrhythmic agent is limited by the potential for proarrhythmia and negative inotropic effects.

THE MANAGEMENT OF ATRIAL FIBRILLATION

As mentioned previously, the onset of atrial fibrillation is an important negative prognostic sign in patients with CHF *(3)*. There are at least three factors that contribute to this observation. The loss of atrial contribution to ventricular filling and irregular ventricular response during atrial fibrillation results in significantly decreased ventricular function. Even more importantly, there is growing evidence that high-ventricular rates during atrial fibrillation frequently cause at least some degree of superimposed tachycardia-related myopathy *(46)*. Finally, prior to the realization of the potential for harm with many antiarrhythmic drugs, the onset of atrial fibrillation often prompted inappropriate antiarrhythmic drug therapy.

The foundations of treatment for recurrent paroxysmal or permanent (requiring cardioversion to restore sinus rhythm) atrial fibrillation in heart failure are similar to those in patients without structural heart disease; the risks of adverse events are considerably higher, however. Warfarin anticoagulation (international normalized ratio [INR] 2.0–3.0) should be maintained indefinitely in all patients with atrial fibrillation and structural heart disease without a clear contraindication *(1)*. Considerable controversy exists regarding additional treatment, specifically to the superiority of strategies to restore sinus rhythm (rhythm control) vs those that control the rapid ventricular response (rate control). Results of the Atrial Fibrillation Follow-Up Investigation of Rhythm Management (AFFIRM) trial *(47)* will help to determine preferred strategy. The Strategies of Treatment of Atrial Fibrillation (STAF) trial, demonstrated that patients who were successfully maintained in sinus rhythm were significantly less likely to suffer endpoints of death and major cardiovascular events than patients in a rate-control strategy *(48)*. However, maintenance of sinus rhythm was achieved in only 23% of the cohort at 3 years, even with amiodarone. Furthermore, this treatment response may suggest a selection bias (healthier patients more likely to respond to antiarrhythmic drugs) than a true benefit of rhythm control treatment strategy. At present, deciding between these treatment strategies depends on degree of symptoms, patient preference and initial success of therapy.

Rate Control Strategy

Central to this strategy is control of the ventricular response, both at rest and with exercise, without regard to continuing fibrillation in the atrium. Although guidelines for appropriate rate control are scarce, the resting rate should be consistently below 80 bpm and the rate during casual exertion should only occasionally exceed 100–110 bpm. Holter monitoring may be helpful in assessing heart rate response in ambulatory patients after rate control at rest is demonstrated to be adequate. Rate control agents all affect conduction at the level of the atrioventricular (AV) node and include β-blockers, calcium-channel antagonists, and digitalis. Although clearly indicated in the treatment of atrial fibrillation in systolic heart failure, digitalis monotherapy is no more effective than placebo in control of exercise heart rate (49). Digitalis in combination with other agents does exert an additive effect. Amiodarone is occasionally used as a rate control agent after failure as a rhythm control agent. Although amiodarone does provide effective rate control and has less negative inotropic effects than many other rate control agents, in general, the cost and fear of long-term extracardiac side effects argue against this practice.

Most patients receive symptom relief and are successfully treated by a rate control strategy. In fact, one of the arguments for this strategy is its relative convenience for patients, avoiding admission, cardioversion procedures and exposure to antiarrhythmic drugs. However, side effects are also possible in this strategy; rate control drugs may have negative inotropic effects or may cause episodic symptomatic bradycardia. In patients whose ventricular response cannot be controlled with the maximum tolerated doses of AV nodal blocking agents, catheter ablation of the AV junction is often extremely effective. Catheter ablation not only controls ventricular rate, but also provides a regular ventricular rate which further improves symptoms and ventricular performance. Success rates for this procedure are greater than 95%. Randomized comparisons of ablation vs pharmacologic rate control therapy have demonstrated better symptomatic control and improvement in left-ventricular function in patients with severe symptoms (50,51). Nonetheless, it is important to consider that AV junction ablation results in permanent pacemaker dependence. In addition, right-ventricular pacing with the resultant pacing-induced left-bundle branch block may result in worsened ventricular synchrony; biventricular pacing may obviate this problem. There have been reports of sudden cardiac death following AV junctional ablation because of bradycardia-dependent *torsade de pointes*, presumably due to abrupt heart rate reduction (52). This complication can be avoided by high rate (80–90 beats/min) ventricular pacing for 4–6 weeks following ablation. Despite appropriate pacing intervention, there remains a 1–2% risk of late sudden death, which most likely represents the natural history of advanced heart disease rather than complications of the procedure (53).

Rhythm Control Strategy

Most physicians have a bias that restoring sinus rhythm provides a hemodynamically superior solution to control of heart rate, particularly in patients with advanced structural heart disease. It is important to emphasize that the rhythm control strategy, even when successful, does not mitigate the need for long-term anticoagulation and exposes patients to the risks of drug therapy. In general, any single antiarrhythmic drug is only 50% likely to completely prevent atrial fibrillation recurrence at 6 months (1); although not specifically tested, drug efficacy in the setting of heart failure may be even worse. Tiered therapy with several different doses or medications coupled with serial cardioversions may be necessary. More often, the use of drugs to decrease the frequency of rather than totally prevent recurrent atrial fibrillation episodes is a reasonable goal. As discussed above, Class I antiarrhythmic drugs are contraindicated in patients with structural heart disease *(1,17,18)*. This limits antiarrhythmic drug choice to sotalol, amiodarone and dofetilide, although several other agents (azimilide and "second-generation" forms of amiodarone) are on the horizon.

Although generally considered safe and moderately effective, sotalol has several important disadvantages in treating atrial fibrillation in heart failure. Anecdotally, sotalol seems to be less well tolerated than other β-blockers and may exacerbate congestive failure. In addition, *torsade de pointes* proarrhythmia, which is more frequent in the setting of ventricular dysfunction and renal insufficiency, requiring constant attention to electrolyte control and other drugs that further increase risk. For these reasons, sotalol is generally avoided in our practice.

Amiodarone is the main-stay of rhythm control therapy for atrial fibrillation in the setting of ventricular dysfunction. In addition to having greater efficacy than other drugs in controlling atrial fibrillation *(54)*, amiodarone has no important negative inotropic effects, minimal risk of torsade de pointes type proarrhythmia and provides effective ventricular rate control during arrhythmia recurrence. After a variable loading dose, chronic therapy is usually instituted at 200 mg/day. Limitations to amiodarone therapy include interactions with warfarin and digitalis therapy (typically requiring dose reduction of both agents by 50%), sinus node dysfunction (particularly in the setting of concomitant β-blocker therapy), and dose and time-dependent risk of pulmonary and hepatic toxicity. Amiodarone effects thyroid gland function in approximately 10% of treated patients. Hypothyroidism is much more common than hyperthyroidism and is usually managed with thyroid hormone supplements.

Dofetilide was recently approved for treatment of atrial fibrillation, and may provide an alternative to amiodarone therapy in patients with advanced heart failure. The Danish Investigations of Arrhythmia and Mortality on Dofetilide in Congestive Heart Failure (DIAMOND-CHF) study demonstrated that dofetilide was more effective than placebo in conversion of atrial fibrillation and maintenance of sinus rhythm in patients with symptomatic heart failure. There was no effect of dofetilide on survival, but there was a 3.3% incidence of *torsade de pointes* in the dofetilide group *(55)*. The risk of torsade with dofetilide is dose dependent, and initiation of therapy and subsequent dosage adjustments must be performed in the hospital with careful telemetry monitoring. Electrolyte disorders and many other medications exacerbate dofetilide's effect on QT prolongation and increase the risk of *torsade de pointes*. For these reasons, and for our own anecdotal experience, which suggests relatively low efficacy in prevention of recurrent atrial fibrillation, dofetilide is seldom used in our practice.

In summary, atrial fibrillation frequently exacerbates chronic heart failure. In addition to warfarin anticoagulation, relief of symptoms and prevention of high-ventricular rates can be accomplished with rate control or rhythm control strategies. In our experience, amiodarone is the antiarrhythmic agent of choice in this setting.

THE MANAGEMENT OF ASYMPTOMATIC VENTRICULAR TACHYCARDIA

As was discussed in the first section, antiarrhythmic drug therapy for asymptomatic ventricular ectopy is not indicated. Although direct evidence of harm in all etiologies of heart failure is lacking, this tenet is held on the basis of the CAST study in patients with ischemic heart disease (17), the retrospective SPAF analysis (although this focused on treatment of atrial fibrillation) (18), and the lack of consistent benefit in primary prevention trials using amiodarone (22–27). Although often considered as a harbinger of sustained arrhythmias, frequent ventricular ectopy is not sufficiently predictive of arrhythmic death as opposed to progressive pump failure (12–14). Furthermore, with the possible exception of amiodarone (in GESICA [24] and CAMIAT [27], but not in other trials; see above for discussion), no specific antiarrhythmic drug has been demonstrated helpful in this setting. Amiodarone is indicated for use in symptomatic ventricular ectopy unresponsive to β-blocker therapy. Preliminary experience suggests that dofetilide may provide a reasonable alternative.

The treatment of nonsustained ventricular tachycardia depends on heart failure etiology. Two important recent studies have verified that patients with prior myocardial infarction, nonsustained VT, depressed left-ventricular function (ejection function < 35-40%) and inducible sustained VT at electrophysiologic study represent an extremely high-risk group (55% mortality at 5 years). In the Multicenter Automatic Defibrillator Implantation Trial (MADIT), patients who fit these characteristics and whose VT was not suppressed by intravenous procainamide were randomized to antiarrhythmic drug therapy (usually amiodarone) vs implantable cardioverter defibrillators (ICD) therapy. The trial was terminated prematurely when a significant survival benefit was recognized in the ICD group (56). A major criticism of the MADIT trial was the limited and unequal use (favoring the ICD group) of β-blockers. The Multicenter UnSustained Tachycardia Trial (MUSTT), although originally conceived as a controlled trial of the strategy of programmed stimulation-guided antiarrhythmic drug therapy, provided compelling data for the superiority of ICD therapy in this setting. Patients with inducible VT were randomized to no antiarrhythmic therapy or guided drug therapy; patients who remained inducible after several attempts could be offered ICD implantation. After a median follow-up of 39 months, there was a significant reduction in overall mortality in patients who received ICD therapy in comparison to both the groups receiving EPS guided antiarrhythmic drug therapy or no antiarrhythmic therapy (24 vs 55%, $p <$ 0.001) *(57)*. Because of these trials, patients ischemic cardiomyopathy and NSVT should be risk-stratified with EPS testing; patients with inducible sustained VT should be treated with ICD implantation.

Similar data are not available to guide treatment for patients with nonischemic cardiomyopathy and asymptomatic NSVT. Again, NSVT in this setting does not clearly distinguish risk of future ventricular arrhythmias *(12–14)*. EPS in nonischemic heart failure is not sufficiently sensitive or specific to guide therapy *(58)*. Many heart failure experts treat such patients with amiodarone empirically, based on the supposition that this therapy should at very least do no harm.

It is feasible that the benefits observed with ICD therapy in higher risk patient subsets may extend more generally in patients with heart failure. The second Multicenter Automatic Defibrillator Implantation Trial (MADIT II) compared ICD therapy vs standard care in otherwise unselected patients with healed MI and LVEF below 30%. The trial was terminated prematurely when a 31% reduction in all-cause mortality (14.2 vs 19.8% at 20-month follow-up) was demonstrated for the ICD group *(14a)*. Prophylactic implantation of a defibrillator in patients with MI and reduced ejection fraction *(14a)*. Interestingly, this mortality benefit occurred at the expense of an increase in need for heart failure hospitalization (19.9 vs 14.4%); some investigators believe this may be due to the harmful effects of right-ventricular pacing from the ICD.

Data from several multicenter studies may provide important insight into primary prevention in such patients *(59)*. The Sudden Cardiac Death–Heart Failure Trial (SCD-HeFT, presently closed to enrollment), is a randomized comparison of placebo, amiodarone, and ICD therapy patients with NHYA Class II–III heart failure without any qualifying arrhythmia variables. DEFINITE is a similar study, focusing only on patients with nonischemic cardiomyopathy, comparing placebo to ICD therapy. The results of these trials will hopefully better define the role of both ICD and amiodarone therapy and the utility of several risk stratification strategies in subsets of patients with heart failure with no evidence of prior sustained ventricular arrhythmias.

THE MANAGEMENT OF SYNCOPE

Syncope, independent of mechanism, confers a dire prognosis in the setting of advanced heart failure. In a study by Middlekauff and coworkers, the actuarial incidence of sudden death at 1 year was 45% in heart failure patients with syncope, in comparison to 12% without *(60)*. Obviously, syncope can be multifactorial, and excessive medication induced hypotension or orthostasis must be considered. Nonetheless, a high index of suspicion for arrhythmic causes of syncope should be maintained. Many investigators feel that a careful history for the events immediately preceding loss of consciousness or events that are sufficiently abrupt to result in significant injury verify the diagnosis of arrhythmic cause with some degree of certainty. Although EPS are used to determine the mechanism of syncope, and though the success of this strategy has been established in patients with healed infarction *(58)*, the sensitivity of EPS in other etiologies of ventricular dysfunction is uncertain but assumed to be poor. On the basis of the proven efficacy of ICD therapy in patients with sustained arrhythmias (most notably in the antiarrhythmics vs implantable defibrillators [AVID] study *[61]*) and the lack of consistent efficacy of antiarrhythmic drugs, ICD therapy is indicated in patients who have prior syncope with inducible VT at EPS.

Present American Heart Association/American College of Cardiology (AHA/ACC) guidelines require inducible VT at EP study to justify ICD implantation in patients with an episode of syncope *(62)*. Although these guidelines are presently in review, the limited sensitivity of EPS in nonischemic cardiomyopathy presents a management problem. Knight and collegeaues began to address this conundrum with a small case-control study of patients with syncope who were treated with ICD therapy despite negative EPS (63). They found a significant incidence of appropriate ICD therapy in follow-up, which approximated that observed in patients who received ICDs for more traditional indications.

In summary, syncope confers a poor prognosis in the setting of advanced heart failure. In patients who have syncope that appears to be arrhythmic in nature, EPS is performed in our practice independent of heart failure etiology. Unless other causes (such as conduction system disease, or rarely, supraventricular tachycardia) can be confirmed, our strong bias leads to ICD therapy in patients who have reasonable treatment options from a heart failure standpoint.

SUMMARY

Arrhythmia management is critical to the success of caring for patients with heart failure. Although specific antiarrhythmic therapy has not proven useful in the primary prevention of sudden death in this setting, improvements in heart failure therapy have resulted in achieving this goal. Certainly symptomatic arrhythmias often require therapy, and both trial data and extensive clinical experience have demonstrated the safety and efficacy of amiodarone. Patients at the highest degree of risk (infarct survivors with EF less than 30% or those with LV dysfunction and NSVT, patients with arrhythmic syncope or sustained ventricular arrhythmias) are best treated with defibrillator therapy, unless prognosis from a heart failure standpoint countermands *(64)*.

REFERENCES

1. Prystowsky EN, Benson DW, Foster V, et al. Management of patients with atrial fibrillation. Circulation 1996;93:1262–1277.
2. Ryder KM, Benjamin EJ. Epidemiology and significance of atrial fibrillation. Am J Cardiol 1999;84(9A):131R–138R.
3. Middlekauff HR, Stevenson WG, Stevenson LW. Prognostic significance of atrial fibrillation in advanced heart failure: a study of 390 patients. Circulation 1991;84:40–48.
4. Aronow WS, Ahn C, Kronzon I. Prognosis of congestive heart failure after prior myocardial infarction in older persons with atrial fibrillation versus sinus rhythm. Am J Cardiol 2001;87:224,225.
5. DiMarco JP, Haines DE. Sudden Cardiac Death. Curr Probl Cardiol. 1990: 187–232.
6. Gradman A, Deedwania P, Cody R, et al. Predictors of total mortality and sudden death in mild to moderate heart failure. Captopril-Digoxin Study Group. J Amer Coll Cardiol 1989;14:564–570.
7. Kjekshus J: Arrhythmias and mortality in congestive heart failure. Am J Cardiol 1990;65:42–48.
8. Hinkle LE Jr. Thaler HT. Clinical classification of cardiac deaths. Circulation. 1982;65:457–464.
9. Kim SG, Fisher JD, Furman S, et al. Benefits of implantable defibrillators are overestimated by sudden death rates and better represented by the total arrhythmic death rate. J Am Coll Cardiol 1991;17:1587–1592.
10. Luu M, Stevenson WG, Stevenson LW, Baron K, Walden J. Diverse mechanisms of unexpected cardiac arrest in advanced heart failure. Circulation 1989;1675–1680.
11. Uretsky BF, Thygesen K, Armstrong PW, et al. Acute coronary findings at autopsy in heart failure patients with sudden death: results from the assessment of treatment with lisinopril and survival (ATLAS) trial. Circulation 2000;102:611–616.
12. Doval HC, Nul DR, Grancelli HO, et al: Nonsustained ventricular tachycardia in heart failure: Independent marker of increased mortality due to sudden death. Circulation 1996;94:3189–3203.
13. Packer M. Lack of relation between ventricular arrhythmias and sudden death in patients with chronic heart failure. Circulation 1992;85:I50–I56.
14. Teerlink JR, Jalaluddin M, Anderson S, et al. Ambulatory ventricular arrhythmias in patients with heart failure do not specifically predict an increased risk of sudden death. Circulation 2000;101:40–46.
14a. Moss AJ, Zareba, W, Itall WJ, et al. Prophylactic implantation of a defribrillator in patients with myocardial infarction and reduced ejection fraction. N Engl J Med 2002;346:877–883.
15. Stevenson WG, Stevenson LW, Middlekauff HR, Saxon LA. Sudden death prevention in patients with advanced ventricular dysfunction. Circulation 1993;88:2953–2961.
16. Wilbur DJ. Ventricular tachycardia in patients with heart failure. In: Zipes DP, Jalife J (eds) Cardiac Electrophysiology: From Cell to Bedside. 3rd edition. W.B. Saunders Company, Philadelphia, PA: 1999, pp, 569–579.

17. Echt DS, Liebson PR, Mitchell LB, et al. Mortality and morbidity in patients receiving encainide, flecainide, or placebo. The Cardiac Arrhythmia Suppression Trial. N Engl J Med 1991;324:781–788.

18. Flaker GC, Blackshear JL, McBride R, et al. Antiarrhythmic drug therapy and cardiac mortality in atrial fibrillation. J Am Coll Cardiol 1992;20:527–532.

19. Teo K, Yusuf S, Furber C. Effects of prophylactic antiarrhythmic drug therapy in acute myocardial infarction: an overview of results from randomized controlled trial. JAMA 1993;270:1589–1595.

20. Waldo A, Camm A, deRuyter H, et al. For the survival with oral d-sotalol (SWORD) investigators. Effect of d-sotalol on mortality in patients with left ventricular dysfunction after recent and remote myocardial infarction. Lancet 1996;348:7–12.

21. Stevenson WG, Stevenson LW, Middlekauff HR, et al. Improving survival for patients with advanced heart failure: a study of 737 consecutive patients. J Amer Coll Cardiol 1995;26:1417–1423.

22. Singh SN, Fletcher RD, Fisher SG, et al: Amiodarone in patients with congestive heart failure and asymptomatic ventricular arrhythmia. N Engl J Med 1995;333:77–82.

23. Burkart F, Pfisterer M, Kiowski W, et al. Effect of antiarrhythmic therapy on mortality in survivors of myocardial infarction with asymptomatic complex ventricular arrhythmias: Basel Anti-arrhythmic Study of Infarct Survival (BASIS). J Am Coll Cardiol 1990;16:1711–1718.

24. Doval IIC, Nul DR, Grancelli HO, et al. Randomised trial of low-dose amiodarone in severe congestive heart failure. Grupo de Estudio de la Sobrevida en la Insuficiencia Cardiaca en Argentina (GESICA). Lancet. 1994;344:493–498.

25. Singh S, Fletcher R, Fisher S, et al. for the Survival Trail of Antiarrhythmic Therapy in Congestive Heart Failure (CHF-STAT) Investigators. Amiodarone in patients with congestive heart failure and asymptomatic ventricular arrhythmia. N Engl J Med 1995;333:77–82.

26. Julian D, Camm A, Frangin G, et al. for the European Myocardial Infarct Amiodarone Trial (EMIAT) Investigators. Randomized trial of effect of amiodarone on mortality in patients with left ventricular dysfunction after recent myocardial infarction: EMIAT. Lancet 1997;349:667–674.

27. Cairns J, Connolly S, Roberts R, et al. for the Canadian Amiodarone Myocardial Infarction Arrhythmia Trial (CAMIAT) Investigators. Lancet 1997;349:675–682.

28. The B-Blocker Heart Attack Trial Research Group, A randomized trial of propranolol in patients with acute myocardial infarction. JAMA 1982;247:1707–1714.

29. The Norwegian Multicenter Study Group. Timolol-induced reduction in mortality and reinfarction in patients surviving acute myocardial infarction. N Engl J Med 1981;304:801–807.

30. The MERIT-HF Study Group. Effect of metoprolol CR/XL in chronic heart failure: Metoprolol CR/XL Randomised Intervention Trial in Congestive Heart Failure (MERIT-HF). Lancet 1999; 353:2001–2007.

31. Packer M, Bristow MR, Cohn JN, et al. for the U.S. Carvedilol Heart Failure Study Group. The effect of carvedilol on morbidity and mortality in patients with chronic heart failure. N Engl J Med 1996;334:1349–1355.

32. Packer M, Coats AJ, Fowler MB, et al: Prospective Randomized Cumulative Survival Study Group. Effect of carvedilol on survival in severe chronic heart failure. N Engl J Med 2001;344(22):1651–1658.

33. Domanaski M. for The BEST Steering Committee. BEST (Beta-Blocker Evaluation Survival Trial). Paper presented at:1999 Scientific Sessions of the American Heart Association; November 7-10, 1999; Atlanta, GA.

34. Teerlink JR, Massie BM. Beta-adrenergic blocker morality trials in congestive heart failure. Am J Cardiol 1999;84:94R–102R.

35. Hjalmarson A. Prevention of sudden cardiac death with beta blockers. Clin Cardiol 1999;22:VII–5.
36. The CONSENSUS Trial Study Group. Effects of enalapril on mortality in severe congestive heart failure: Results of the Cooperative North Scandinavian Enalapril Survival Study (CONSENSUS). N Engl J Med 1987;316:1429–1435.
37. The SOLVD Investigators. Effect of enalapril on survival in patients with reduced left ventricular ejection fractions and congestive heart failure. N Engl J Med 1991;325:293–302.
38. Cohn J, Johnson G, Ziesche S, et al. A comparison of enalapril with hydralazine-isosorbide dinitrate in the treatment of chronic congestive heart failure. N Engl J Med 1991;325:303–310.
39. Kober L, Torp-Pedersen C, Carlsen J, et al. for the Trandolapril Cardiac Evaluation (TRACE) Study Group. A clinical trial of the angiotensin-converting-enzyme inhibitor trandolapril in patients with left ventricular dysfunction after myocardial infarction. N Engl J Med 1995;333:1670–1676.
40. The Acute Infarction Ramipril Efficacy (AIRE) Study Investigators. Effect of ramipril on mortality and morbidity of survivors of acute myocardial infarction with clinical evidence of heart failure. Lancet 1993;342:821–828.
41. Cleland J, Erhardt L, Murray G, et al. on behalf of the AIRE Study Investigators. Effect of ramipril on morbidity and mode of death among survivors of acute myocardial infarction with clinical evidence of heart failure. Eur Heart J 1997;18:41–51.
42. Pfeffer M, Braunwald E, Moye L, et al., for the Survival and Ventricular Enlargement Trial (SAVE) Investigators. Effect of captopril on mortality and morbidity in patients with left ventricular dysfunction after myocardial infarction. N Engl J Med 1992;327:669–677.
43. Pitt B, Segal R, Martinez FA, et al. on behalf of ELITE Study Investigators. Randomised trial of losartan versus captopril in patients over 65 with heart failure (Evaluation of Losartan In the Elderly Study, ELITE). Lancet 1997;349:747–752.
44. Pitt B, Poole-Wilson P, Segal R, et al. Effect of losartan compared with captopril on mortality in patients with symptomatic heart failure: randomized trial - the Losartan Heart Failure Survival Study - ELITE II. Lancet 2000;355:1582–1587.
45. Pitt B, Zannad F, Remme WJ, et al. for the Randomized Aldactone Evaluation Study Investigators. The effect of spironolactone on morbidity and mortality in patients with severe heart failure. N Engl J Med. 1999;341:709–717.
46. Grogan M, Smith HC, Gersh BJ, Wood DL. Left ventricular dysfunction due to atrial fibrillation in patients initially believed to have idiopathic dilated cardiomyopathy. Am J Cardiol 1992;69:1570.
47. The Planning and Steering Committees of the AFFIRM study for the NHLBI AFFIRM Investigators. Atrial fibrillation follow up investigation of rhythm management-the AFFIRM study design. Am J Cardiol 1997;79:1198–1202.
48. Carlsson J. Strategies of treatment of atrial fibrillation. Paper presented at the 2001 Scientific Session of the American College of Cardiology, Orlando, FL.
49. David D, Di Segni E, Klein HO, Kaplinskhy E. Inefficacy of digitalis in the control of heart rate in patients with chronic atrial fibrillation. Beneficial effect of an added beta adrenergic blocking agent. Am J Cardiol 1979;44:1378–1382.
50. Kay GN, Bubien RS, Epstein AE, Plumb VJ. Effect of catheter ablation of the atrioventricular junction on quality of life and exercise tolerance in paroxysmal atrial fibrillation. Am J Cardiol 1988;62:741.
51. Brignole M, Gianfranchi L, Menozzi C, et al. Influence of atrioventricular junction radiofrequency ablation in patients with chronic atrial fibrillation and flutter on quality of life and cardiac performance. Am J Cardiol 1994;74:242.

52. Conti JB, Mills RM Jr, Woodard DA, Curtis AB. QT dispersion is a marker for life-threatening ventricular arrhythmias after atrioventricular nodal ablation using radiofrequency energy. Am J Cardiol 1997;79:1412.

53. Wood MA. Brown-Mahoney C. Kay GN. Ellenbogen KA. Clinical outcomes after ablation and pacing therapy for atrial fibrillation: a meta-analysis. Circulation. 2000;101:1138-44.

54. Gosselink ATM, Crijns HJ, Van Gelder IC, et al. Low-dose amiodarone for maintenance of sinus rhythm after cardioversion of atrial fibrillation or flutter. JAMA 1992;267:3289–3293.

55. Torp-Pedersen C, Moller M, Bloch-Thomsen PE, et al. Dofetilide in patients with congestive heart failure and left ventricular dysfunction. N Engl J Med 1999;341:857–865.

56. Moss A, Hall W, Cannom D, et al., for the Multicenter Automatic Defibrillator Implantation Trial (MADIT) Investigators. Improved survival with an implanted defibrillator in patients with coronary disease at high risk for ventricular arrhythmia. N Engl J Med 1996;335:1933–1940.

57. Buxton AE, Lee KL, Fisher JD et al. for the Multicenter Unsustained Tachycardia Trial Investigators. A randomized study of the prevention of sudden death in patients with coronary artery disease. N Engl J Med 1999;341:1882–1890.

58. Poll DS. Marchlinski FE. Buxton AE. Josephson ME. Usefulness of programmed stimulation in idiopathic dilated cardiomyopathy. Am J Cardiol 1986;58:992–997.

59. Naccarelli GV, Wolbrette DL, Dell'Orfano JT, Patel HM, Luck JC. A decade of clinical trial developments in post-myocardial infarction, congestive heart failure and sustained tachyarrhythmia patients: from CAST to AVID and beyond. J Cardiovasc Electrophysiol 1998;9:864.

60. Middlekauff HR. Stevenson WG. Stevenson LW. Saxon LA. Syncope in advanced heart failure: high risk of sudden death regardless of origin of syncope. J Am Coll Cardiol 1993;21:110–116.

61. The Antiarrhythmics versus Implantable Defibrillator Investigators. A comparison of antiarrhythmic-drug therapy with implantable defibrillators in patients resuscitated from near-fatal ventricular arrhythmias. N Engl J Med 1997;337:1576–1583.

62. Gregoratos G, Cheitlin MD, Conill A, Epstein AE, Fellows C, et al. ACC/AHA guidelines for implantation of cardiac pacemakers and antiarrhythmia devices: a report of the ACC/AHA Task Force on Practice Guidelines (Committee on Pacemaker Implantation). J Am Coll Cardiol. 1998,31:1175–1206.

63. Knight BP, Goyal R, Pelosi F, et al. Outcome of patients with nonischemic dilated cardiomyopathy and unexplained syncope treated with an implantable defibrillator. J Am Coll Cardiol 1999;33:1964–1970.

64. Josephson ME, Callans DJ, Buxton AE. The role of the implantable cardioverter-defibrillator for prevention of sudden cardiac death. Ann Int Med 2000;133:901–910.

16 Emerging Therapies in Heart Failure

David Zeltsman, MD and Michael A. Acker, MD

Traditionally, heart failure has been thought secondary to impaired left ventricular pump performance. According to this view, systolic dysfunction is secondary to contractile failure. Recently, a new view of heart failure has been developed where systolic dysfunction is thought secondary to a structural increase in ventricular chamber volume. Instead of contractile failure leading to chamber dilatation, chamber dilatation occurs as an early response that results in decreased wall motion that is mandated to generate a normal stroke volume from a larger end-diastolic volume. Remodeling is the term used to refer to the pathologic change in chamber length and shape, not related to a preload-mandated increase in sacromere length. As the heart remodels and dilates, the radius of curvature increases, increasing wall tension, leading to increased myocardial oxygen consumption, decreased subendocardial blood flow, impaired energetics, and increased arrhythmias. Overall, poor prognosis directly correlates with the degree of remodeling (1).

According to this view, remodeling, not contractile failure, is the key to the severity of depression of ejection fraction and poor prognosis. The process has also been shown to be reversible. Current therapies that improve mortality, such as angiotensin-converting enzyme (ACE) inhibitors and new generation β-blockers, can inhibit progressive chamber remodeling and improve survival. Nevertheless, despite the significant advances in the pharmacological support of failing heart, the results remain far from perfect. The mortality continues to be high and hospitalization costly. There is a growing understanding that old, as well as new and evolving surgical therapies, that in the past were contraindi-

From: *Contemporary Cardiology: Heart Failure:*
A Clinician's Guide to Ambulatory Diagnosis and Treatment
Edited by: M. L. Jessup and E. Loh © Humana Press Inc., Totowa, NJ

cated for the failing heart, can be used successfully to impact on the process of ventricular remodeling and improve cardiac function.

Cardiac transplantation remains the gold standard of surgical therapies for advanced and end-stage heart failure. However, the Achilles heel of heart transplantation is the persistent and worsening shortage of organ donors. Although 4296 patients were on the UNOS national patient waiting list as of April 2001, only 49% will proceed to heart transplantation. Because of the unavailability of a donor heart, 709 patients died while on the cardiac transplant waiting list *(2)*. Despite its success, transplantation is epidemiologically trivial. It will remain a very limited option that trades one disease for another and can only be applied to a small number of patients who potentially could benefit. Therefore, aggressive search for alternative surgical management of end-stage heart disease must be sought.

Surgical revascularization for patients with ejection fractions less than 20% to recruit hibernating myocardium is becoming commonplace *(3)*. These patients are generally sicker with more perioperative risk factors and, though having increased hospital mortality of approximately 4–6% *(4)*, they enjoy 90% and 64% survival at 1 and 5 years, respectively *(4)*. Patients with ischemic cardiomyopathy, evidence of viable myocardium, and presence of bypassable vessels can be revascularized with permissible risk achieving 88% perioperative survival with 72% of the patients alive at 1 year. These results are reproducible and have been reported by different authors *(5–8)*.

Mitral valve repair for both primary and secondary severe mitral regurgitation in dilated cardiomyopathic ventricles with ejection fraction less than 30% is being actively pursued. Mitral insufficiency is an important complication of dilative cardiomyopathy, resulting from enlargement of the mitral annular-ventricular apparatus with ensuing loss of valve leaflet coaptation *(9–11)*. As the annular dilation progresses, centrally located functional regurgitant jet develops despite structural preservation of chordal and papillary muscle complex *(11)*. Ischemic mitral regurgitation appears to be more complex and is multifactorial resulting from deformational changes in the ventricular geometry, annular dilatation, and papillary muscles dysfunction. Often the posterior leaflet becomes functionally restricted as a result of ventricular enlargement. In patients with significant (>2+) secondary mitral regurgitation, mitral valve repair should be considered in New York Heart Association (NYHA) Class III/IV patients with dilated cardiomyopathies. Bolling has demonstrated operative mortality <5% with significant improvement in NYHA class symptoms, as well as good survival rates at 1 and 2 years *(10,11)*. The annuloplasty is performed with complete ring and undersizing the mitral annulus and offers effective correction of mitral regurgitation in heart failure patients. The procedure is well tolerated and the elimination of mitral regurgitation contributes to reversed remodeling with restoration of elliptical left-ventricular contour and decreased sphericity (11). If mitral valve repair is not possible, it is essential that mitral valve replacement be performed with retention of the subchordal attachments. Preservation of both the anterior and posterior chorded attachments to the papillary muscles helps to maintain normal ventricular geometry and function following mitral valve replacement (12–15).

The concept of surgically reversing the remodeling process—partial left ventriculectomy—for patients with Class IV idiopathic-dilated cardiomyopathies was introduced by Batista in 1996. He described an operation in which normal muscle between the anterior and posterior papillary muscles is resected along with mitral valve repair/replacement so to restore the ventricle to a more normal volume/mass/diameter relationship. The reduction in ventricular diameter, according to LaPlace's law results in decreased ventricular wall tension and thus improved systolic performance (16,17). Though many patients improved markedly, perioperative mortality was high (>20%) in many reports. In the largest and best controlled series from the Cleveland Clinic, perioperative mortality was only 3.2%, but 16% required left ventricular assist devices (LVAD) following the procedure. Many patients improved to allow removal from the transplant list but freedom from death, need for LVAD, need for transplant or return to Class IV heart failure symptoms was 50% and 37% at 1 and 2 years. After initial success, many patients would redilate (18,19). Overall enthusiasm for the procedure has waned. Selection criteria needs to improve before the role of partial left-ventriculectomy for end-stage heart failure patients can be determined.

Direct surgical restoration of left-ventricular geometry with reduction in left-ventricular size and shape has evolved over the last few years from partial left-ventriculectomy to a modification of the Dor procedure for left-ventricular aneurysm (20) called endoventricular circular patch plasty or surgical ventricular restoration (SVR). This procedure is considered for patients with ischemic cardiomyopathies with post-large anterior wall myocardial infarctions resulting in dilated spherical left ventricles associated with an area of anterior akinesia or dyskinesia. An endoventricular dacron patch is used to exclude akinetic or dyskinetic portions of the anterior wall and septum, so to restore a more normal size and shape to the left ventricle. This then results in more normal ventricular geometry (elliptical instead of a spherical ventricle) and improved systolic performance. A recent report on the results of this procedure, combined usually with coronary artery bypass grafting in 586 patients, reported overall mortality of 7.7%, left ventricular and systolic volume index decreased from 98 ± 95 to 64 ± 40 ml/m^2, whereas left-ventricular ejection function improved from 29.5 to 40% postoperatively *(21–23)*. Carefully controlled studies need to be performed to determine if decreased ventricular size results in diastolic compromise, if the increase in ejection fraction in smaller ventricles translates to an increase stroke volume, and whether further remodeling occurring after the operation limits its overall long-term success *(23)*. A National Institutes of Health (NIH)-sponsored, multicentered randomized trial is planned for patients with heart failure and coronary artery disease amenable to surgical revascularization (STICH). In patients with reported left-ventricular dysfunction, SVR and surgical revascularization will be randomized to either surgical revascularization alone or to surgical revascularization and SVR to determine its impact on cardiac function and overall survival.

Recently, new girdling devices have been evaluated to limit or to reverse ventricular remodeling. Lessons learned from the clinical experience with dynamic cardiomyoplasty revealed that much of its benefit was derived from the girdling effect of the muscle wrap and not from an increase in stroke volume as originally conceived. Evaluation of the prosthetic external constraint CardioCor (Acorn Cardiovascular, Inc.) is currently under active clinical investigation and is based on the belief that heart failure is primarily the result of ongoing ventricular remodeling. Preclinical evaluation in canine models of chronic-dilated cardiomyopathy and heart failure have demonstrated a halting or reversal of ventricular remodeling and preservation or improved cardiac function. In addition, improved myocyte contraction and relaxation, enhance inotropic response, as well as altered gene expression have been demonstrated *(24–29)*. In more than 60 patients who have had the Acorn jacket placed in Europe, no evidence of coronary or ventricular constriction has been seen for up to 2 years *(30)*. Currently, a randomized prospective multicentered Phase II Food and Drug Administration (FDA) study is underway in patients with NYHA Class III heart failure comparing the efficacy of the Acorn jacket in dilated left ventricles with and without mitral insufficiency. Recently, in a chronic animal model of heart failure following acute myocardial infarction, placement of the Acorn jacket following the infarction prevented further ventricular remodeling compared to control animals at 2 months. Further ventricular dilatation was halted, infarct size was decreased, and systolic function was improved. In this model, the Acorn jacket was effective in preventing the progression of heart failure owing to acute myocardial infarction *(31,32)*. In the future, this device, or something similar, may be used prophylactically in patients with large myocardial infarctions to prevent subsequent remodeling and heart failure.

Mechanical ventricular assistance as a bridge to transplantation is an established therapy. A 70% success to transplantation after implantation of a LVAD can be expected. The TCI HeartMate is the most successful device with the lowest incidence of stroke despite patients managed on only one aspirin daily. Patients can be sent home to wait for a suitable heart to become available. These devices allow patients in cardiogenic shock from a variety of causes, not only to live but to be mobile and rehabilitated prior to their transplant. The expert use of a variety of different ventricular assist devices for left, right, and biventricular support is mandatory for any cardiac transplant center today *(33–36)*.

Recently, there have been a number of published reports of prolong (weeks to months) LVAD support used as a bridge to recovery. Muller reports a number of patients with dilated cardiomyopathy improving after weeks to months of left-ventricular unloading *(37)*. Others feel that this approach in patients with chronic heart failure is very unpredictable and rarely successful *(38)*. In patients presenting with fulminant acute myocarditis, however, such support has been particularly successful resulting in full cardiac recovery in many cases *(39,40)*.

The success of the TCI HeartMate as a bridge to transplantation has led to its consideration as a permanent or destination device. This is currently being studied in Class IV patients that are not transplant candidates in a multicentered prospective randomized study (REMATCH) *(41)*. Though this study is still ongoing, the Achilles heel of this and other present day devices, may turn out to be a high incidence of infection—driveline exit site, pump pocket, or true endocarditis. Until this complication is drastically reduced, these devices cannot be considered for permanent placement *(42)*.

A new generation of assist devices will soon be entering initial Phase I and II studies. Axial flow pumps have been developed that are tiny compared to present general pulsatile pumps though still capable of up to 10 L of flow. The LionHeart (Arrow International), currently undergoing Phase I FDA evaluation, is a destination device that is totally intracorporeal, powered by transcutaneous energy transmission, with no driveline crossing the skin. Within the very near future, total artificial hearts (Abiocor – Abiomed) will also be entering clinical trials *(43)*.

In summary, an aggressive approach to surgical revascularization, correction of mitral insufficiency, or reversal of left-ventricular remodeling by new girdling devices, or the Dor procedure in end-stage heart failure, should be considered in any patient who has exhausted current pharmacologic therapy. The development and clinical use of a new generation of totally intracorporeal assist devices, permanently implanted in patients with end-stage heart failure that are not transplant candidates, that overcome present day problems of thromboembolism, infection, and large size, will be a clinical reality within the near future.

REFERENCES

1. Cohn JN, Ferrari R, Sharpe N, on behalf of an International Forum on Cardiac Remodeling. Cardiac remodeling—concept and clinical implications: a consensus paper. J Am Coll Cardiol 2000;35:569–582.
2. Transplant Patient Data Source (2001, May 11). Richmond, VA. United Network for Organ Sharing. Retrieved May 11, 2001 from the World Wide Web: http://www.patients.unos.org/data.htm
3. Pagano D, Bonser RS, Camici PG. Myocardial revascularization for the treatment of post-ischemic heart failure. Curr Opin Cardiol 1999;14:506–509.
4. Trachiotis GD, Weintraub WS, Johnston TS, et al. Coronary artery bypass grafting in patients with advanced left ventricular dysfunction. Ann Thorac Surg 1998;66:1632–1639.
5. Dreyfus GD, Duboc D, Blasco A, et al. Myocardial viability assessment in ischemic cardiomyopathy: benefits of coronary revascularization. Ann Thorac Surg 1994;57:1402–1407.
6. Tjan TD, Kondruweit M, Scheld HH, et al. The bad ventricle—revascularization versus transplantation. Thorac Cardiovasc Surg 2000;48:9–14.
7. Lansman SL, Cohen M, Galla JD, et al. Coronary bypass with ejection fraction of 0.20 or less using centigrade cardioplegia: long-term follow-up. Ann Thorac Surg 1993;56:480–485.
8. Kaul TK, Agnihotri AK, Fields BL, et al. Coronary artery bypass grafting in patients with an ejection fraction of twenty percent or less. J Thorac Cardiovasc Surg 1996;111:1001–1012.
9. Hendren WG, Nemec JJ, Lytle BW, et al. Mitral valve repair for ischemic mitral insufficiency. Ann Thorac Surg 1991;52:1246–1251.
10. Bolling SF, Pagani FD, Deeb GM, Bach DS. Intermediate-term outcome of mitral reconstruction in cardiomyopathy. J Thorac Cardiovasc Surg 1998;115:381–386.
11. Smolens IA, Pagani FD, Bolling SF. Mitral valve repair in heart failure. Eur J Heart Fail 2000;2:365–371.
12. Sintek CF, Pfeffer TA, Kochamba G, et al. Preservation of normal left ventricular geometry during mitral valve replacement. J Heart Valve Dis 1995;4:471–475.
13. Sarris GE, Cahill PD, Hansen DE, et al. Restoration of left ventricular systolic performance after reattachment of the mitral chordae tendineae. The importance of valvular-ventricular interaction. J Thorac Cardiovasc Surg 1988;95:969–979.
14. Natsuaki M, Itoh T, Tomita S, et al. Importance of preserving the mitral subvalvular apparatus in mitral valve replacement. Ann Thorac Surg 1996;61:585–590.
15. Komeda M, David TE, Rao V, et al. Late hemodynamic effects of the preserved papillary muscles during mitral valve replacement. Circ 1994;90:II190–194.
16. Batista RJ, Santos JL, Takeshita N, et al. Partial left ventriculectomy to improve left ventricular function in end-stage heart disease. J Card Surg 1996;11:96,97.
17. Batista RJ, Verde J, Nery P, et al. Partial left ventriculectomy to treat end-stage heart disease. Ann Thorac Surg 1997;64:634–638.

18. McCarthy JF, McCarthy PM, Starling RC, et al. Partial left ventriculectomy and mitral valve repair for end-stage congestive heart failure. Eur J Cardiothorac Surg 1998;13:337–343.

19. Etoch SW, Koenig SC, Laureano MA, et al. Results after partial left ventriculectomy versus heart transplantation for idiopathic cardiomyopathy. J Thorac Cardiovasc Surg 1999;117:952–959.

20. Dor V, Saab M, Coste P, et al. Left ventricular aneurysm: a new surgical approach. Thorac Cardiovasc Surg 1989;37:11–19.

21. Athanasuleas CL, Stanley AW Jr, Buckberg GD, et al. Surgical anterior ventricular endocardial restoration (SAVER) in the dilated remodeled ventricle after anterior myocardial infarction. RESTORE group. Reconstructive Endoventricular Surgery, returning Torsion Original Radius Elliptical Shape to the LV. J Am Coll Cardiol 2001;37:1199–1209.

22. Dor V, Sabatier M, Di Donato M, et al. Efficacy of endoventricular patch plasty in large postinfarction akinetic scar and severe left ventricular dysfunction: comparison with a series of large dyskinetic scars. J Thorac Cardiovasc Surg 1998;116:50–59.

23. Di Donato M, Sabatier M, Dor V, et al. Effects of the Dor procedure on left ventricular dimension and shape and geometric correlates of mitral regurgitation one year after surgery. J Thorac Cardiovasc Surg 2001;121:91–96.

24. Sabbah HN, Sharov VG, Chaudhry PA, et al. Chronic therapy with the Acorn Cardiac Support Device in dogs with chronic heart failure: three and six months hemodynamic, histologic and ultrastructural findings (abstr). J HeartLung Transplant 2001;20:189.

25. Sabbah HN, Gupta RC, Sharov VG, et al. Prevention of progressive left ventricular dilation with the Acorn Cardiac Support Device down regulates stretch response proteins and improves sarcoplasmic reticulum recycling in dogs with chronic heart failure (abstr). J Am Coll Cardiol 2001;1:37:474A.

26. Saavedra F, Tunin R, Mishima T, et al. Reverse remodeling and enhanced adrenergic reserve from a passive external ventricular support in experimental dilated heart failure (abstr). Circulation 2000;102:11:501.

27. Sabbah HN, Gupta RC, Sharov VG, et al. Prevention of progressive left ventricular dilation with the Acorn Cardiac Support Device (CSD) down regulates stretch-mediated p21ras. attentuates myocyte hypertrophy and improves sarcoplasmic reticulum calcium cycling in dogs with heart failure (abstr). Circulation 2000;102:11–683.

28. Chaudry PA, Mishima T, Sharov VG, et al. Passive epicardial containment prevents ventricular remodeling in heart failure. Ann Thor Surg 2000;70:1275–1280.

29. Gupta RC, Sharov VG, Mishra S, et al. Chronic therapy with the Acorn Cardiac Support Device (CSD) attentuates cardiomyocyte apoptosis in dogs with heart failure (abstr) J Am Coll Cardiol 2001;1:37:478A.

30. Kleber FX, Sonntag S, Krebs H, et al. Follow-up on passive cardiomyoplasty in congestive heart failure: influence on the Acorn Cardiac Support Device on left ventricular function (abstr) J Am Coll Cardiol 2001;3737:143A.

31. Pilla JJ, Brockman DJ, Blom AS, et al. Prevention of dilatation using the Acorn cardiac support devise (CSD) results in reversed remodeling and improvement of function. (Poster) American Heart Association, Scientific Session 2001, Anaheim, CA, Nov. 2001.

32. Pilla JJ, Blom AS, Brockman DJ, et al.. Ventricular constraint using the Acorn cardiac support device (CSD) limits infarct expansion. (Poster) American American Heart Association, Scientific Session 2001, Anaheim, CA, Nov. 2001.

33. Goldstein DJ, Oz MC. Mechanical support for postcardiotomy cardiogenic shock. Semin Thorac Cardiovasc Surg 2000;12:220 228.

34. McCarthy PM, Portner PM, Tobler HG, et al. Clinical experience with the Novacor ventricular assist system. Bridge to transplantation and the transition to permanent application. J Thorac Cardiovasc Surg 1991;102:578–586.

35. Levin HR, Chen JM, Oz MC, et al. Potential of left ventricular assist devices as outpatient therapy while awaiting transplantation. Ann Thorac Surg 1994;58:1515–1520.

36. Sun BC, Catanese KA, Spanier TB, et al. 100 long-term implantable left ventricular assist devices: the Columbia Presbyterian interim experience. Ann Thorac Surg 1999;68:688–694.

37. Muller J, Wallukat G, Weng YG, et al. Weaning from mechanical cardiac support in patients with idiopathic dilated cardiomyopathy. Circulation 199715;96:542–549.

38. Mancini DM, Beniaminovitz A, Levin H, et al. Low incidence of myocardial recovery after left ventricular assist device implantation in patients with chronic heart failure. Circulation 1998;98:2383–2389.

39. McCarthy RE, Boehmer JP, Hruban RH, et al. Long-term outcome of fulminant myocarditis as compared with acute (nonfulminant) myocarditis. N Engl J Med 2000;342:690–695.

40. Acker MA. Mechanical circulatory support for patients with acute/fulminant myocarditis. Ann Thorac Surg discussion S82–85, 2001;71:S73–76.

41. Rose EA, Moskowitz AJ, Packer M, discussion S82-5, The REMATCH trial: rationale, design, and end points. Randomized evaluation of mechanical assistance for the treatment of congestive heart failure. Ann Thorac Surg 1999;67:723–730.

42. Mann DL, Willerson JT. Left ventricular assist devices and the failing heart: a bridge to recovery, a permanent assist device, or a bridge too far? Circulation 1998;98:2367–2369.

43. Frazier OH. Future directions of cardiac assistance. Semin Thorac Cardiovasc Surg 2000;12:220–228.

17 Current Concepts of Biventricular Pacing in Heart Failure

Robert W. Rho, MD, Vickas V. Patel, MD, PhD, and Dusan Z. Kocovic, MD

INTRODUCTION

It is estimated that 4.8 million Americans carry the diagnosis of heart failure. As nearly 600,000 new cases are diagnosed every year, it is the leading cause of hospitalizations in patients over 65 years of age *(1)* and a significant source of health care expenditures *(2)*. The incidence of heart failure doubles with every decade of life *(3)*. With the aging of the general population and enhanced survival afforded by modern medical treatment, the incidence of heart failure is increasing *(4)*.

Intraventricular conduction delay (IVCD) manifesting as a left-bundle branch block (LBBB) or right-bundle branch block (RBBB) is observed in as many as 53% of patients with dilated cardiomyopathy. The presence of intraventricular conduction delay in patients with dilated cardiomyopathy prolongs left-ventricular contraction and

From: *Contemporary Cardiology: Heart Failure:*
A Clinician's Guide to Ambulatory Diagnosis and Treatment
Edited by: M. L. Jessup and E. Loh © Humana Press Inc., Totowa, NJ

decreases left-ventricular filling time. A lack of coordinated contraction of all segments of the left-ventricular results in impairment in overall systolic function. A delay in relaxation owing to left-ventricular intraventricular dysynchrony and right-ventricular to left-ventricular interventricular asynchrony results in impaired diastolic filling *(6)*. The presence of a left-ventricular to left-atrial diastolic gradient seen in patients with elevated left-ventricular filling pressures and exacerbated by an intraventricular conduction delay, may result in or worsen diastolic mitral regurgitation (MR). Prolonged mitral regurgitation contributes to the deleterious effects of intraventricular conduction delay upon hemodynamics *(7)*. Furthermore, the presence of intraventricular conduction delay is an independent predictor of mortality in patients with dilated cardiomyopathy *(8)*. Despite significant advancements in the medical treatment of heart failure, patients continue to suffer from symptomatic heart failure and remain at high risk of death from arrhythmias and progressive heart failure.

In 1994, Cazeau et al. *(9)* reported a patient with refractory heart failure who responded to four-chamber pacing. Since then, several studies have shown significant improvement in acute hemodynamic parameters and long-term functional improvement with atriobiventricular pacing. This chapter provides an overview of biventricular pacing in symptomatic patients with heart failure and intraventricular conduction delay.

LBBB AND LEFT-VENTRICULAR EJECTION FRACTION (LVEF)

Conduction through the specialized conduction system (His-purkinje system) allows for brisk distribution of the cardiac impulse to all segments of the left ventricle, resulting in the simultaneous contraction (within 40 milliseconds) of all segments of the left ventricle. Patients with conduction abnormalities in one or more fascicles of the His-purkinje system suffer from a temporal imbalance in the distribution of the cardiac electrical impulse resulting in asynchronous left-ventricular and right-ventricular filling and contraction. Bramlet et al. reported that the development of rate-related LBBB is associated with a significant delay in contraction of the lower septum and apical segments of the left ventricle in normal subjects with normal mechanical left-ventricular function at baseline. This apical septal delay resulted in a significant decrease in regional and global ejection fraction *(10)*. Grines et al. compared two groups of patients with normal left-ventricle function. The study group included 18 patients with isolated LBBB and the control group included 10 patients with no intraventricular conduction delay.

Echocardiograms and radionuclide ventriculograms were compared between the two groups. In patients with LBBB, a shortening of the left-ventricular diastolic filling phase was observed. Assessment of regional ejection fractions via radionuclide ventriculography revealed a significant decrease in regional septal ejection fraction in the LBBB group. This loss of septal contribution resulted in a reduction in global LVEF in the LBBB group *(11)*. The author concluded that a LBBB results in a reduction in the diastolic filling time and offsets the timing of left-ventricular septal contraction with the rest of the left ventricle resulting in a reduction in global left-ventricular function.

In patients with normal left-ventricular function, these alterations in left-ventricular function are well tolerated, but in patients with severe left-ventricular dysfunction and symptomatic heart failure, the consequences of LBBB on hemodynamics and functional capacity may be more significant. The degree of mechanical dysynchrony in this patient population may be profound *(12)*. Dysynchronous left-ventricular contraction significantly shortens the diastolic filling phase of the left ventricle *(13)*. Furthermore, asynchrony between the left ventricular and right-ventricular in the setting of elevated diastolic filling pressures may offset the relationship between the left-ventricular and the right-ventricular in the confined space of the pericardium and further restrict left-ventricular filling.

Pre-ejection MR occurs in a significant number of patients with left-ventricular dysfunction and intraventricular conduction delay. Doppler ultrasound studies have revealed that preejection MR occurs commonly in patients with first degree atrioventricular (AV) block *(14,15)*. Furthermore, elevated left-ventricular end-diastolic pressure in patients with heart failure contributes significantly to the severity of MR because of a persistent gradient between the left-ventricular and left atrium *(16)*.

Dyssynchronous contraction of the left ventricle may result in significant regional wall tension from regional stretch that results from inefficient contraction of "late" segments, whereas left-ventricular systolic pressure is rising rapidly following contraction of "early" segments. This increase in wall tension is energetically unfavorable and may result in an elevation in myocardial oxygen demand. Short-term studies have revealed a decrease in sympathetic activity and improved cardiac efficiency (decreased myocardial oxygen consumption) with biventricular pacing *(17,18)*. In summary, LBBB results in significant intraventricular (left-ventricular) and interventricular (right-ventricular and left-ventricular) dyssynchrony. This results in significant impairment in systolic and diastolic function and may cause or aggravate MR. Dyssynchrony decreases cardiac efficiency and increases sympathetic activity. These findings may possibly contribute to the increased mortality observed in patients with IVCD and heart failure.

HEMODYNAMICS OF RIGHT-VENTRICULAR PACING

Right-ventricular pacing results in a functional LBBB with resultant ventricular dysnchrony. Several studies have demonstrated a deterioration in left-ventricular systolic and diastolic function during right-ventricular pacing. Rosenqvist et al. reported lower cardiac outputs and paradoxic septal motion using radionuclide ventriculography in 12 patients during right-ventricular pacing in comparison to atrial pacing. A 25% impairment in regional septal ejection fraction was reported in this study (19). Betocchi et al. reported an upward shift in the left-ventricular diastolic pressure-volume relationship, decreased left-ventricular peak filling rate, increased time constant of isovolumic relaxation, and decreased cardiac index during right-ventricular pacing (20).

The negative impact of right-ventricular pacing on ventricular performance may offset any benefit that might be derived from improved AV timing from conventional atrioventricular synchronous pacing. Prospective studies of dual-chamber pacing in patients with drug refractory heart failure and no pacing indication have failed to show hemodynamic or functional improvement despite "atrioventricular optimization" on echocardiography. Linde et al. reported the acute and long-term effects of dual-chamber pacing with AV optimization performed individually using Doppler echocardiography. A short-term improvement in stroke volume and cardiac output was reported, however, LVEF and functional class did not improve significantly during a 1-, 3-, and 6-month follow-up period. The lack of benefit from AV optimization with dual chamber pacing is most likely a result of the deleterious effect of right-ventricular apical pacing and the resultant ventricular asynchrony associated with this mode of pacing in this patient population. The lack of benefit of dual-chamber pacing dampened the interest in pacing for heart failure until the advent of biventricular pacing.

ACUTE HEMODYNAMIC EFFECTS
OF BIVENTRICULAR PACING

In 1994, Cazeau et al. implanted the first four-chamber cardiac pacing system in a patient with refractory heart failure and intraventricular conduction delay. Significant hemodynamic and functional improvement was observed in this patient. Shortly after this initial case report, several investigators have reported the efficacy of biventricular pacing on the hemodynamics of patients with heart failure and intraventricular conduction delay. Foster et al studied the acute hemodynamic effects of four different modes of pacing therapy (right-atrial pacing [AAI], dual-chamber pacing-right atrium and right ventricle [RV-DDD], dual-chamber pacing-left atrium and left ventricle [LV-DDD], and atrial-biventricular pacing [BiV-DDD]) on 18 patients with LVEF below 40%. A significant increase in cardiac output was observed with BiV-DDD pacing in comparison with AAI, RV-DDD, and LV-DDD (3.26 ± 0.18 vs 3.03 ± 0.14, 2.98 ± 0.16, and 3.07 ± 0.18 L/min, respectively, p < 0.05) and a significant decrease in systemic vascular resistance was reported (981 ± 80 vs 1078 ± 81, 1057 ± 86, and 1038 ± 96 dynes•S•cm ^{5}, p < 0.05) (22). Cazeau et al. subsequently reported the acute hemodynamic effects of several pacing modes in eight patients with severe heart failure and widened QRS. Invasive hemodynamic parameters were measured during right-ventricular pacing and biventricular pacing. Biventricular pacing increased the mean cardiac index by 25% (from a baseline of 1.83 ± 0.3 L/min/m², p < 0.006), decreased the mean V wave by 26% (from a baseline of 36 ± 12 mm Hg, p < 0.004), and decreased the pulmonary capillary wedge pressure by 17% (from a baseline of 31 + 10 mm Hg, p < 0.01) (23). Leclercq et al. studied the acute hemodynamic effects of four-chamber pacing compared to biatrial pacing and RV-DDD pacing in 18 patients with severe heart failure and a wide QRS. A significant improvement in cardiac index (2.7 ± 0.7 L/min/m² [four chamber] vs 2.0 ± 0.5 L/min/m² [biatrial], and 2.4 ± 0.6 L/min/m² [RV-DDD], p < 0.001) and pulmonary artery wedge pressure (22 ± 8 mmHg [four chamber] vs 27 ± 9 mm Hg [RV-DDD], p < 0.001)was observed with biventricular pacing (24). Blanc et al. also evaluated the acute hemodynamic effects of biventricular pacing in 23 patients with severe heart failure. Both left ventricular pacing and biventricular pacing was associated with a significant decrease in pulmonary arterial pressure and pulmonary arterial wedge pressure (25). Aside from the consistent improvement in acute hemodynamics reported in these studies, an interesting observation was that in many cases, left-ventricular pacing alone improved hemodynamics equally to that of biventricular pacing. Furthermore, acute hemodynamic improvement has been observed with biventricular pacing in patients with chronic atrial fibrillation (26) suggesting that the improvement in hemodynamics is independent of AV temporal optimization.

Clinical Trials of Biventricular Pacing

The benefits of biventricular pacing have been reported in several randomized controlled prospective trials. These trials targeted patients with medically refractory symptomatic heart failure, prolonged QRS duration (>120–150 ms), and depressed LVEF (ejection fraction < 35%).

The PATH-CHF trial, which utilized epicardial pacing leads and two separate pacemakers, included an acute hemodynamic study and a chronic study. In the acute study, hemodynamics were assessed for right atrial-right-ventricular, right atrial-left-ventricular, and right atrial-biventricular pacing. Left-ventricular pacing was found to be superior to right-ventricular and biventricular pacing and the importance of AV optimization was emphasized. In the chronic study, patients were given 4 weeks of active pacing, followed by 4 weeks of no pacing and then by a second 4-week active pacing period. Improvement in exercise tolerance was observed only during periods of active left-ventricular or biventricular pacing *(27,28)*.

The Multisite Stimulation in Cardiomyopathy (MUSTIC) trial is a randomized prospective, crossover study of biventricular pacing therapy in heart failure. The inclusion criteria included all patients with severely symptomatic congestive heart failure (CHF) (New York Heart Association [NYHA] Class III and IV), an ejection fraction of less than 35%, and significant intraventricular conduction delay (QRS duration > 150 ms). This single-blind randomized, controlled crossover study compared the responses of the patients during two periods: a 3-month period of inactive pacing and a 3-month period of active atriobiventricular pacing. In 48 patients who completed both phases of the study, biventricular pacing significantly improved VO_2 max (8% increase; $p < 0.03$) and 6-minute walk test (23% greater with biventricular pacing [399 ± 100 m vs 326 ± 134 m] $p < 0.001$). Significant improvements in quality-of-life score (32% improvement; $p < 0.001$), and a decrease in number of hospitalizations by two-thirds ($p < 0.05$) was also reported. At the end of the crossover phase, 86% of patients (blinded to mode of therapy) preferred biventricular pacing over no pacing *(29)*.

The MIRACLE trial was recently reported at the 50th annual American College of Cardiology (ACC) meeting in 2001 *(30)*. The MIRACLE trial was a randomized controlled double- blind multicenter trial comparing biventricular pacing and no pacing. In this study, the biventricular pacing system is randomized to "on" or "off" mode for the first 6 months. After a 6-month follow-up, all patients were switched to biventricular pacing and followed every 6 months. A significant improvement in NYHA functional class, quality of life, 6-minute walk, and peak VO^2 max was observed in patients randomized to biventricular pacing. The MUSTIC trial, MIRACLE trial, and PATH-CHF trials have demonstrated a significant improvement in functional capacity and quality of life in patients with drug refractory symptomatic CHF with intraventricular conduction delay. To date, there has been no clinical trial that has shown a reduction in mortality with biventricular pacing *(see* Table 1).

Nonhemodynamic Benefits of Biventricular Pacing

In addition to the improvement in systolic and diastolic performance associated with biventricular pacing, other benefits of biventricular pacing have been reported including: (1) reduction in serum norepinephrine levels *(18)* and sympathetic activity *(31)*, (2) a possible reduction in ventricular arrhythmias *(32)*, and (3) reverse left-ventricular remodeling with chronic biventricular pacing *(33)*. Although the positive effects of biventricular pacing on each of these factors may potentially effect mortality, the clinical significance of these findings requires further investigation.

Biventricular Pacing in Atrial Fibrillation

The acute hemodynamic benefit of biventricular pacing has been observed in atrial fibrillation, as well as in sinus rhythm *(26)*. The second study group of the MUSTIC trial evaluated biventricular pacing in patients with chronic atrial fibrillation. This study failed to show a difference with biventricular pacing in atrial fibrillation, however, limitations of the study including lack of effective pacing in several patients may have contributed to this finding *(34)*. Leclercq et al. reported a comparison of biventricular pacing in patients with atrial fibrillation vs patients in sinus rhythm. A significant improvement in VO^2 max, NYHA class, and LVEF was reported in the atrial fibrillation group ($n = 15$ patients). A limitation of this study was that patients in the atrial fibrillation group underwent His-bundle ablation at the time of implantation, and some of the benefit may have been attributed to improved ventricular rate control. To address this issue Leon et al. reported the effect of biventricular pacing in 20 consecutive patients with atrial fibrillation who had undergone His-bundle ablation and chronic right-ventricular pacing (±6-month duration) by upgrading them from RV-VVI pacing to biventricular pacing. At 3–6 months follow-up a significant improvement in NYHA functional class (29%, $p < 0.001$), LVEF (44%, $p < 0.001$), number of hospitalizations (81% reduction, $p < 0.001$), and quality-of-life (33% improvement in Minnesota Living with Heart Failure survey, $p < 0.01$) was reported *(35)*. These studies suggest that the benefits derived from biventricular pacing are extended to patients with atrial fibrillation, and that the hemodynamic and clinical benefits are independent of AV optimization.

Biventricular Pacing in RBBB

The efficacy of biventricular pacing in RBBB is less clear. Patients with RBBB may have concomitant left-sided intraventricular conduc-

Table 1
Randomized Clinical Trials of Biventricular Pacing

Clinical trial	NYHA class	Follow-up	6-Minute walk test	QOL	VO² max	Other
MIRACLE (30)	III–IV	6 months	+ 13%	+ 13%	NA	Implant success = 93%; NYHA III to II with BiV
MUSTIC (29)	III	3 months	+ 23%	+ 32%	+ 8%	2/3 less hospitalizations; 86% preferred BiV pacing
PATH CHF (28)	III–IV	3 months	+ 22%	+ 43%	+ 20%	

tion delay, which may be masked by the RBBB on the surface 12-lead EKG. Garrigue et al. studied 12 patients with RBBB (QRS > 140 ms). Four of these patients had atrial fibrillation. LVEF, exercise tolerance (maximal treadmill test), echocardiography, and Doppler tissue imaging was measured before implantation and at 1-, 6-, and 12-month follow-up. Variations of the left-intraventricular delay were quantified by measuring the time difference from the electromechanical delay of the left-ventricular free wall to that of the left-ventricular septal wall. A significant improvement in NYHA functional class, maximum treadmill performance (6.1 ± 1.9 METS vs 4.7 ± 2.1 preimplant; $p = 0.019$), degree of mitral regurgitation (2.1 ± 0.8 before vs 1.2 ± 0.6 after implant; $p < 0.01$), reduction in left-ventricular end-diastolic diameter (72 ± 7 mm before vs 68 ± 6mm after implant; $p = 0.04$), and LV electromechanical delay (67 ± 38 ms before implant vs 26 ± 8 ms after implant; $p < 0.01$) was observed. Three patients (25%) did not improve at the end of follow-up (no change in NYHA functional class and treadmill test performance). Two of these patients were in atrial fibrillation but two of four patients with atrial fibrillation in the study were responders. The three patients with no improvement had no significant difference in QRS duration compared to the responders but had a smaller degree of left-ventricular electromechanical delay at baseline assessed by tissue Doppler analysis (36). In patients with RBBB, biventricular pacing may provide hemodynamic and clinical benefit in patients with concomitant left-ventricular asynchrony. Patient selection may include patients with more significantly prolonged QRS duration or EKG evidence of concomitant left anterior or posterior fascicular block. However, EKG criteria to identify patients with RBBB who are likely to respond have not been established. Future investigations in identifying echocardiographic assessment of left-ventricular asynchrony may be the key to identifying responders in this population.

PATIENT SELECTION FOR BIVENTRICULAR PACING

Although biventricular pacing affords hemodynamic and symptomatic benefit to the majority of patients, some patients do not improve. To date, consistent clinical factors predicting hemodynamic improvement from biventricular pacing therapy has not been elucidated. Leclercq et al. compared responders ($n = 12$) and nonresponders ($n = 6$) in 18 patients who received biventricular pacing therapy. By univariate analysis, a lower baseline LVEF was the only predictive factor associated with acute hemodynamic improvement. The PR interval, QRS duration, and presence of left-axis deviation did not predict a positive hemodynamic response *(24)*. Aurucchio et al. reported that 5 of 27 patients who did not have significant hemodynamic improvement with biventricular pacing had significantly shorter QRS width compared to the other 22 patients (128 ± 12 ms vs 180 ± 22 ms, respectively) *(37)*. Kass et al. also reported that baseline QRS width was predictive of improvement in left-ventricular contractile function from biventricular pacing. The degree of QRS narrowing with biventricular pacing was not predictive of hemodynamic improvement *(38)*. More recent investigations have focused on echocardiographic assessment of left-ventricular asynchrony indexed by tissue Doppler imaging with M-mode analysis, regional velocities and tissue tracking, and strain rate analysis *(39,40)*. Currently, no definite criteria exists, but tissue Doppler imaging's high temporal and spatial resolution makes it the ideal tool for identifying biventricular pacing candidates. Based on these measurements, the development of an "asynchrony index" may provide a valuable tool for patients who would most likely benefit from resynchronization therapy.

Implantation Procedure

The early biventricular pacing systems were implanted by placing the LV lead in the epicardium via a limited thoracotomy *(41)*. This procedure was associated with significant morbidity and mortality. In 1998, Daubert et al. introduced a transvenous left-ventricular lead system that was implanted retrograde into a lateral tributary cardiac vein of the coronary sinus. This approach is safe and was associated with preserved long-term lead performance *(42,43)*.

The coronary sinus and cardiac veins differ anatomically from individual to individual. Meisel et al. performed retrograde venography in 86 patients who were referred for an implantable cardiac defibrillator. The anterior interventricular vein and the middle cardiac vein was present in 85/86 (99%) patients and 86/86 (100%) of patients, respectively. Between these two veins, at least one additional cardiac vein was present in 85/86 (99%) patients. Just one vein was present in 44/86 (51%) of patients, two were present in 40/86 (46%), and more than two veins were present in 2/86 (2%) patients *(44)*. Cannulation of the coronary sinus may be technically difficult owing to the increased size of the right atrium and angulation of the coronary sinus. Furthermore, different degrees of coronary sinus stenosis may be present in patients with prior cardiac surgery making implantation of a coronary sinus lead difficult or impossible *(45)*. The ideal site for the left-ventricular lead is in a lateral cardiac vein *(46)*. Poor thresholds may be encountered at "ideal" anatomic coronary sinus lead positions. High but "acceptable" thresholds may be significantly worse when connected with the RV lead

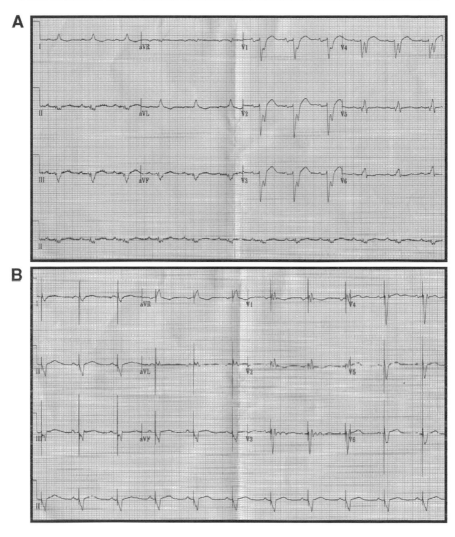

Fig. 1. (A) 12-Lead electrocardiogram of a patient with wide complex QRS (QRS duration = 210 ms). (B) 12-Lead electrocardiogram of the same patient after successful implantation of a biventricular pacing system. Note the short AV delay and significantly narrowed QRS with pacing (QRS duration = 145 ms).

through a Y adaptor or a first-generation biventricular pacemaker (these devices split a single-ventricular output from the can to two outputs within the header), as a result of differences in pacing configurations during threshold testing *(47)*. Despite these challenges, the overall success rate of coronary sinus lead implant in the MIRACLE trial was 93%. Complications rates from coronary sinus lead implantation are low.

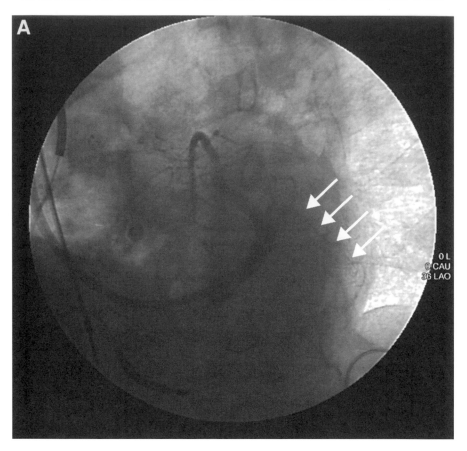

Fig. 2. (A and **B)** Venograms of the coronary sinus and its tributaries. The flouroscopic images in LAO **(A)** and RAO **(B)** are shown. In **A** thread-like lateral cardiac vein is present (arrows).

Ricci et al. reported a 0.9% (*n* = 190 patients) rate of coronary sinus perforation resulting in cardiac tamponade *(48)*. Leclercq et al. reported that the rate of coronary sinus dissection was 2% (*n* = 102) with none of these incidences leading to adverse outcomes *(49)*. In summary, implantation of biventricular pacing system is technically difficult and time consuming. A significant learning curve exists among operators, but improvements in lead design, coronary sinus lead delivery systems, and "over the wire" lead systems combined with increased operator experience should ensure equal success rates to that observed in MIRACLE with reduced implantation times (Figs. 2 and 3).

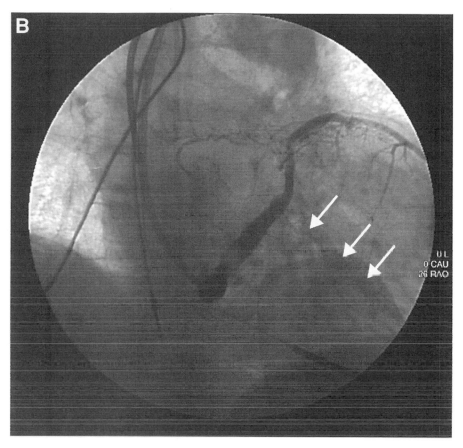

Fig. 2 (B). (Continued) RAO fluoroscopic projection of lateral cardiac vein.

CONCLUSION

Biventricular pacing is an exciting and effective adjunctive treatment option for patients with severe heart failure symptoms and intraventricular conduction delay. Significant improvement in quality of life and functional capacity can be expected in the majority of patients who receive biventricular pacing systems. Acute hemodynamic effects of biventricular pacing can be seen immediately. With chronic biventricular pacing, patients can expect to have a significant improvement in functional class, increase their 6-minute walk distance by up to

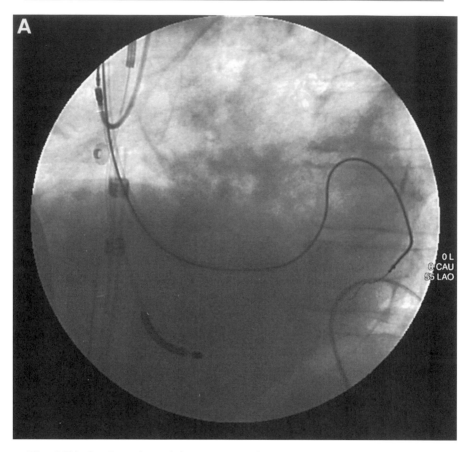

Fig. 3(A). Implantation of the coronary sinus lead using an "over-the-wire" system. The fluoroscopic images in the LAO (**A**) and RAO (**B**) projections are shown (Model 4512 Easy Track CS lead [Guidant Corp.]). In this example, the small caliber vein is successfully wired and the lead is advanced into an optimal lateral position.

23% and improve quality of life by up to 43%. Identification of clinical and echocardiographic predictors of responders to biventricular pacing will be useful in ensuring implantation of the device in only those patients who are most likely to improve with therapy, and therefore save patients from needless morbidity with improved overall cost effectiveness. Although biventricular pacing decreases sympathetic activity, improves cardiac efficiency, improves functional class, promotes reverse left-ventricular remodeling, and may decrease the incidence of ventricular arrhythmias, a direct impact on mortality has not yet been shown in clinical trials. Some of the questions that remain unanswered in biventricular pacing are: (1) what is the optimal left-ventricular and

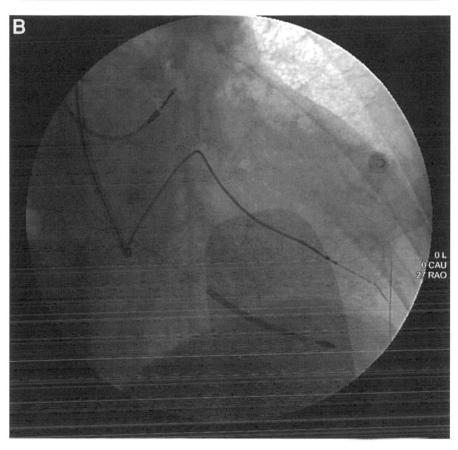

Fig. 3(B). RAO fluoroscopic projection of lateral cardiac vein with successfully implanted lead.

right-ventricular stimulation site? (2) Is left-ventricular pacing better, equal to, or worse than biventricular pacing in achieving long-term clinical results? (3) Is AV delay important and if so, what is the optimal AV delay with biventricular pacing? How should it be determined? (4) Can the improvements in functional status and quality of life last? Future randomized controlled studies with long-term follow-up should shed light on these questions.

REFERENCES

1. Graves EG, Gillum BS. 1994 Summary: National Hospital Discharge Survey: advance data. National Center for Health Statistics. 1996;278:1.
2. Havranek EP, Abraham WT. The healthcare economics of heart failure. 1998;14:10–18.
3. Hoes AW, Mosterd A, Grobbee DE. An epidemic of heart failure? Recent evidence from Europe. Eur Heart J 1998;19:L2–9.

4. Ho KK, Pinski JL, Kannel WB, et al. The epidemiology of heart failure: the Framingham study. J Am Coll Cardiol 1993;22:6A–13A.
5. Aaronson K, Schwartz J, Chen TM, et al. Development and prospective validation of a clinical index to predict survival in ambulatory patients referred for cardiac transplant evaluation. Circulation 1997;95:2660–2667.
6. Xiao H, Roy C, Fujimoto S, et al. Natural history of abnormal conduction and its relation to prognosis in patients with dilated cardiomyopathy. Int J Cardiol 1996;53:163–170.
7. LeclercQ C, Daubert JC. Why biventricular pacing might be of value in refractory heart failure? Heart 2000;84:125,126.
8. Venkateshawar K, Gottipaty K, Krelis P, et al. The resting electrocardiogram provides a sensitive and inexpensive marker of prognosis in patients with chronic congestive heart failure. J Am Coll Cardiol 1999;33:145A.
9. Cazeau S, Ritter P, Bakdach S, et al. Four chamber pacing in dilated cardiomyopathy. PACE 1994;17:1974–1979.
10. Bramlet DA, Morris KG, Coleman RE, et al. Effect of rate-dependent left bundle branch block on global and regional left ventricular function. Circulation 1983;67:1059–1065.
11. Grines C, Bashore T, Boudoulas H, et al. Functional abnormalities in isolated left bundle branch block: the effect of interventricular asynchrony. Circulation 1989;79:845–853.
12. Curry CW, Nelson GS, Wyman BT, et al. Mechanical dyssynchrony in dilated cardiomyopathy with intraventricular conduction delay as depicted by 3D tagged magnetic resonance imaging. Circulation 2000;1-1:e2.
13. Xiao H, Lee CH, Gibson DG. Effect of left bundle branch block on diastolic function in dilated cardiomyopathy. Br Heart J 1991;66:443–447.
14. Panidis IP, Ross J, Munley B, et al. Diastolic mitral regurgitation in patients with atrioventricular conduction abnormalities: a common finding by Doppler echocardiography. Am Coll Cardiol 1986,7:768–774.
15. Schnittger I, Appleton CP, Hatle LK, et al. Diastolic mitral and tricuspid regurgitation by Doppler echocardiography in patients with atrioventricular block: a new insight into the mechanism of atrioventricular valve closure. J Am Coll Cardiol 1988,11:83–88.
16. Ishikawa T, Kimura K, Nihei T, et al. Relationship between diastolic mitral regurgitation and PQ intervals or cardiac function in patients implanted with DDD pacemakers. Pacing Clin Electrophysiol 1991, 14:1797–1802.
17. Nelson G, Berger R, Fetics B, et al. Left and biventricular resynchronization pacing in patients with dilated cardiomyopathy and intraventricular conduction delays achieves systolic benefit at reduced energetic cost. Europace 2000;1:212.
18. Saxon LA, De Marco T, Chatterjee K, et al. Chronic biventricular pacing decreases serum norepinephrine in dilated heart failure patients with the greatest symptathetic activation at baseline. PACE 1999;22:830.
19. Rosenqvist M, Isaaz K, Botvinick EH, et al. Relative importance of activation sequence compared to atrioventricular synchrony in left ventricular function. Am J Cardiol 1991;67:148–156.
20. Betocchi S, Piscione F, Villari B, et al. Effects of induced asynchrony on left ventricular diastolic function in patients with coronary artery disease. J Am Coll Cardiol 1993,21:1124–1131.
21. Linde C, Gadler F, Edner M, et al. Results of atrioventricular synchronous pacing with optimized delay in patients with severe congestive heart failure. Am J Cardiol 1995;75:919–923.
22. Foster AH, Gold MR, McLauglin JS. Acute hemodynamic effects of atriobiventricular pacing in humans. Ann Thorac Surg 1995;59:294–300.

23. Cazeau S,. Ritter P, Lazarus A, et al. Multisite pacing for end-stage heart failure: early experience. Pacing Clin Electrophysiol 1996;19:1748–1757.

24. Leclercq C, Cazeau S, Breton HL, et al. Acute hemodynamic effects of biventricular DDD pacing in patients with end-stage heart failure. J Am Coll Cardiol 1998;32:1825–1831.

25. Blanc JJ, Etienne Y, Gilard M, et al. Evaluation of different ventricular pacing sites in patients with severe heart failure. Circulation 1997;96:3273–3277.

26. Etienne Y, Mansourati J, Gilard M, et al. Evaluation of left ventricular based pacing in patients with congestive heart failure and atrial fibrillation. Am J Cardiol 1999;83:1138–1140.

27. Auriccio A, Stellbrink C, Sack S, et al. The Pacing Therapies for Congestive Heart Failure (PATH-CHF) study: rationale, design, and endpoints of a prospective randomized multicenter study. Am J Cardiol 1999,83:130D–135D.

28. Salo R, Auricchio A, Sack S, et al. Chronic benefit index (CBI) summarizes PATH CHF chronic results. Pacing Clin Electrophysiol 2000;23:681.

29. Cazeau S, Leclercq C, Lavergne T, et al. Effects of multisite biventricular pacing in patients with heart failure and intraventricular conduction delay. N Eng J of Med 2001;344:873 880.

30. Abraham WT. Late breaking clinical trials: results from late breaking clinical trial sessions at ACC 2001. J Am Coll Cardiol 2001;38:604,605.

31. Hamdan MH, Zagrodzky JD, Joglar JA, et al. Biventricular pacing decreases sympathetic activity compared with right ventricular pacing in patients with depressed ejection fraction. Circulation 2000;102:1027–1032.

32. Walker S, Levy TM, Rex S, et al. Usefulness of suppression of ventricular arrhythmia by biventricular pacing in severe congestive cardiac failure. Am J Cardiol 2000;86:231–233.

33. YU CM, Chau E, Sanderson JE, et al. Tissue Doppler echocardiographic evidence of reverse remodeling and improved synchronicity by simultaneously delaying regional contraction after biventricular pacing therapy in heart failure. Circulation 2002;105:438–445.

34. Daubert JC, Linde C, Cazeau S, et al. Clinical effects of biventricular pacing in patients with severe heart failure and chronic atrial fibrillation: results from the Multisite Stimulation in Cardiomyopathy (MUSTIC) study group II (abst). Circulation 2000;102:3349A.

35. Leon AR, Greenburg JM, Kanuru N, et al. Cardiac resynchronization in patients with congestive heart failure and chronic atrial fibrillation: effect of upgrading to biventricular pacing from chronic right ventricular pacing. J Am Coll Cardiol 2002;17:1258–1263.

36. Garrigue S, Reuter S, Labeque JN, et al. Usefulness of biventricular pacing in patients with congestive heart failure and right bundle branch block. Am J Cardiol 2001;88:1436–1441.

37. Aurricchio A, Stellbrink C, Block M, et al. Effect of pacing chamber and atrioventricular delay on acute systolic function of paced patients with congestive heart failure. Circulation 1999;99:2993–3001.

38. Kass DA, Chen CH, Curry C, et al. Improved left ventricular mechanics from acute VDD pacing in patients with dilated cardiomyopathy and ventricular conduction delay. Circulation 1999;99:1567–1573.

39. Pan C, Hoffmann R, Kuhl H, et al. Tissue tracking allows rapid and accurate visual evaluation of left ventricular function. Eur J Echocardiogr 2001;2:197–202.

40. Sogaard P, Kim WY, Jensen HK, et al. Impact of acute biventricular pacing on left ventricular performance and volumes in patients with severe heart failure. A tissue Doppler and three dimensional echocardiographic study. Cardiology 2001;95:173–182.

41. Bakker P, et al. Complications associated with chronic biventricular pacing for severe congestive heart failure. J Cardiac Failure 1998;4:1–28.
42. Daubert JC, Ritter P, Le Breton H, et al. Permanent left ventricular pacing with transvenous leads inserted into the coronary veins. PACE 1998;21:239–245.
43. Gras D, et al. Permanent left ventricular pacing via coronary sinus leads: early results and long term follow up. Archives des maladies du Coeur des vaisseaux. Cardiostim 1998;91:245.
44. Meisel E, Pfeiffer D, Engelmann L, et al. Investigation of coronary venous anatomy by retrograde venography in patient with malignant ventricular tachycardia. Circulation 2001;104:442–447.
45. Kocovic DZ, Pavri BB, Hsia H, et al. Coronary sinus abnormalities in patients with congestive heart failure and previous cardiac surgery.
46. Butter C, Auricchio A, Stellbrink C, et al. Should stimulation site be tailored in the individual heart failure patient? Am J Cardiol 2000;86:K144–151.
47. Rho RW, Patel V, Gerstenfeld E, et al. Elevations in left ventricular thresholds with the use of Y adaptors: implications for biventricular pacing. PACE 2002;in press.
48. Ricci R, Ansalone G, Tasacano, et al. Cardiac resynchronization: materials, techniques, results. The INSYNC Italian Registry. Eur Heart J 2000;2:J6–15.
49. Leclercq C, Kass DA. Retiming the failing heart: principles and current clinical status of cardiac resynchronization. J Am Coll Cardiol 2002;16;39:194–201.

18 Alternate Therapies for Congestive Heart Failure

Shashank Desai, MD

Contents

INTRODUCTION

Despite optimal medical therapy, congestive heart failure (CHF) remains a progressive disease. Thus, patients and their physicians search for new and alternative therapies. The term alternative therapy indicates that a potential agent still needs to be methodically studied before being accepted as standard of care. Anecdotes and small observational studies are how many new options for heart failure have been discovered. For example foxglove, first used 200 years ago, started as an herbal treatment and today its derivative has become standard therapy for heart failure.

More popular alternative therapies for the treatment of CHF include coenzyme Q10, thyroid hormone, hawthorn, and growth hormone. Each agent has conflicting evidence surrounding its use. In addition, only weakly powered, small-scale studies have been performed on these

From: *Contemporary Cardiology: Heart Failure:*
A Clinician's Guide to Ambulatory Diagnosis and Treatment
Edited by: M. L. Jessup and E. Loh © Humana Press Inc., Totowa, NJ

potential agents. As a result, these agents have not gained widespread acceptance for use as standard medical therapy for heart failure. Future studies are needed before these therapies are part of the repertoire of accepted treatment.

COENZYME Q10

Coenzyme Q10, appropriately named ubiquinone, is a coenzyme found throughout the body. It is an obligatory member of the mitochondrial electron transport chain, used for mitochondrial oxidative phosphorylation. It acts as an antioxidant and free radical scavenger. Because the weakened myocardium of patients with CHF demonstrates increased oxidative stress, it is conceivable that coenzyme Q10 may prevent further stress and deterioration *(1)*. It has been found in increased concentrations in the heart *(2)*. The density of coenzyme Q10 is decreased in patients with advanced heart failure and the deficiency correlates with the severity of heart failure *(3)*. This provides the rationale for its proposal as a treatment for heart failure.

In 1974, the Japanese government approved marketing of coenzyme Q10 for the treatment of heart failure. This was based on more than 30 clinical reports describing the favorable effects with coenzyme Q10. Further trials in the United States and Europe uncovered more controversial results. A 1985 randomized study revealed an improvement in cardiac function on coenzyme Q10 *(4)*. In a 1999 study, 22 patients enrolled in a randomized, double-blind, placebo-controlled, crossover trial demonstrated coenzyme Q10 to increase stroke work and a decreased pulmonary capillary wedge pressure *(5)*. However, another study evaluated 30 patients in the same randomized, double-blind, placebo-controlled, crossover method, and found no difference in systolic function *(6)*. In another randomized trial of 79 patients, exercise tolerance and quality of life improved, but no significant change in ejection fraction was observed *(7)*. Because this dissociation between ejection fraction and exercise has been previously observed in heart failure patients, the findings may be credible. A recent meta-analysis of clinical trials from 1984 to 1994 included 14 studies where comparable improvement in stroke volume, ejection fraction, cardiac output, and end-diastolic ventricular volumes were all seen to improve in patients treated with coenzyme Q10 *(8)*.

The severity of heart failure further complicates analysis of the results. An Italian multicenter study in 1994 studied 2664 patients with New York Heart Association (NYHA) Class II–III CHF reported efficacy in treating the many symptoms of heart failure including edema, pulmonary rales, enlargement of liver, dyspnea, and jugular distention *(9)*. A 1999 study of NYHA Class II-III patients showed that cardiac output and wedge pressures improved after 12 weeks of treatment with coenzyme Q vs placebo *(5)*. An Italian multicenter study in 1993 evaluated 640 patients in NYHA Class III–IV CHF in a randomized study *(10)*, which concluded that hospitalizations for worsening heart failure and episodes of pulmonary edema were significantly reduced in the group treated with coenzyme Q10.

In contrast, other studies have failed to show significant benefit of this treatment modality. A 1999 study published in the *Journal of the American College of Cardiology* (ACC), revealed little change in left-ventricular function, cardiac volumes, hemodynamics or quality of life indicies *(6)*. One criticism of this study is that the 3-month study period was too short to detect a significant difference with coenzyme Q10. Furthermore, the dose of 100 mg/day of coenzyme Q10 may not have achieved significant concentration in the blood. Dosages approximating 240 mg/day may be needed to achieve optimal blood concentrations. A second study randomized patients with NYHA Class III–IV CHF to 200 mg/day of coenzyme Q10 and failed to show a difference in exercise testing and ejection fraction at 6 months *(11)*. Again, questions arose regarding the efficacy of this therapy on classic CHF surrogate endpoints. Criticism focused on length of follow up and serum levels of coenzyme Q10 not being adequate to treat severe CHF adequately *(12)*.

Thus, there is conflicting evidence over the use of coenzyme Q10 in NYHA Class II–IV CHF. On one hand, there have been improvements seen in a variety of surrogate markers such as exercise tolerance, ejection fraction, cardiac output, pulmonary capillary wedge pressure, and ventricular volumes. However, no study has yet determined a true mortality benefit of coenzyme Q10. Dosage is debated in the literature with dosages ranging from 50–60 mg/day to 100–240 mg/day. With this information coenzyme Q10 may be appropriate for adjunctive therapy for CHF. Minimal side effects have been seen with the use of coenzyme Q10.

THYROID HORMONE

Studies of left-ventricular function in hypothyroid patients have revealed abnormal contractility with lengthening of systolic time intervals, reduced ejection fractions, and decreased left-ventricular shortening *(13–15)*. Echocardiography proven improvements in cardiac contractility have been seen upon conversion to a euthyroid state *(16)*. Hypothyroidism also caused a delay of left-ventricular relaxation that normalized with thyroid replacement.

After discovering this association between thyroid hormone, and cardiac systolic and diastolic performance, studies were directed to demonstrate a clear benefit in treating cardiac dysfunction with supplemental thyroid hormone. A 1999 study looked at the use of intravenous thyroxine as an adjunctive salvage measure for cardiogenic shock *(17)*. Hemodynamic parameters improved including cardiac output and pulmonary capillary wedge pressure. A thyroid hormone analog DITPA has also been shown to increase systolic and diastolic function *(18)*.

Support for the use of thyroxine in heart failure of patients without thyroid disease remains controversial. However, its use appears to have some scientific support as evidenced by improved hemodynamic and echocardiographic parameters. This is difficult to translate to improved quality and quantity of life without larger studies centered on these endpoints. In addition, thyroid hormone has potent side effects and is not a therapy that should be entered into lightly.

HAWTHORN

The hawthorn plant contains pharmacologically active flavinoids that inhibit vasoconstriction and actively dilate blood vessels. One of these flavinoids has been shown in animal and in vitro experiments to have effects on the cardiovascular system. It seems to have cAMP-independent positive inotropy, peripheral and coronary vasodilation, protection against ischemia-induced ventricular arrhythmias, antioxidant properties and anti-inflammatory effects *(19)*. The blocking of vasoconstriction appears to occur by inhibiting angiotensin-converting enzyme (ACE). Increased $Ca+2$ transit and increased force of contraction gives hawthorn its theoretic basis for use in CHF *(20)*.

The extract has been studied in Germany and is being used as treatment for NYHA Class II heart failure *(21)*. A recent study, in which 136 patients in NYHA Class II heart failure were randomized to receive 160 mg Hawthorne special extract WS 1442 vs placebo, demonstrated a significant increase in cardiac function *(22)*. In addition, patients also reported improvement in subjective symptoms of heart failure and quality of life.

Hawthorne is a prescription medication in Europe and Asia for the treatment of mild cardiac insufficiency. SPICE is an international, randomized, blinded study which is studying the effect of Crataegus Special Extract WS 1442 on morbidity and mortality in CHF *(23)*. In this study, 2300 patients with NYHA Class II and III heart failure will be evaluated in centers throughout seven countries in Europe. The study was expected to be completed by the end of 2002 and may provide conclusive evidence as to the clinical use of this agent.

Hawthorn may potentiate the action of cardiac glycosides and thus may interfere with digoxin. Although no clinical studies have clearly documented this potential interaction, their concomitant use is not recommended. Otherwise, no significant side effects have been seen with the use of hawthorn.

GROWTH HORMONE

Both growth hormone (GH) and insulin-like growth factor (IGF-1) have primary regulatory effects on the developmental growth of the heart by controlling the maintenance of its structure. A relationship between GH/IGF-1 and the cardiovascular system has long been suggested *(24)*. An increased risk for cardiovascular morbidity and mortality has been documented both in GH excess and deficiency. Wide fluctuations in plasma volume also occur in both GH excess and deficiency. GH deficiency correlates with decreased extracellular volume and plasma volume that is restored by GH replacement *(25)*. IGF-1 has been implicated in an autocrine and paracrine effect on the heart. Both the epicardium and coronary vessels of human fetuses express mRNA for IGF-1 *(26)*. Additionally, increased IGF-1 activity has been seen in the inner layers of the left ventricle where the wall stress is highest and decreases closer to the epicardium *(27,28)*. IGF-1 expression has been associated with the development of left-ventricular hypertrophy *(27,29)*. Clinically, patients with acromegaly and elevated levels of GH, have a cardiomyopathy secondary to myocardial hypertrophy with interstitial fibrosis, lymphomononuclear infiltrate, and areas of necrosis resulting in biventricular hypertrophy. In contrast, patients with GH deficiency suffer from structural cardiac abnormalities such as narrowing of cardiac walls and functional impairment of diastolic filling and peak systolic function. Furthermore, these patients have evidence of atheromatous plaque development *(30)*.

Rat studies performed in chronic postinfarction heart failure revealed those treated with GH to have increased contractility. By augmenting calcium in myocytes, ejection and, thus, cardiac function improved *(31–33)*. Further studies demonstrated treatment with IGF-1 and GH increased cardiac output and decreased systemic vascular resistance *(34)*.

In humans, a 1996 study evaluated patients with idiopathic-dilated cardiomyopathy and moderate to severe heart failure *(35)*. These patients were treated with human GH for 3 months. Based on echo, catheterization, and exercise testing there was an improvement in hemodynamics, clinical symptoms, exercise capacity, and quality of life. There was partial reversibility of the cardiac shape and size, systolic function, and exercise capacity even after the discontinuation of the GH. Another randomized study evaluated the efficacy of recombinant human GH *(36)*. An increase in myocardial mass without a reciprocal increase in wall stress was seen. Two studies in 1999, looked at recombinant growth hormone in patients with an ischemic cardiomyopathy *(37,38)*. Both of these studies reveal an increase in exercise capacity, wall thickness, and cardiac output with the administration of GH. Clinical symptoms also improved significantly.

THALIDOMIDE—NEW DIRECTION IN THE SEARCH FOR ALTERNATIVES

Thalidomide's original use ended in the 1960s to its association with severe birth defects. However, since then it has been found to be effective in treating a variety of conditions including cancers, HIV, cachexia, and leprosy. Its best-recognized action has been to suppress tumor necrosis factor (TNF)-α activity.

Paracrine and cytokine elements such as endothelin, bradykinin, nitric oxide (NO), TNF-α, and interleuin (IL)-10 have been implicated in the evolution of heart failure. Novel thoughts about TNF as a mediator in CHF have recently evolved *(39)*. Animal models have shown that overexpression of TNF-α leads to CHF. The underlying mechanism is possibly mediated by direct immunotoxicity, NO-mediated damage, increased toxic calcium oscillations, apoptosis via specific receptors, transcription of factors that disrupt sarcolemma function, or a decrease in effectiveness of β adrenergic stimulation. This may be controlled by the modulation of other detrimental cytokines, such as IL-6 and IL-10, that exacerbate heart failure.

Attempts to artificially reduce endogenous TNF levels are underway. The development of a protein that mimics the TNF receptor, Etanercept, was studied in the treatment of decompensated heart failure and was eagerly anticipated. However, problems such a rapid breakdown of the drug and a paradoxic increase in TNF levels have obscured data analysis.

Further amino substituted thalidomide analogs have an even greater TNF-α suppressing activity. Although they have biologic plausibility, they have not been studied clinically in CHF.

CONCLUSION

Alternative therapies to heart failure are simply those that have not accumulated enough scientific data to convince the existing medical establishment for their consistent use in heart failure patients. Many of today's widely accepted drugs have shared this historical perspective.

Several decades ago, ACE inhibitors in their infancy, were likely considered alternative therapies for heart failure. Today, they are an accepted modality in the repertoire of therapy offered to patients. However, further advanced studies are needed on the above compounds before they are inaugurated into routine use.

REFERENCES

1. Keith M, Geranmayegan A, Sole M, et al. Increased oxidative stress in patients with congestive heart failure. J Am Coll Cardiol 1998;31:1352–1356.
2. Folkers K, Vadhanavikit S, Mortensen S. Biochemical rationale and myocardial tissue data on the effective therapy of cardiomyopathy with coenzyme Q10. Proc Natl Acad Sci 1985;82:901–904.
3. Mortensen S. Perspectives on therapy of cardiovascular diseases with coenzyme Q10. Clin Invest 1993;71:s116–123.
4. Langsjoen P, Vadhanavikit S, Folkers K. Response of patients in classes III and IV of cardiomyopathy to therapy in a blind and crossover trial with coenzyme Q10. Proc Natl Acad Sci USA 1985;82:4240–4244.
5. Munkholm H, Hansen H, Rasmussen K. Coenzyme Q10 treatment in serious heart failure. Biofactors 1999;9:285–289.
6. Watson P, Scalia G, Gallbraith A, et al. Lack of effect of coenzyme Q10 on left ventricular function in patients with congestive heart failure. J Am Coll Cardiol 1999;33:1549–1552.
7. Hofman-Bang C, Rehnqvist N, Swedberg K, et al. Coenzyme Q10 as an adjunctive in the treatment of chronic congestive heart failure. J Cardiac Failure 1995;1.101–107.
8. Soja A, Mortensen S. Treatment of congestive heart failure with coenzyme Q10 illuminated by meta-analyses of clinical trials. Molec Aspects Med 1997;18:s159–168.
9. Baggio E, Gandini R, Plancher A, et al. Italian multicenter study on the safety and efficacy of coenzyme Q10 as adjunctive therapy in heart failure. CoQ10 Drug Surveillance Investigators. Molec Aspects Med 1994;15:s287–294.
10. Morisco C, Trimarco B, Condorelli M. Effect of coenzyme Q10 therapy in patients with congestive heart failure: A long-term multicenter randomized study. Clin Invest 1993;71:s116–123.
11. Khatta M, Alexander B, Krichten C, et al. The effect of coenzyme Q10 in patients with congestive heart failure. Ann Intern Med 2000;132:636–640.
12. Sinatra S. Coenzyme Q10 and congestive heart failure. Ann Intern Med 2000;133:745.
13. Crowley W, Ridgway E, Bough E, et al. Non-invasive evaluation of cardiac function in hypothyroidism: response to gradual thyroxine replacement. N Engl J Med 1977;296.
14. Forfar J, Muir A, Toft A. Left ventricular function in hypothyroidism. Responses to exercise and beta adrenoceptor blockade. Br Heart J 1982;48:278–284.
15. Cohen M, Schulman I, Spenillo A, Surks M. Effects of thyroid hormone on left ventricular function in patients treated for myxoedema. Am J Cardiol 1981;48:33–36.
16. Kahaly G, Mohr-Kahaly S, Beyer J, Meyer J. Left ventricular function analyzed by doppler and echocardiographic methods in short-term hypothyroidism. Am J Cardiol 1995;75:645–648.
17. Malik F, Mehra M, Uber P, Park M, Scott R, VanMeter C. Intravenous thyroid hormone supplementation in heart failure with cardiogenic shock. J Cardiac Failure 1999;5:31–37.

18. Spooner P, Morkin E, Goldman S. Thyroid hormone and thyroid hormone analogues in the treatment of heart failure. Coronary Artery Dis 1999;10:395–399.
19. Gildor A. Crataegus oxyacantha and heart failure. Circulation 1998;98:2098.
20. Schwinger R, Pietsch M, Frank K, Brixius K. Crataegus special extract WS 1442 increases force of contraction in human myocardium cAMP - independently. J Cardiovasc Phar 2000;35:700–707.
21. Leuchtgens H. Crataegus special extract WS 1442 in NYHA II heart failure. A placebo controlled randomized double-blind study. Fortschritte der Medizin 1993;111:352–354.
22. Weikl A, Assmus K, Neukum-Schmitz J, Zapfe G, Noh H, Siegrist J. Crataegus special extract WS 1442. Assessment of objective effectiveness in patients with heart failure (NYHA II). Fortschritte der Medizin 1996;114:291–296.
23. Holubarsch C, Colucci W, Meinertz T, Gaus W, Tendera M. Survival and prognosis: investigation of crataegus extract WS 1442 in congestive heart failure (SPICE) - rationale, study design and study protocol. Eur J Heart Failure 2000;2:431–437.
24. Huchard H. Anatomie pathologique, lesions et trouble cardiovasculaires de l'acromegalie. J Practiciens 1895;9:249,250.
25. Moller J, Moller N, Frandsen E, Wolthers T, JOL J, Christiansen J. Blockade of the renin-angiotensin-aldosterone system prevents growth hormone induced fluid retention. Am J Physiol 1997;272:E803–808.
26. Han V, D'ercole A, PK L. Cellular localization of somatomedin (insulin-like growth factor) messenger RNA in the human fetus. Science 1987;236:193–197.
27. Wahlander H, Isgaard J, Jennische E, Friberg P. Left ventricular insulin-like growth factor-I increases in early renal hypertension. Hypertension 1992;19:25–32.
28. Mirsky J. Elastic properties of the myocardium: a quantitative approach with physiological and clinical applications. Handbook of Physiology American Physiology Society I 1979;14:497–531.
29. Guron G, Friberg P, Wickman A, Branstsing C, Gabrielsson B, Isgaard J. Cardiac insulin-like growth factor I and growth hormone receptor expression in renal hypertension. Hypertension 1996;27:636–642.
30. Colao A, Marzullo P, DiSomma C, Lombardi G. Growth hormone and the heart. Clin Endocrinol 2001;54:137–154.
31. Tajima M, Weinberg E, Bartunek J, et al. Treatment with growth hormone enhances contractile reserve and intracellular calcium transients in myocytes from rats with postinfarction heart failure. Circulation 1999;99:127–134.
32. Yang R, Bunting S, Gillett N, Clark R, Jin H. Congestive heart failure: growth hormone improves cardiac performance in experimental heart failure. Circulation 1995;92:262–267.
33. Ross J. Growth hormone, cardiomyocyte contractile reserve, and heart failure. Circulation 1999;99:15–17.
34. Duerr R, McKirnan M, Gim R, Clark R, Chien K, Ross J. Cardiovascular effects of insulin-like growth factor-1 and growth hormone in chronic left ventricular failure in the rat. Circulation 1995;93:2188–2196.
35. Fazio S, Sabatini D, Capaldo B, et al. A preliminary study of growth hormone in the treatment of dilated cardiomyopathy. N Engl J Med 1996;334:809–814.
36. Osterziel K, Strohm O, Schuler J, et al. Randomised, double-blind, placebo-controlled trial of human recombinant growth hormone in patients with chronic heart failure due to dilated cardiomyopathy. Lancet 1998;351:1233–127.
37. Genth-Zotz S, Zotz R, Geil S, Voigtlander T, Meyer J, Darius H. Recombinant growth hormone therapy in patients with ischemic cardiomyopathy: effects on hemodynamics, left ventricular function, and cardiopulmonary exercise capacity. Circulation 1999;99:18–21.

38. Spallarossa P, Rossettin P, Minuto F, et al. Evaluation of growth hormone administration in patients with chronic heart failure secondary to coronary artery disease. Am J Cardiol 1999;84:430–433.

39. Davey P, Ashrafian H. New therapies for heart failure: Is thalidomide the answer? QJM 2000;93:305–311.

19 Established Therapies for Advanced Heart Failure

Lee R. Goldberg, MD, MPH, FACC

INTRODUCTION

Heart failure is a chronic, progressive disease. Despite advances in the management of heart failure over the past 30 years, many patients will progress to an advanced stage of the disease that negatively impacts their quality of life and ultimately leads to death. As our success in managing acute coronary syndromes and sudden cardiac death has improved, more patients are surviving to end-stage heart failure. Understanding the etiology of the progression and eliminating other causes of dyspnea or edema is the first step in the management of this challenging population. For younger patients without serious comorbidities, cardiac transplantation is an alternative that may extend the quantity and improve the quality of life. For those who are not transplant candidates, there are limited options, and often the focus becomes one of maintaining function and controlling symptoms, occasionally at the expense of mortality. In truly refractory heart failure, hospice care may be appropriate in order to maintain comfort and dignity.

From: *Contemporary Cardiology: Heart Failure:*
A Clinician's Guide to Ambulatory Diagnosis and Treatment
Edited by: M. L. Jessup and E. Loh © Humana Press Inc., Totowa, NJ

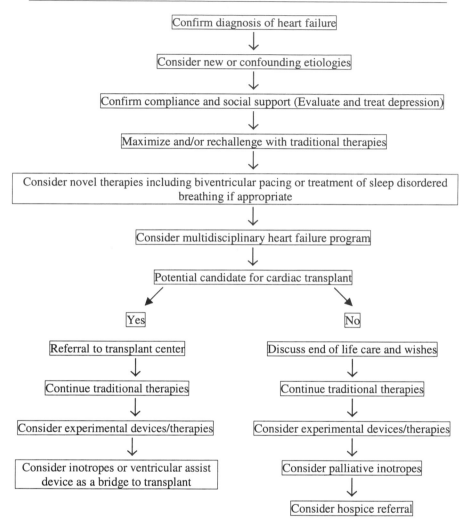

Fig. 1. Approach to the patient with advanced heart failure.

The recent American College of Cardiology/American Heart Association (ACC/AHA) treatment guidelines for the management of chronic heart failure classify patients with refractory or end-stage heart failure as stage D *(1)*. Patients at this stage may benefit from care at specialized centers focusing on advanced heart failure and may be candidates for cardiac transplant or experimental therapies. Figure 1 presents an overview to the approach of a patient with advanced heart failure.

ESTABLISHING THE DIAGNOSIS

In approaching any patient with advanced or refractory heart failure, the first step is to re-evaluate the etiology of the heart failure. For a patient who had previously been stable with chronic heart failure, the development of worsening symptoms may indicate that a new, superimposed process has occurred. In a patient who has had a nonischemic myopathy for many years, the development of subsequent coronary disease may precipitate worsening failure. In a subset of these patients, repeating a coronary angiogram or stress test in order to rule out potentially reversible disease is often appropriate. Several clinical trials have shown that in selected patients, revascularization may improve or stabilize ventricular function and symptoms and improve mortality, especially in patients with low ejection fractions (2).

The development of valvular heart disease can also lead to progression and clinical decompensation, especially for those patients with already impaired ventricular function. The natural history of heart failure often involves progressive ventricular dilatation and alterations in ventricular and annular geometry, causing worsening valvular regurgitation. Repeating an echocardiogram or re-evaluating hemodynamics can effectively evaluate valvular function and lead to consideration of surgical or experimental therapies. In the appropriate clinical context, subacute bacterial endocarditis should be excluded. Careful reassessment of the underlying structure and function of the heart may identify new therapeutic avenues that can improve functional capacity and symptoms and potentially delay or obviate the need for cardiac transplantation.

The symptoms and signs of heart failure often overlap with other clinical disease states. Dyspnea can be a manifestation of pulmonary disease, whereas volume overload, fatigue, and dyspnea may be symptoms of advanced renal disease. Although the initial approach to a patient with a history of ventricular dysfunction is to assume that the patient is suffering from worsening heart failure, it is critical to confirm the validity of this assumption. Re-evaluating laboratory values including renal and thyroid function can confirm that the symptoms are not a result of another cause. Recent studies have suggested that the use of brain natriuretic peptide (BNP) may help to differentiate cardiac from noncardiac causes of dyspnea (3,4). This can be especially useful in the setting of concurrent pulmonary disease when both the symptoms and physical examination findings can be very misleading. Other factors that may impact patients with advanced heart failure include alcohol consumption, new onset atrial fibrillation, anemia, and pulmonary emboli. Consideration of these disorders is important so they can be either ruled out or treated in appropriate patients (5).

In a previously stable heart failure patient who becomes refractory, it is critical to ensure that the patient has been compliant with recommended medications, diet, and lifestyle modifications. A change in insurance carriers may make previously available medications prohibitively expensive. Changes in the social situation of the patient, including the death of a spouse, may lead to loss of social or physical support. Identifying and correcting these barriers can often re-establish stability. Meticulous focus on maintaining salt and fluid balance in this population is critical. Multidisciplinary care models can often provide additional support to patients and their families, which, in turn, may stabilize heart failure symptoms. Multidisciplinary disease management models have been shown to be effective in reducing the rehospitalization rate and quality of life of older patients with heart failure (6).

Depression is common in patients with cardiovascular disease including those with heart failure (7). Depressed patients are less likely to be compliant with diet, exercise, and medications and several studies have indicated that depression is an independent risk factor for mortality in this population (8–10). Several researchers are evaluating the effectiveness of treating depression in this population in the hopes of impacting cardiovascular outcomes as well as mortality.

Several medications can exacerbate heart failure and cause a previously stable patient to become much more difficult to manage. The thiazolidinediones are used to treat insulin resistance in type II diabetics. This class of medications has many potentially beneficial effects on the cardiovascular system beyond glucose lowering. One side effect impacting patients with heart failure is fluid retention that can significantly worsen heart failure symptoms (11,12). Although β-blockers have been shown to improve morbidity and mortality in patients with heart failure, their use may transiently worsen heart failure symptoms, and they may be poorly tolerated by patients with advanced heart failure. Nonsteroidal anti-inflammatory drugs may inhibit the benefit of heart failure medications and may lead to worsening renal function and salt and water retention (13,14). Nutritional supplements and herbals can occasionally cause dangerous drug interactions, including digoxin and coumadin toxicity. Identification of all medications including prescription, over-the-counter, and nutritional agents, will allow for potential interactions to be identified.

Evaluation of the patient with advanced heart failure should also include a careful review of current and prior medications to confirm that all possible medical therapies have been attempted. Most medications approved for use in heart failure patients provide both morbidity and mortality benefits. The side effects of the common medications are often similar to the presenting symptoms of heart failure. For example, many patients are labeled as having experienced a cough when taking angiotensin-converting enzyme (ACE) inhibitors. Unfortunately, cough is a common symptom for patients with heart failure. Differentiating the two often can be difficult and for this reason, patients should be rechallenged with ACE inhibitors once their heart failure symptoms are stable. β-blockers can also present challenges. Many patients with heart failure experience fatigue, which may be caused by low-cardiac output, sleep-disordered breathing, depression, or may be a side effect of the β-blocker. In general, cautious rechallenge to medications that provide a morbidity and mortality benefit is appropriate in the majority of patients with advanced heart failure. There is increasing evidence that these medications, including β-blockers, can be tolerated and provide benefits even in the most advanced heart failure patients *(15,16)*.

Nohria et al. *(5)* developed a system to categorize patients based on their filling pressures and cardiac output state. This system relies on a bedside assessment, including variables obtained from patient history, as well as a focused clinical examination. The focus is on improving volume status to lower filling pressures while maintaining an adequate cardiac output. There has been significant controversy regarding the use of invasive hemodynamic monitoring for patients with advanced heart failure who do not respond to the traditional therapies. Several clinicians have reported that physical findings can be misleading in this population of patients, leading to inappropriate management *(17)*. There are several situations in which invasive monitoring may be useful. These include failure to respond despite appropriate therapy, inability to determine clinical status by noninvasive means, concomitant pulmonary or renal disease, critical situation in which restoring hemodynamic stability rapidly is paramount and in any patient in whom inotropes cannot be weaned. There are data indicating that following adjustment of oral therapies using invasive hemodynamic monitoring, long-term stability can then be maintained *(18)*.

Multidisciplinary heart failure disease management programs are effective in improving the outcomes of patients with advanced heart failure *(19)*. Additional resources enable these programs to provide more support to this high-risk patient group than an individual practitioner would be able to provide. Frequent contact with nurses using care algorithms can prevent subsequent admissions *(6)*. Focused education considering the patient's and family's needs and level of understanding can also improve outcomes. The availability of a social worker specializing in heart failure can help meet the many psychosocial needs of patients and their families. Referral to community services, identifying insurance resources and providing counseling and support are all integral to providing effective care. If necessary, referral to hospice or "pre-hospice" is an important service that can coordinate community resources to the needs of the patient and their caregivers. Dieticians, pharmacists, and physical therapists can provide additional support in their respective disciplines to reinforce diet, medication compliance, and physical activity goals *(20)*.

The use of a technology-driven heart failure disease management system has recently been shown to improve outcomes in patients with advanced heart failure. This technology transmitted daily weights and symptoms using an electronic scale to a central monitoring station staffed by trained nurses. These nurses then confirmed the data and notified physicians based on pre-established treatment algorithms. As these technologies continue to improve, they may provide a cost-effective extension to the traditional multidisciplinary team approach to heart failure disease management.

CARDIAC TRANSPLANTATION

Cardiac transplantation is an option for selected patients with advanced heart failure. Unfortunately, the supply of donor organs is far outweighed by the number of potential recipients. In the United States, approximately 2300 transplants are performed annually *(21)*. This number has remained essentially constant for several years despite increased public awareness of organ donation and the use of "marginal donor" hearts. For this reason, it is critical to select patients who will benefit most from cardiac transplantation. The ideal candidate must have advanced heart failure that is not responsive to the traditional medical and surgical therapies, but must also be free of significant noncardiac comorbid diseases and end-organ dysfunction. These patients must be able to survive the transplant surgery and should be expected to have a reasonable quality of life following recovery.

An initial approach for most centers is to screen patients for the absolute contraindications to transplant prior to completing the remainder of the evaluation. Table 1 contains a list of the absolute contraindications to cardiac transplant *(22)*. The absolute contraindications are factors known to increase the risk of the transplant surgery itself, severely limit life expectancy after transplant, or limit quality of life, despite a normally functioning cardiac allograft *(23)*. Over the past decade, factors that had previously been felt to be absolute contraindications have now become relative contraindications to be considered in the context of other risk factors *(24)*. These factors are listed in Table 2. In particular, some centers have had success in transplanting older patients who do not have many comorbid illnesses. Age over 65 years has become a relative contraindication for many centers assuming an otherwise healthy candidate *(24)*. A limited number of transplant centers will

Table 1
Contraindications to Isolated Cardiac
Transplantation[a]

Active or recent malignancy
Irreversible significant pulmonary disease
Irreversible significant renal disease
Irreversible hepatic dysfunction
Severe vascular disease—peripheral or cerebral
Irreversible pulmonary hypertension
Severe osteoporosis
Severe obesity
Unstable psychiatric disease
Active infection
Co-existent systemic illness with poor prognosis
HIV infection

[a]Adapted from ref. 22.

Table 2
Relative Contraindications to Isolated Cardiac Transplantation

Diabetes Mellitus
Vascular disease
Moderate obesity
Peptic ulcer disease
Age over 65 years
Poor psychosocial support
History of medical noncompliance
Renal insufficiency
Hepatitis C infection
Active Hepatitis B infection
Presence of anti-human antibodies (positive panel reactive antibodies [PRA])

perform multiple organ transplants including heart–lung, heart–kidney, and heart–liver in highly selected patients. For example, this allows dialysis-dependent patients with end-stage heart failure to receive combined heart–kidney transplants. Candidates for multiple organ transplantation typically need to meet the criteria of each organ's program separately.

In considering a patient for cardiac transplant, understanding the process during the waiting phase, as well as the post-transplant phase, is essential. Early referral to a transplant center for a potential candidate for cardiac transplantation is important, as it allows the entire transplant evaluation to be completed, and all problems to be appropriately identified and resolved. The waiting list for cardiac transplant, although very variable, is influenced by blood type, body size, and location of the transplant center. Most patients wait months on the transplant list. Continuing aggressive management of heart failure is obviously necessary during the waiting phase to allow survival until a donor organ becomes available *(25)*. As part of a transplant evaluation, anti-human antibodies are screened to identify high-risk patients for early severe rejection. Patients at risk of having high antibody levels include those who have received multiple blood transfusions and women who have had multiple pregnancies. Therefore, avoidance of blood transfusions for a potential cardiac transplant recipient is prudent unless absolutely necessary.

The most potent predictor of heart failure outcome is functional capacity as measured by peak exercise VO_2 during a metabolic exercise test. Most centers use this objective measure of functional capacity to decide if a candidate is at high risk of poor outcomes without transplant *(26)*. The 1-year average survival with transplant is approximately 80–85% *(21)*. A peak measured VO_2 of less than 14 mL/kg/min is correlated to a 1-year survival rate of approximately 85% *(27)*. Therefore, many transplant centers use a threshold peak VO_2 of less than 14 mL/kg/min to move forward with listing for cardiac transplant. Once the transplant evaluation has been completed, serial metabolic exercise testing can help to monitor patient status and determine the effectiveness of therapies as well as the progression of the disease. Nearly all cardiac transplant recipients have advanced New York Heart Association (NYHA) Class III or Class IV heart failure as manifest by dyspnea with minimal exertion or at rest.

Once listed, many patients require support or "a bridge" to transplant. Common bridging strategies include the use of intravenous inotropes and mechanical support using ventricular assist devices. Continuous intravenous inotropic support with milrinone or dobutamine has successfully been used to enable a patient with poor cardiac output to survive to transplant. Inotropes are associated with excess mortality in multiple trials and therefore appropriate precautions are necessary including continuous electrocardiographic monitoring or the placement of a functioning implantable defibrillator *(28)*. Selected centers will manage patients awaiting transplant at home on intravenous milrinone under very closely supervised conditions and with the placement of an implantable defibrillator prior to discharge. Ventricular assist devices are currently approved only for use as a bridge to transplant. Although these devices carry the up-front risk of surgery and are invasive, they offer the advantage of allowing patients to rehabilitate and potentially become a better transplant candidate once a donor organ becomes available. Patients who had received ventricular assist devices before transplant had improved renal function, improved functional capacity and had a slightly improved 6-month survival after transplant than those managed only with inotropes. Most of the benefit with the ventricular assist device appears to accrue in the first 6 weeks after which a plateau is reached. Transplant in the first few weeks after ventricular assist device placement has been associated with increased complications. Theoretically, these patients have yet to receive the full benefit of their ventricular assist device and are still recovering from its placement when subjected to transplant *(29)*.

After cardiac transplantation, patients are exposed to multiple drugs that inhibit the immune system to prevent rejection of the cardiac allograft *(30)*. These medicines include the calcineurin inhibitors (cyclosporine or tacrolimus), antiproliferatives (mycophenolate mofetil or azathioprine) and corticosteroids. The side effects of these medications often limit the quality of life for patients after transplant. The calcineurin inhibitors often cause hypertension and worsening renal insufficiency. They can cause resting tremors and can lead to a neuropathy or amplify a pre-existing neuropathy. Mycophenolate mofetil can cause bone marrow suppression and is associated with gastrointestinal side effects including nausea and occasionally diarrhea. Azathioprine is associated with bone marrow suppression and diarrhea. The corticosteroids are associated with worsening insulin resistance, making diabetes much more difficult to manage. Most patients with diabetes after transplant will require treatment with insulin. Steroids can also lead to weight gain, peptic ulcer disease, and osteoporosis. They can cause emotions to become more labile and in patients with a history of psychiatric disease may make previously stable patients unstable. All of the immunosuppressants can increase the risk of malignancy especially of the skin, bone marrow, and lymph nodes. In addition, patients are at increased risk of infection, especially in the early post-transplant phase when the doses of the immunosuppression drugs are the highest. Patients who come to transplant evaluation with pre-existing renal insufficiency, diabetes, neuropathy, or obesity often find these medical conditions worse after transplant as a result of the confounding effects of the necessary immunosuppressant medications. This can clearly effect quality of life and survival after transplant.

Ventricular assist devices have recently been studied as a permanent solution for patients with advanced heart failure instead of just a temporary bridge to transplant. A recent multicenter clinical trial designed to evaluate an implantable left-ventricular assist device vs continued medical therapy showed that quality of life and survival was improved in those randomized to the device *(31)*. Despite this, overall mortality was still very high at 2 years, and concerns about the long-term durability of the device, as well as complications, including infection and bleeding, indicate that there are still shortcomings to this technology. The next generation of devices promises transcutaneous power transmission to reduce the risk of infection and more durable parts. The ultimate goal is to find a reliable, long-term mechanical replacement for the human heart that would make transplantation obsolete. Patients in the study had very advanced heart failure but were not transplant candidates. To date, no device has been able to achieve better long-term outcomes than cardiac transplantation.

PALLIATIVE CARE

For most patients, cardiac transplantation is not an option. Once all possible therapies have been evaluated, clinicians should discuss with their patients goals for ongoing therapy. For many patients and their families, the focus of care often becomes preserving comfort, minimizing symptoms, avoiding hospitalization, and maintaining dignity. Many patients with advanced heart failure prefer not to be resuscitated should they suffer a cardiac arrest *(32)*. Detailed discussions about the patient's wishes while the patient can actively participate are critical. Most authors, including the recent consensus ACC/AHA guidelines for the management of chronic heart failure, emphasize that patients and their families should be candidly told about the course of advanced heart failure so that they can weigh the various options and decide about palliative and end-of-life care *(1)*.

One controversial area in the management of patients with advanced heart failure is the use of inotropic agents. Inotropes clearly improve hemodynamics and symptoms in patients with heart failure. Unfortunately, multiple studies evaluating oral and intravenous inotropes given either chronically or intermittently have shown increased mortality *(28,33–36)*. Many researchers believe that chronic exposure to inotropes may accelerate the "negative" remodeling of the ventricle in patients with heart failure and therefore lead to more rapid deterioration. Despite this, some studies have shown improved quality of life and decreased costs because of fewer hospitalizations, although total length of life may be shortened *(28,37)*. Many centers have reported success in using continuous intravenous inotropes in palliating those with refractory advanced heart failure *(37)*. The key elements to success include an experienced multidisciplinary team and family and community support.

Patients and their families must be informed of the risks of continuous inotropes and the alternative therapies available. Whenever continuous inotropes are considered for a patient who is not a transplant candidate, it must be made clear that the therapy is being used for palliation, and a discussion about end-of-life care should be included.

As functional capacity deteriorates, hospitalizations may occur more frequently. A referral to hospice can provide additional community support to enable patients to remain at home. Many hospice providers have care plans to accommodate those with advanced heart failure. Pain management may be less important initially as in comparison with treating dyspnea and volume overload. As the disease progresses, the use of narcotics and anxiolytics are often necessary to maintain comfort. Hospice programs also provide support for families including bereavement counseling. Early referral for hospice care enables a patient and family to develop a trusting relationship with the hospice provider and the physician. It is these relationships that provide comfort when medical care has little more to offer.

One of the most difficult decisions for patients and clinicians is when to turn off a previously placed implantable defibrillator. The purpose of an implantable defibrillator is to extend life by treating potentially fatal arrhythmias. For those with a poor quality of life at baseline, multiple defibrillator firings may be seen as only worsening their quality of life without adding any significant benefit. In this context, deactivating a defibrillator may allow for a peaceful death as opposed to progressive suffering with end-stage heart failure. Placement of an implantable defibrillator into a patient with end-stage heart failure should be undertaken only if the symptoms of heart failure are manageable, and the baseline quality of life is reasonable (38).

Decisions regarding readmission to the hospital or the use of specific technologies like ventilators, dialysis or CPR should be discussed. Do not resuscitate orders are critical in establishing the goals of therapy. Durable power of attorney and a health care proxy for decision making enables a smoother transition should the patient later be unable to participate in care discussions. These decisions should occur in the presence of family members, be clearly documented in the medical record, and a copy should be given to the patient and/or his or her family. Shifting the focus of discussions to emotional and spiritual needs can often provide significant comfort when therapies to alleviate heart failure symptoms are limited (39).

As our therapies for the treatment of heart failure improve, more patients will survive to an advanced form of the disease. Meticulous guideline driven multidisciplinary care can improve outcomes and quality of life. For a selected few, cardiac transplant is currently the best long-term therapy. For the rest, newer technologies and experimental protocols hold promise for the future. In the interim, clinicians must recognize the limitations in therapeutic options for this challenging group of patients and have the courage to discuss end-of-life care.

REFERENCES

1. Hunt HA, Baker DW, Chin MH, et al. ACC/AHA Guidelines for the Evaluation and Management of Chronic Heart Failure in the Adult: Executive Summary A Report of the American College of Cardiology/American Heart Association Task Force on Practice Guidelines (Committee to Revise the 1995 Guidelines for the Evaluation and Management of Heart Failure): Developed in Collaboration With the International Society for Heart and Lung Transplantation; Endorsed by the Heart Failure Society of America. Circulation 2001;104:2996–3007.
2. Mock MB, Ringqvist I, Fisher LD, et al. Survival of medically treated patients in the coronary artery surgery study (CASS) registry. Circulation 1982;66:562–568.
3. Morrison LK, Harrison A, Kirishraswamy P, Kazanegra R, Clapton P, Maisel A. Utility of a rapid B-natriuretic peptide assay in differentiating congestive heart failure from lung disease in patients presenting with dyspnea. J Am Coll Cardiol 2002;39:202–209.
4. Cabanes L, Richard-Thiriez B, Fulla Y, et al. Brain natriuretic peptide blood levels in the differential diagnosis of dyspnea. Chest 2001;120:2047–2050.
5. Nohria A, Lewis E, Stevenson LW. Medical management of advanced heart failure. JAMA 2002;287:628–640.
6. Rich MW, Beckham V, Wittenberg C, Leven CL, Freedland KE, Carney RM. A multidisciplinary intervention to prevent the readmission of elderly patients with congestive heart failure. N Engl J Med 1995;333:1190–1195.
7. Hawthorne MH, Hixon ME. Functional status, mood disturbance and quality of life in patients with heart failure. Prog Cardiovasc Nursing 1994;9:22–32.
8. Vaccarino V, Kasl VA, Abramson J, Krumholz HM. Depressive symptoms and risk of functional decline and death in patients with heart failure. J Am Coll Cardiol 2001;38:199–205.
9. MacMahon KM, Lip GY. Psychological factors in heart failure: a review of the literature. Arch Intern Med 2002;162:509–516.
10. Carney RM, Freedland KE, Eisen SA, Rich MW, Jaffe AS. Major depression and medication adherence in elderly patients with coronary artery disease. Health Psychol 1995;14:88–90.
11. Mudaliar S, Henry RR. New oral therapies for type 2 diabetes mellitus: the glitazones or insulin sensitizers. Ann Rev Med 2001;52:239–257.
12. Schoonjans K, Auwerx J. Thiazolidinediones: an update. Lancet 2000;355:1008–1010.
13. Page J, Henry D. Consumption of NSAIDs and the development of congestive heart failure in elderly patients: an underrecognized public health problem. Arch Intern Med 2000;160:777–784.
14. Dzau VJ, Packer M, Lilly IS, Swartz SL, Hollenberg NK, Williams GH et al. Prostaglandins in severe congestive heart failure. Relation to activation of the renin—angiotensin system and hyponatremia. N Engl J Med 1984;310:347–352.
15. The CONSENSUS Trial Study Group. Effects of enalapril on mortality in severe congestive heart failure. Results of the Cooperative North Scandinavian Enalapril Survival Study (CONSENSUS). N Engl J Med 1987;316:1429–435.
16. Packer M, Coats, AJ, Fowler MB, et al. Effect of carvedilol on survival in severe chronic heart failure. N Engl J Med 2001;344:1651–1658.

17. Badgett RG, Lucey CR, Mulrow CD. Can the clinical examination diagnose left-sided heart failure in adults? JAMA 1997;277:1712–1719.

18. Stevenson LW, Tillisch JH, Hamilton M, et al. Importance of hemodynamic response to therapy in predicting survival with ejection fraction less than or equal to 20% secondary to ischemic or nonischemic dilated cardiomyopathy. Am J Cardiol 1990;66:1348–1354.

19. McAlister FA, Lawson FM, Teo KK, Armstrong PW. A systematic review of randomized trials of disease management programs in heart failure. Am J Med 2001;110:378–84.

20. Rich MW. Heart failure disease management programs: efficacy and limitations. Am J Med 2001;110:410–412.

21. Hosenpud JD, Bennett LE, Keck BM, Boucek MM, Novick RJ. The Registry of the International Society for Heart and Lung Transplantation: eighteenth Official Report-2001. J Heart Lung Transplant 2001;20:805–815.

22. Mudge GH, Goldstein S, Addonizio LJ, et al. 24th Bethesda conference: Cardiac transplantation. Task Force 3: recipient guidelines/prioritization. J Am Coll Cardiol 1993;22:21–31.

23. Dec GW, Semigran MI, Vlahakes GJ. Cardiac transplantation. current indications and limitations. Transplant Proc 1991;23:2095–2106.

24. Miniati DN, Robbins RC. HEART TRANSPLANTATION: a thirty year perspective. Annu Rev Med 2002;53:189–205.

25. Stevenson WG, Stevenson LW, Middlekauff HR, et al. Improving survival for patients with advanced heart failure: a study of 737 consecutive patients. J Am Coll Cardiol 1995;26:1417–1423.

26. Stevenson LW. Selection and management of candidates for heart transplantation. Curr Opin Cardiol 1996;11.166 173.

27. Mancini DM, Eisen H, Kussmaul W, Mull R, Edmunds LH Jr., Wilson JR. Value of peak exercise oxygen consumption for optimal timing of cardiac transplantation in ambulatory patients with heart failure. Circulation 1991;83:778–786.

28. Felker GM, O'Connor CM. Inotropic therapy for heart failure: an evidence-based approach. Am Heart J 2001;142:393–401

29. Morrone TM, Buck LA, Catanese KA, et al. Early progressive mobilization of patients with left ventricular assist devices is safe and optimizes recovery before heart transplantation. J Heart Lung Transplant 1996;15:423–429.

30. Kobashigawa JA. Advances in immunosuppression for heart transplantation. Adv Cardiac Surg 1998;10:155–174.

31. Rose EA, Gelijns AC, Moskowitz AJ, et al. Long-term mechanical left ventricular assistance for end-stage heart failure. N Engl J Med 2001;345:1435–1443.

32. Krumholz HM, Phillips RS, Hamel MB, et al. Resuscitation preferences among patients with severe congestive heart failure: results from the SUPPORT project. Study to Understand Prognoses and Preferences for Outcomes and Risks of Treatments. Circulation 1998;98:648–6655.

33. Ewey GA. Inotropic infusions for chronic congestive heart failure: medical miracles or misguided medicinals? J Am Coll Cardiol 1999;33:572–575.

34. Hatzizacharias A, Makris T, Krespi P, et al. Intermittent milrinone effect on long-term hemodynamic profile in patients with severe congestive heart failure. Am Heart J 1999;138:241–246.

35. Nieminen MS, Akkila J, Hasenfuss, G, et al. Hemodynamic and neurohumoral effects of continuous infusion of levosimendan in patients with congestive heart failure. J Am Coll Cardiol 2000;36:1903–1912.

36. O'Connor C, Gattis W, Uretsky B, et al. Continuous intravenous dobutamine is associated with an increased risk of death in patients with advanced heart failure: insights from the Flolan International Randomized Survival Trial (FIRST). Am Heart J 1999;138:78–86.
37. Mehra MR, Uber PA. The dilemma of late-stage heart failure. Rationale for chronic parenteral inotropic support. Cardiol Clin 2001;19:627–636.
38. Stevenson WG, Stevenson LW. Prevention of sudden death in heart failure. J Cardiovasc Electrophysiol 2001;12:112–114.
39. Albert NM, Davis M, Young J. Improving the care of patients dying of heart failure. Cleveland Clin J Med 2002;69:321–328.

20 Diastolic Heart Failure

A Clinician's Approach to Diagnosis and Management

Martin G. Keane, MD

INTRODUCTION

Signs and symptoms of congestive heart failure (CHF) frequently occur in the presence of normal left-ventricular systolic function. Clinical findings mimic those of systolic failure, making confirmation of preserved ventricular systolic performance essential for accurate diagnosis and therapeutic intervention (1). Although occasionally secondary to valvular or coronary disease superimposed on otherwise normal left-ventricular function, clinical heart failure in these cases is most commonly caused by abnormalities of diastolic performance. So-called "diastolic dysfunction" is a most important etiology of the overall syndrome of "diastolic heart failure." Impaired ventricular relaxation during diastole results in poor ventricular filling, diminished forward cardiac output, and retrograde elevation of left atrial and pulmonary pressures as a result of increased ventricular end-diastolic pressure.

From: *Contemporary Cardiology: Heart Failure:*
A Clinician's Guide to Ambulatory Diagnosis and Treatment
Edited by: M. L. Jessup and E. Loh © Humana Press Inc., Totowa, NJ

In population studies, it is apparent that heart failure because of diastolic dysfunction represents a major portion of the overall heart failure burden, particularly in geriatric populations. The overall incidence of heart failure is estimated at 550,000 cases/year (2). Between 30–50% of these individuals have heart failure in the absence of systolic dysfunction or valvular disease (3,4), presumably owing to primary abnormalities of diastolic function. Recognition of this large population problem has grown over the past several decades, resulting from improvements in the assessment of ventricular systolic and diastolic function and valvular disease.

Overall morbidity and mortality from primary diastolic heart failure have traditionally been considered to be less than that from systolic left ventricular failure (5,6). However, recent studies have demonstrated 4- to 5-year mortality of 24–40% (7,8), and a combined cardiovascular morbidity and mortality up to 75% (9). Clinical heart failure is the most common reason for admission in patients over the age of 65, a population where diastolic heart failure is endemic (10,11). Given the high prevalence of morbidity in this syndrome, the economic significance of diastolic heart failure is exceedingly high. It is estimated that this represents an economic burden on the health system of up to $10 billion annually (12,13).

Clearly, diastolic heart failure is a clinical entity that cannot be treated with complacency. Accurate diagnosis and effective therapy are of great importance. The lack of large population studies specifically addressing the clinical syndromes caused by diastolic dysfunction might therefore be surprising. Unfortunately, diagnostic techniques used in day-to-day practice are often imprecise in identifying the presence of diastolic abnormalities (14), and there is a concomitant lack of an explicit clinical diagnostic definition for the entity (15,16). Identification of uniform populations of diastolic heart failure subjects for prospective clinical trials is therefore exceedingly difficult (13). Furthermore, the group of disorders that cause isolated diastolic dysfunction is heterogeneous. Combined with a diverse group of superimposed secondary exacerbants, the selection of an "optimal" single- or multiagent therapeutic strategy for large population studies is nearly impossible.

PATHOPHYSIOLOGY

A common error in understanding diastolic dysfunction relates to the misconception of diastole as a strictly passive phenomenon. Innate left-ventricular myocardial resilience is a major factor in determining the effectiveness of filling during diastole. However, the relaxation process is also an active phenomenon, dependent on orchestrated inactivation of the contractile elements to allow extension of sarcomeres to their resting/precontraction length. This process is intimately dependent on reuptake of calcium ions, an ATP/energy-dependent process. Alterations in both passive and active qualities of the left-ventricular myocardium result in impairment of diastolic performance (17).

Abnormality of the *passive* qualities of the myocardial tissues typically result from thickening of the ventricular walls because of myocyte hypertrophy, as well as from increases in the fibrous interstitial component (18,19). These changes are compounded by alterations in the normal collagen structure and crosslinking that accompanies most cases of diastolic heart failure (20,21). Changes in passive compliance are found in the most common causes of diastolic heart failure: hypertensive heart disease and the "normal" aging ventricle (22). Infiltrative diseases such as amyloid can affect passive relaxation via deposition of abnormal protein components within the interstitium (1). Increases in wall thickness and the interstitial component result in alteration of the relationship between left-ventricular volume and pressure. The increase in intraventricular pressure with diastolic filling becomes exaggerated. Small increases in diastolic volume, usually easily accommodated by the normal ventricle, result in very large pressure increases in the ventricle with diastolic dysfunction. This limits the amount of volume that the ventricle can accept during diastole and increases dependence on the atrial phase (atrial "kick").

Changes in the function of intracellular components of the myocytes can impair diastolic relaxation through their effects on the *active* relaxation process. The contractile process is dependent on calcium release from the sarcoplasmic reticulum. Inactivation of contraction is therefore dependent on the reuptake of the calcium ions within the cytosol (23). During hypertrophic processes and the senescence of myocytes, the volume of sarcoplasmic reticulum is increased, but is characterized by impaired calcium ion uptake by abnormal calcium channels (24). This is further exacerbated by impaired myocardial oxygen exchange through the hypertrophic/fibrotic myocardium. Myocyte ischemia results with impaired adenosine triphosphate (ATP) production and further decline in active calcium reuptake. Transient impairment of myocyte function occurs during ischemic episodes from coronary artery disease or in stunned or hibernating myocardium (14). Episodes of tachycardia significantly shorten the diastolic period and diminish time and efficacy of calcium reuptake (25). Furthermore, atrial fibrillation results not only in diminished diastolic filling time, but also in loss of atrial "kick"—so essential to the overall filling of the nondistensible ventricle *(17)*. Superimposed active and passive relaxation abnormalities compound failure of normal relaxation and further limit diastolic filling.

Maintenance of normal left-ventricular filling and cardiac output in diastolic dysfunction therefore requires elevated left-ventricular pressures throughout diastole, which is transmitted retrograde to the left atrium and pulmonary veins. Concurrent volume overload of the left atrium and pulmonary circulation exists in more advanced cases, due to the excess blood volume that cannot flow naturally into the left ventricle during diastole. These diastolic abnormalities are often well-tolerated at rest, when left ventricular filling times are long and relaxation is at its optimum. However, perturbations of the resting state cause more pronounced atrial and pulmonary overload, resulting in dyspnea or pulmonary edema. Impairment of left-ventricular filling is most commonly pronounced during exercise, with resulting excessive increases in left atrial and pulmonary capillary wedge pressure *(26)*. Dyspnea on exertion is therefore a predominant feature of early diastolic heart failure. Volume overload from excessive salt intake or retention by the kidneys can result in dyspnea at rest, and if significant enough, pulmonary edema.

In addition to such changes in preload, significant increase in afterload is poorly tolerated by the ventricle with diastolic dysfunction. During periods of substantial hypertension or hypertensive crisis, increase in end-diastolic volume is an important ventricular compensatory mechanism *(6)*. As described earlier, this is associated with significant increases of intracavitary pressure in ventricles with diastolic dysfunction. This is a common cause of flash pulmonary edema in patients with otherwise normal systolic function and with normal coronary perfusion *(27)*. Limitation of ventricular diastolic reserve can be a feature of more subtle degrees of impaired forward cardiac output associated with diminished diastolic compliance.

ETIOLOGY

In clinical practice, heart failure symptoms in the presence of apparent normal systolic function should not immediately equate to truly "diastolic" heart failure. Transient systolic or diastolic abnormalities may be responsible, or signs and symptoms may be related to other coexisting pathophysiology. The differential diagnostic profile for diastolic dysfunction vs "imitators" is described in Table 1.

Cardiac valvular or ischemic heart diseases frequently have attendant normal baseline systolic function. Although co-existing diastolic abnormalities may augment the underlying hemodynamic disturbances,

Table 1
Etiologies for Isolated Diastolic Heart Failure

Intrinsic ventricular abnormalities ("true" diastolic dysfunction)	Normalventricular aging
	Left-ventricular hypertrophy (LVH)
	Hypertrophic cardiomyopathy
	Infiltrative disease
	Myocardial storage diseases
	Endomyocardial disease
Superimposed exacerbants of diastolic dysfunction	Hypertension
	Arrhythmia—tachycardia
	Arrhythmia—loss of atrial phase
	Volume/salt overload
	High-output states
Imitators—cardiac	Measured ejection fraction is inaccurate
	Ischemic heart disease
	Valvular heart disease
	Pericardial disease
	Congenital heart disease
	High-output states (severe anemia)
Imitators—noncardiac	COPD
	Obesity
	Physical deconditioning
	Venous insufficiency
	Medication effects (Norvasc)
	Severe volume overload

native valvular diseases frequently present with CHF in the absence of diastolic abnormalities. Ischemic heart disease may present with intermittent CHF or "flash" pulmonary in the face of what appears to be baseline normal systolic and diastolic function. Thus, evaluation for coronary disease is important in those with coronary risk factors and CHF. Pericardial disease often presents with heart failure symptoms a result of extrinsic diastolic constriction, but therapy is entirely different for these individuals and should not be mistaken for intrinsic diastolic abnormality.

Noncardiac diseases such as chronic obstructive pulmonary disease, significant obesity, and chronic venous insufficiency are associated with signs and symptoms similar to right- or left-sided CHF. Patients with these disorders frequently have normal systolic, diastolic, and valvular function. Treatment of the primary noncardiac problem is essential in these individuals for symptomatic relief. These imitators must be ruled out before a diagnosis of diastolic dysfunction is considered.

In those with intrinsic, isolated diastolic dysfunction, the normal aging process of the heart is by far the most common cause. Diastolic heart failure is increasingly recognized as a prevalent phenomenon in the elderly population *(10,28)*. Myocyte attrition and progressive myocardial fibrosis contribute to increased passive stiffness of the ventricle in the elderly *(10,21)*. Ongoing hypertrophic process of the remaining myocytes as a result of prevalent systolic hypertension also contributes to abnormalities of both active and passive relaxation. Senile abnormalities of calcium handling have also been demonstrated to play an additional role *(10)*. Superimposed valvular regurgitation and stenosis merely exacerbate underlying diastolic dysfunction, as does a high prevalence of atrial dysrhythmias.

The second most common etiology is hypertensive heart disease, characterized by varying degrees of left-ventricular hypertrophy. Hypertrophic thickening of the left-ventricular walls reduces the myocardial wall stress imposed by volume and pressure loads *(18,19)*. In its early stages, hypertrophy allows more effective ventricular function at reduced myocardial oxygen consumption. The process becomes maladaptive, however, because the synthetic process stimulated during hypertrophy is not identical to normal myocyte growth. Abnormal forms of myocardial components accumulate, including fetal myoglobin and α troponin, abnormal mitochondria, and poorly functioning sarcoplasmic reticulum *(21)*. Whereas systolic function may be maintained in the normal range for long periods of time, diastolic abnormalities appear far more early.

Similar diastolic abnormalities are also present in congenital hypertrophic cardiomyopathies, both obstructive and nonobstructive forms. In these cases, congenitally abnormal cellular structural and functional abnormalities are to blame. Highly eccentric and abnormal myocardial architecture with marked disarray of myocyte placement also contributes. Other less common etiologies of diastolic dysfunction include infiltrative diseases such as amyloid and hemochromatosis *(29,30)*. Infiltration of the interstitial connective tissue by abnormal proteins increases myocardial stiffness and interferes with normal intercellular signalling. Abnormalities of passive and active relaxation processes frequently appear early in the course of such diseases and usually precede overt systolic dysfunction *(30)*. Extremely rare causes of isolated diastolic dysfunction also include the myocardial storage diseases and endomyocardial fibrosis. These are exceedingly uncommon in routine clinical practice.

DIAGNOSTIC STRATEGY

The Framingham group and the European Society of Cardiology have both recently proposed formal diagnostic criteria for diastolic heart

Table 2
Diagnostic Strategies

Rule out obvious noncardiac etiologies of symptoms		
	Vasan	*ESC*
Symptoms	Confirmed HF signs/sx	Confirmed HF signs/sx
Normal systolic function	EF ≥ 50%	EF ≥ 45%
Abnormal diastolic function	Hemodynamic	Hemodynamic
		Echocardiographic

failure *(13,31)*. These are helpful not only from a clinical epidemiology and research standpoint, but also provide the clinician with a reasonably cogent method to organize a diagnostic strategy. As outlined in Table 2, confirmation of the diagnosis of CHF is the first (and perhaps most important) priority. Signs and symptoms are not specific, and a diagnosis of CHF may be inaccurate *(32)*. Noncardiac imitators described earlier (Table 1) must be ruled out at this stage. If the signs of heart failure are predominantly right-sided (elevated JVP, edema, fatigue), then right-heart pathology or failure must also be evaluated *(1)*.

Subsequently, confirmation of normal left-ventricular systolic function is essential *(13,31)*. Angiographic ventriculography, echocardiography, and radionuclide blood pool scans can all be utilized to assess systolic function. In typical clinical practice, echocardiographic visualization of the ventricle is typically the most advantageous. This approach provides a reasonably complete noninvasive assessment, and valvular, pericardial, and congenital disease can also be ruled out simultaneously. Presence of regional wall motion abnormalities or scarring may also indicate coexisting coronary artery disease. Evaluation of heart failure upon presentation can be key in detecting transient ischemic wall motion abnormalities or ischemic mitral regurgitation. Such anomalies would be absent on echoes performed 12–24 hours after the event, prohibiting differentiation of these reversible etiologies from primary diastolic functional abnormalities *(27)*. These situations being ruled out, a diagnosis of primary diastolic heart failure may be seriously considered.

The final portion of the proposed diagnostic strategies—proof of underlying diastolic dysfunction—is frequently the most difficult to accomplish definitively. The most certain diagnostic assessment of diastolic function comes from measurement of intracardiac hemodynamics during cardiac catheterization *(13)*. Mapping left-ventricular pressure against concurrent ventricular volume throughout the cardiac cycle allows precise demonstration of the abnormal features of the ventricular pressure-volume relationship (Fig. 1) *(33)*. Performing routine

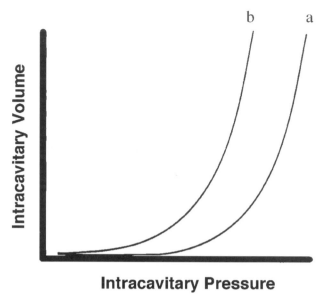

Intracavitary Pressure

Fig. 1. Left-ventricular pressure is intimately related to the volume within the ventricular cavity. (**A**) In the normal ventricle, there is a wide range of end-diastolic volume over which the ventricle can fill at very low pressures. It is only at very high diastolic volumes that ventricular pressure rises precipitously. (**B**) This relationship of pressure and volume is shifted in the ventricle with diastolic dysfunction. In this case, even at low diastolic volumes, there is a more significant increase in intracavitary pressure.

cardiac catheterization in the large population of elderly or hypertensive patients with probable diastolic heart failure is excessively invasive and not cost effective *(13)*. In most cases, noninvasive assessment of diastolic function is more appropriate. By Framingham criteria, this would be considered indicative of "probable" diastolic heart failure *(13)*. Nonetheless, invasive hemodynamic assessment may be necessary for CHF with normal systolic function in the absence of obvious risk factors for diastolic heart failure. Simultaneous coronary angiography can assess potential ischemic etiologies of failure.

Assessment of diastolic function by echocardiography has traditionally relied on Doppler measurements of the left-ventricular inflow through the mitral valve *(34,35)*. As demonstrated in Fig. 2, in the pres-

Fig. 2. Pulsed wave Doppler flow patterns through the mitral valve during diastole are illustrated. (**A**) In the normal ventricle, a majority of filling occurs during early (passive) filling phase. This larger volume flow results in a tall E wave, with a large overall area (velocity-time integral). Atrial contraction represents <25% of the flow across the mitral valve, resulting in a more diminutive

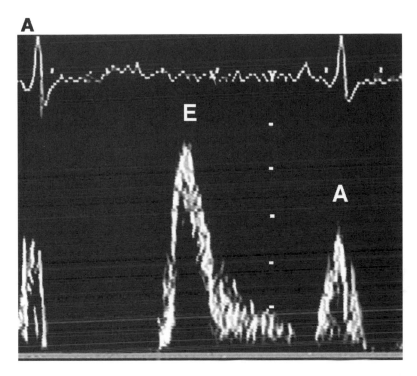

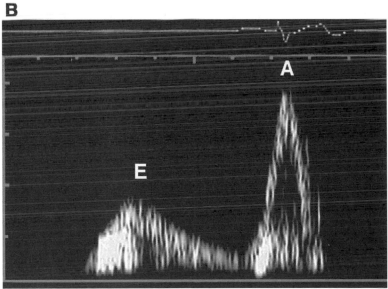

Fig. 2. *(continued)* A wave **(B)** In a ventricle with diastolic dysfunction, a far smaller amount of blood flows across the mitral valve during early, passive filling, due to rapid equalization of the pressure gradient between the chambers. This results in a diminutive E wave. A far more significant A wave is generated by the larger volume of flow during atrial contraction.

ence of normal cardiac physiology, the peak velocity (and velocity time integral) is greater during early, passive filling of the ventricle. Thus, the Doppler measurement of early filling (E-wave) is typically of higher amplitude than that of late filling or atrial kick (A-wave) (Fig. 2A). In "classic" diastolic dysfunction, the volume of blood flow across the mitral inlet during early passive filling diminishes, and a greater volume of blood crosses during late, atrial phase. Thus, the E-wave Doppler velocity becomes small and the A-wave velocity more prominent (Fig. 2B). This reversal of velocity between early and late filling stages has been considered the hallmark defining of diastolic dysfunction.

This velocity ratio is highly sensitive to loading conditions, heart rate, and particularly to the degree of left-atrial pressure elevation. Left-atrial dilatation and dysfunction may progress to a level that left-atrial pressures surpass elevated ventricular diastolic pressures. The newly elevated atrial driving pressure allows enhancement of early diastolic filling. The Doppler measurement of flow velocity can appear normal, despite the presence of advancing diastolic dysfunction. This "pseudonormalization" of Doppler inflow can sometimes be differentiated from truly normal filling by Valsalva maneuver. In patients with normal filling, the Doppler inflow pattern remains normal. In those with advanced diastolic dysfunction, the "pseudonormal" pattern reverts to a reversal of E and A wave of classic diastolic dysfunction during Valsalva.

Several newer echocardiographic techniques have been developed to augment the accuracy of diastolic functional assessment. Use of tissue Doppler to measure velocity of mitral annular motion during diastole has proven to be a highly accurate method for the detection of diastolic dysfunction (36,37). These measurements are not sensitive to changes in loading conditions or left-atrial pressure (36). Assessment of pulmonary venous flow patterns (38), and color Doppler patterns during diastolic filling via color M-mode (39) can also assess diastolic dysfunction. A synthesis of the data from two or more of these techniques with Doppler velocity analysis can further enhance the accuracy of diastolic assessment (40). Radionucleotide blood pool scans may also be utilized to assess diastolic filling, but these are less commonly used in routine clinical practice (41).

TREATMENT

Given the lack of clinical data for treatment of diastolic heart failure as a true syndrome, therapy is largely empiric. Treatment of patients with heart failure despite normal systolic function (in the absence of other intrinsic and extrinsic imitators) must be individualized—guided by the patient's underlying condition and comorbid factors.

Table 3
Treatment Strategies

	Treatment goal	Treatment option
Treatment of intrinsic left-ventricular abnormalities	Diminish LVH	ARB, ACE-I, Ca^{++} blockers
	Diminish fibrosis	ACE-I, spironolactone, selective aldosterone antagonists
	Treat infiltrative disorders	Phlebotomy, liver transplant
	Improve active relaxation process	? Digoxin
Treatment of exacerbating factors	Reduce salt/ volume overload	Diuretics, salt restriction
	Prevent hypertensive crisis	Any drug
	Prevent/Rx ischemia	β-blockers, Ca^{++} blockers
	Prevent sinus tachycardia	β-blockers, Ca^{++} blockers
	Maintain atrial kick	β-blockers, Ca^{++} blockers, amiodarone, other anti-arrhythmia medications

ARB, angiotensin receptor blockers; ACE-1, angiotensin-converting inhibitor.

The primary focus of therapy has traditionally been the treatment and prevention of conditions known to exacerbate the diastolic dysfunction of the left ventricle (Table 3). By far, optimal therapy of underlying hypertension and prevention of hypertensive crisis is absolutely essential (27). The most frequent cause of flash pulmonary edema in the presence of diastolic dysfunction is incidental hypertensive crisis (22). Such episodes begin a deadly spiral of deteriorating diastolic filling, excessive increase in left-ventricular diastolic and pulmonary capillary pressures, sympathetic outflow response, further elevations of blood pressure, and intolerable increases in ventricular wall stress. These augment one another and lead to acute, often severe, CHF. Expeditious, aggressive treatment of the hypertensive crisis and diuresis usually lead to rapid improvement and resolution of CHF (27). These episodes represent the most urgent and memorable tasks in treating patients with diastolic dysfunction. The absolute importance of ongoing treatment of more moderate underlying hypertension—both systolic and diastolic— cannot be ignored. Untreated or incompletely treated hypertension is a major cause of progressive myocardial hypertrophy, fibrosis, and increasing diastolic stiffness of the ventricle. Diminishment of hypertrophic processes can prevent augmentation of diastolic dysfunction from normal aging.

Maintenance of a low-sodium diet and treatment of selected patients with cautious diuretic therapy are also indicated *(42)*. Aside from beneficial effects on blood pressure control, such therapy also prevents the excess volume overload that is so poorly tolerated by patients with diastolic dysfunction. Except in heart failure crises, aggressive diuretic therapy is typically unwise. As small elevations of preload above normal can result in CHF, even ostensibly small reductions of preload to the stiffened ventricle can result in severe, symptomatic hypotension. Optimal volume balance in the presence of more severe diastolic dysfunction can be a very delicate issue.

The stiffened ventricle poorly tolerates decrease in the diastolic filling period with increases in heart rate. Thus, prevention or reduction of tachycardia is essential for optimizing ventricular filling and avoiding diastolic heart failure *(43)*. Treatment with β-blockers and calcium-channel blockers not only lower the resting heart rate, but also effectively blunt rate response to exercise and can thereby improve exercise tolerance and symptoms of dyspnea on exertion. Beyond concerns of simple rate control, maintenance of sinus rhythm itself is essential. The atrial contribution to diastolic filling is proportionally higher with advancing degrees of diastolic dysfunction. Loss of atrial "kick" with atrial fibrillation or other atrial dysrhythmias often leads to dramatic decreases in systolic forward flow, in addition to elevation of left-ventricular EDP and pulmonary capillary wedge pressure (PCWP) *(12,17)*. Significant degrees of left- and right-atrial dilatation, common in longstanding diastolic dysfunction, elevate the risk of dysrhythmias. Treatment with β-blockers and Ca^{++}-blockers may be prophylactic against such incidents in patients without prior history *(17)*. However, in those patients with documented atrial dysrhythmias, specific anti-arrhythmic therapy with amiodarone or other agent may be wise.

Transient ischemic dysfunction, systolic and diastolic, has been previously noted as a possible cause of heart failure with otherwise normal baseline systolic (and diastolic) function. Even in obvious cases of resting diastolic abnormality, superimposed coronary artery disease and episodic ischemia can augment the kernel of diastolic heart failure. Thus, it is wise to consider the possibility of superimposed ischemia, especially when baseline therapy directed at diastolic function is ineffective. Treatment with β-blockers, or even coronary revascularization for the prevention of ischemic episodes, can be effective frequently in reducing episodic diastolic heart failure episodes *(44)*.

Ideally, the most direct therapy of diastolic dysfunction would be aimed toward the intrinsic ventricular abnormalities leading to the dysfunction. Targets include the cellular hypertrophic and fibrotic processes themselves, which lead to abnormal wall thickening and increased passive stiffness. Alteration of the intracellular abnormalities associated with the hypertrophy and aging would also be essential to ameliorate the abnormalities of active relaxation in isolated diastolic dysfunction. The tissue and neurohormonal controllers of these processes are complex and only partially understood, but it is clear that modification of the renin-angiotensin-aldosterone (RAA) axis and controlling excess adrenergic stimulation of the ventricle will be key components of such a therapeutic strategy.

Accumulated evidence from numerous, small studies of hypertrophy regression suggests that angiotensin-converting enzyme (ACE) inhibitors may have greater potency for diminishing hypertrophy beyond that predicted by simple lowering of blood pressure alone (45). Similar additional regressive effects have been reported for calcium-channel blockers (46). Thus, although chronic lowering of the blood pressure alone will result in regression of left-ventricular hypertrophy (LVH), the additional regressive benefits of ACE inhibitors and calcium-channel blockers may make them preferable in the treatment of patients with moderate degrees of LVH as the underlying cause of their diastolic dysfunction. However, these data are derived from meta-analyses of numerous smaller trials of questionable methodology and blinding. The only one large, well-controlled clinical trial of hypertension therapy to date has demonstrated that direct blockade of the angiotensin receptor by losartan results in greater regression of hypertrophy than does similar treatment with atenolol (47). There was clear improvement in diastolic filling associated with LVH regression (48). Patients treated with losartan had reduced all-cause mortality as compared with atenolol, particularly diabetics (49). Although ACE inhibitors may have similar effects, this has never been proven.

The RAA system also plays a role in the abnormal remodeling of the interstitial component of the myocardium (50). The beneficial effects of ACE inhibitors and angiotensin receptor blockers on the regression of LVH likely include the reduction of abnormal interstitial fibrosis. This also favors the use of angiotensin II antagonists in the treatment of patients with diastolic dysfunction. The importance of the aldosterone component of the RAA cannot be ignored. Aldosterone also is elevated in the hypertensive/hypertrophic process, and blockade of its tissue effects may improve overall ventricular performance. It is clear that in advanced stages of systolic heart failure, the addition of the aldosterone antagonist spironolactone improves overall clinical status and long-term prognosis *(51)*. There is recent evidence that a selective direct antagonist of aldosterone has a major beneficial effect on the regression of LVH because of hypertension *(52)*. Aldosterone may exert its primary effect on the interstitial component, and aldosterone blockade may ultimately be an important addition to the therapeutic strategy for diastolic dysfunction.

Utilization of digoxin in the treatment of diastolic heart failure is controversial. Traditionally utilized as a positive inotrope in systolic heart failure, digoxin frequently finds its way into the medical regimen of heart failure patients with preserved systolic function. Mechanistically, digoxin should augment diastolic filling abnormalities by its effective elevation of intracellular calcium concentrations *(53)*. Surprisingly, in a subgroup of CHF patients with preserved systolic function in the Digitalis Investigative Group (DIG) trial, there was evidence of a significantly decreased hospitalization frequency among those treated with digoxin *(54)*. Digoxin may have other limited additional benefits based on atrioventricular-nodal blocking effects, particularly in those with atrial fibrillation. This vagally mediated effect is weak, and β-blockers or calcium-channel blockers are preferable. Still, in some patients with diastolic heart failure, digoxin may have its place in the therapeutic armamentarium.

Clearly, treatment of diastolic heart failure is difficult, multifaceted, but exceedingly important. Therapeutic choices and strategies must clearly be made on a patient-to-patient basis. Once the diagnosis of diastolic heart failure has been made, immediate attention to the treatment and prevention of well-known exacerbating factors can diminish symptoms and reduce hospitalizations. Vigilant control of blood pressure with any agent or combination therapy is clearly most essential. To date, no uniform therapeutic strategy can be formulated toward the diverse histopathology underlying multiple etiologies of diastolic heart failure. However, consideration of the underlying pathophysiology of diastolic dysfunction, with a focus on the RAA system may ultimately provide effective diastolic-driven therapy in the future.

REFERENCES

1. Vasan RS, Benjamin EJ, Levy D. Congestive heart failure with normal left ventricular systolic function: clinical approaches to the diagnosis and treatment of diastolic heart failure. Arch Intern Med 1996;156:146–157.
2. American Heart Association, Heart and stroke statistical update. American Heart Association Publications, 2000.
3. Vasan RS, Benjamin EJ, Levy D. Prevalence, clinical features and prognosis of diastolic heart failure: an epidemiologic perspective. J Am Coll Cardiol 1995;26:1565–1574.

4. Kupari M, et al. Congestive heart failure in old age: prevalence, mechanisms and 4-year prognosis in the Helsinki Ageing Study. J Intern Med 1997;241:387–94.
5. Cohn JN, Johnson G. Heart failure with normal ejection fraction: the V-Heft study. Circulation 1990;81:III48–53.
6. Ghali JK, et al. Survival of heart failure patients with preserved versus impaired systolic function: the prognostic implication of blood pressure. Am Heart J 1992;123:993–997.
7. Senni M, Redfield MM. Heart failure with preserved systolic function: a different natural history? J Am Coll Cardiol 2001;38:1277–1282.
8. Vasan RS, et al. Conjestive heart failure in subjects with normal versus reduced left ventricular ejection fraction: prevalence and mortality in a population-based cohort. J Am Coll Cardiol 1999;33:1948–1955.
9. Setaro JF, et al. Long-term outcome in patients with congestive heart failure and intact systolic left ventricular performance. Am J Cardiol 1992;69:1212–1216.
10. Kitzman DW, et al. Importance of heart failure with preserved systolic function in patients ≥65 years of age. Am J Cardiol 2001;87:413–419.
11. McDermott MM, et al. Systolic function, readmission rates, and survival among consecutively hospitalized patients with congestive heart failure. Am Heart J 1997;134:728–736.
12. Dautermann KW, Massie BM, Gheorghiade M. Heart failure associated with preserved systolic function: A common and costly clinical entity. Am Heart J 1998;135: S310 S319.
13. Vasan RS, Levy D. Defining diastolic heart failure: a call for standardized diagnostic criteria. Circulation 2000;101:2118–2121.
14. Grossman W. Defining diastolic dysfunction. Circulation 2000;101:2020–2021.
15. European Society Guidelines on Diagnosis of Heart Failure. How to diagnose diastolic heart failure. Eur Heart J 1998;19:990–1003.
16. Zile MR, et al. Heart failure with normal ejection fraction: is measurement of diastolic function necessary to make the diagnosis of diastolic heart failure? Circulation 2001;104:779–782.
17. Bonow RO, Udelson JE. Left ventricular diastolic dysfunction as a cause of conjestive heart failure. Ann Intern Med 1992;117:502–510.
18. Gaasch WH, et al. Left ventricular compliance: Mechanisms and implications. Am J Cardiol 1976;38:645–653.
19. Grossman W. Diastolic dysfunction in congestive heart failure. N Engl J Med 1991;325:1557–1564.
20. Frohlich ED. Fibrosis and ischemia: the real risks in hypertensive heart disease. Am J Hyperten 2001;14:194S–199S.
21. Varagic J, Susic D, Frohlich E. Heart, aging, and hypertension. Curr Opin Cardiol 2001;16:336–341.
22. Kitzman DW. Heart failure with normal systolic function. Clin Geriatric Med 2000;16:489–511.
23. Brutsaert DI, Sys SU, Gilleert TC. Diastolic failure: pathophysiology and therapeutic implications. J Am Coll Cardiol 1993;22:318–325.
24. Lorell BH, Grossman WE. Cardiac hypertrophy: the consequences for diastole. J Am Coll Cardiol 1987;9:1189–1193.
25. Gwathmey JK, et al. Abnormal intracellular calcium handling in myocardium from patients with end-stage heart failure. Circ Res 1987;61:70–76.
26. Kitzman DW, Higginbotham MB, Cobb FR. Exercise intoleraance in patients with heart failure and preserved left ventricular systolic function: failure of the Frank-Starling mechanism. J Am Coll Cardiol 1991;17:1065–1069.

27. Gandhi SK, et al. The pathogenesis of acute pulmonary edema associated with hypertension. N Engl J Med 2001;344:17–22.
28. Gardin JM, et al. Left ventricular diastolic filling in the elderly: the cardiovascular health study. Am J Cardiol 1998;82:345–351.
29. Hauser SC. Hemochromatosis and the heart. Heart Dis Stroke 1993;2:487–491.
30. McCarthy RE, Kasper EK. A review of the amyloidoses that infiltrate the heart. Clin Cardiol 1998;21:547–552.
31. Remme WJ, Swedberg K. Guidelines for the diagnosis and treatment of chronic heart failure: task force for the diagnosis and treatment of chronic heart failure, European Society of Cardiology. Eur Heart J 2001;22:1527–1560.
32. Remes J, et al. Validity of clinical diagnosis of heart failure in primary health care. Eur Heart J 1991;12:315–321.
33. Mirsky I. Assessmen of diastolic function: suggested methods and future considerations. Circulation 1984;69:836–841.
34. Nishimura RA, et al. Assessment of diastolic function of the heart: background and current applications of Doppler echocardiography. Mayo Clin Proc 1989;64:181–204.
35. Shapiro SM, Bershohn MM, Laks MM. In search of the wholy grail: the study of diastolic ventricular function by the use of Doppler echocardiography. J Am Coll Cardiol 1991;17:517–519.
36. Garcia MJ, Thomas JD, Klein AL. New Doppler echocardiographic applications for the study of diastolic function. J Am Coll Cardiol 1998;32:865–875.
37. Waggoner AD, Bierig SM. Tissue Doppler imaging: a useful echocardiographic method to assess systolic and diastolic ventricular function. J Am Soc Echocardio 2001;14:1143–1152.
38. Firstenberg MS, et al. Doppler echo evaluation of pulmonary venous—left atrial pressure gradients: human and numerical model studies. Am J Physiol: Heart Circ Physiol 2000;279:H594–H600.
39. Garcia MJ, et al. Color M-mode Doppler flow propagation velocity is a preload insensitive index of left ventricular relaxation: animal and human validation. J Am Coll Cardiol 1999;35:201–208.
40. Ommen SR, et al. Clinical utility of Doppler echocardiography and tissue Doppler imaging in the estimation of left ventricular filling pressures: a comparative simultaneous Doppler-catheterization study. Circulation 2000;102:1788–1794.
41. Bonow RO. Radionuclide angiographic evaluation of left ventricular diastolic function. Circulation 1991;84:208–215.
42. Hunt SA, et al. ACC/AHA guidelines for the evaluation and management of chronic heart failure in the adult: executive summary. J Am Coll Cardiol 2001;38:2101–2113.
43. Shah PM, Pai RG. Diastolic heart failure. Curr Prob Cardiol 1992;17:783–868.
44. Humphrey LS, et al. Effects of left ventricular relaxation by coronary artery bypass grafting: intraoperative assessment. Circulation 1988;77:886–896.
45. Dahlof B, Pennert K, Hansson L. Reversal of left ventricular hypertrophy in hypertensive patients: metaanalysis of 109 treatment studies. Am J Hyperten 1992;5:95–110.
46. Schmieder RE, et al. Update on reversal of left ventricular hypertrophy in essential hypertension (a meta-analysis of all randomized double-blind studies until December 1996). Nephrol Dialysis Transplant 1998;13:564–569.
47. Dahlof B, et al. Cardiovascular morbidity and mortality in the Losartan intervention for endpoint reduction in hypertension study (LIFE): a randomised trial against atenolol. Lancet 2002;359:995–1003.
48. Wachtell K, et al. Change in diastolic left ventricular filling after one year of antihypertensive treatment. Circulation 2002;105:1071–1076.

49. Lindholm LH, et al. Cardiovascular morbidity and mortality in patients with diabetes in the Losartan intervention for endpoint reduction in hypertension study (LIFE): a randomised trial against atenolol. Lancet 2002;359:1004–1010.
50. Dostal DE. Regulation of cardiac collagen: angiotensin and cross-talk with local growth factors. Hypertension 2001;37:841–844.
51. RALES Group. Effectiveness of spironolactone added to an angiotensin-converting enzyme inhibitor and a loop diuretic for severe chronic congestive heart failure. Am J Cardiol 1996;78:902–907.
52. Pitt B, et al. Efficacy and safety of eplerenone, enalapril, and eplerenone/enalapril combination therapy in patients with left ventricular hypertrophy. American College of Cardiology, 51st Annual Scientific Session, 2002: Oral Presentation, Late-Breaking Clinical Trials III.
53. Gheorghiade M, Pitt B. Digitalis Investigation Group (DIG) trial: a stimulus for further research. Am Heart J 1997;134:3–12.
54. Garg R, et al. The effect of digoxin on mortality and morbidity in patients with heart failure. N Engl J Med 1997;336:525–533.

21 Disease Management and Practice Guidelines for Heart Failure

A Practical Approach

Jerry Johnson, MD

CONTENTS

INTRODUCTION

Physicians informed about the current recommendations for diagnosis and management of heart failure find significant challenges applying up-to-date recommendations consistently in a population of patients. The first challenge is the chronicity of the disorder. The physician cannot be content to effectively manage the individual through an acute episode; the greater challenge is to prevent decompensations during the

From: *Contemporary Cardiology: Heart Failure:*
A Clinician's Guide to Ambulatory Diagnosis and Treatment
Edited by: M. L. Jessup and E. Loh © Humana Press Inc., Totowa, NJ

course of the illness. The second challenge is the prevalence of heart failure in elderly individuals. The prevalence of heart failure approaches 10% in individuals over age 80. In this age group, comorbidities create significant management challenges for the practicing physician at a significant cost. Whereas physicians may be mindful of the clinical morbidity and mortality associated with heart failure, they may be unaware of the total treatment costs for heart failure, including drugs, physician costs, and nursing home stays, costs estimated at more than $17 billion in health care expenditures yearly. The third challenge is the need to recognize that the physician alone cannot successfully manage heart failure. Because of the chronicity of the disorder, and the complexity of caring for older adults, primary care physicians must incorporate the patient, members of the patient's support network, other physician consultants, and other disciplines in a system of care.

To manage heart failure optimally, the practicing physician should aim to introduce a system that results in early diagnosis, effective monitoring through the acute and chronic phases, appropriate use of consultants, and the appropriate use of tools such as checklists, clinical practice guidelines, disease management systems, and critical pathways. Most offices have a traditional staffing arrangement with a physician, receptionist, and a nurse. In other instances, the physician may have access to advanced practice nurses, physician assistants, dieticians, and social workers. In some communities and hospitals, disease management systems and critical pathways are available to the physician. The following sections illustrate how a practicing physician can take advantage of these opportunities.

CLINICAL PRACTICE GUIDELINES

Clinical practice guidelines, a set of clinical practice statements designed to assist practitioners and patients in choosing appropriate health care for specific clinical conditions (1), were established because of extensive variations in physician practices that cannot be explained by clinical factors or patient preferences. Considerable public and private sector efforts have been invested in development of practice guidelines by federal agencies, physician professional societies, and multidisciplinary health associations. Heart failure guidelines established by the Agency for Health Care Research and Quality and the American College of Cardiology (ACC) in collaboration with the American Heart Association (AHA) review current literature, critique the weight of evidence for various diagnostic and management decisions, and make recommendations (2). Proponents of practice guide-an opportunity to create an internal quality control system to improve practice. Quality control systems are based on the principle that one can establish systematic or routine standards of performance, review the performance standards, and change behavior in response to the performance outcomes. Each practice is charged with coming up with its own system of monitoring or quality control. The advantage of an internal control system is that it is self-directed, but nevertheless, the system must have a structure that delineates who conducts performance checks and provides feedback.

In perhaps the most common practice arrangement, the physician practices with a nurse, probably a baccalaureate or diploma-trained nurse, and a receptionist. The receptionist should make sure that the office records maintain up-to-date phone numbers of persons in the patient's support network, including one person outside the patient's place of residence. It is not enough to have the number of the patient only, because the physician will eventually have to enlist the assistance of a family member or friend.

The heart failure guidelines contain five categories of recommendations: (1) history and examination, (2) laboratory and imaging tests, (3) management (pharmacologic and nonpharmacologic), (4) use of consultants, and (5) patient and family education. All categories are critical and complementary, as inadequate practice in one category has an impact on others.

HISTORY AND EXAMINATION

The critical elements of the history and examination amenable to performance monitoring in the office are the dietary history, patient weight, and patient medications. All three of these elements frequently change over time, necessitating an effective monitoring system. Dietary history, patient weight, and patient medications are often incorporated in progress notes, but monitoring these notes is a tedious and time-consuming process. A simple alternative is to create a flowchart indicating a check of diet and recording weights and medications at each visit. At periodic intervals, the flowcharts can be reviewed to examine trends and up-to-date information. A member of the office staff will have to be assigned to perform the checks. The nurse can obtain dietary data, although most are not able to make detailed dietary recommendations. The nurse should make sure the patient is weighed accurately in a standard manner. The office should adopt the same system for weighing all patients, as a change of 2 or 3 pounds may be an important signal of a pending decompensation. One approach is to weigh all individuals

lines contend that scientifically based and clinically sound criteria lea
to more effective and efficient use of medical resources and improv
outcomes while containing costs *(1,3)*. In one review of 59 publishe
evaluations of the effects of clinical guidelines on the process and out
comes of care, the authors found that 55 out of 59 studies detecte
varying levels of change in the process of care following the introduction of guidelines with improvement in the outcomes of care in 9 out ol
10 studies *(1)*. Successful introduction of guidelines was related to the
appropriateness of the methods of development, dissemination, and
implementation of guidelines.

Others contend that guidelines are ineffective for several reasons *(3)*.
Physicians may be unaware of the guideline recommendations because
the typical method of dissemination relies on publications in academic
journals. They may not accept or believe the recommendations when
developed by an external national organization, rather than a local committee or group. In other instances, they may not believe the guidelines
apply to their patient population. Finally, the busy physician may simply not find the form of the guidelines user-friendly.

Several studies have examined barriers to the use of guidelines. One
of the most extensive studies examined how studies of guidelines were
designed, particularly the characteristics of the populations studied and
the variation in responses to surveys *(3)*. After classifying possible
barriers into common themes, they found that the questions about barriers included seven general categories of barriers. The barriers affected
physician knowledge (lack of awareness or lack of familiarity), atti-
tudes (lack of agreement, lack of self-efficacy, lack of outcome expectancy, or the inertia of previous practice), or behavior (external barriers).
Of most interest, the study determined that of the seven types of barriers,
the majority of surveys (70 [59%] of 120) examined only one type. The
average number examined was 167 (median 2). Thirty (25%) surveys
examined two, 11 (9%) examined three, 8 (7%) examined four, and 1
(0.8%) examined five. None examined six or more types of barriers.
Therefore, most studies do not fully explore the range of barriers.

USING CLINICAL PRACTICE GUIDELINES:
A PRACTICAL APPROACH IN THE OFFICE

Effective use of guidelines requires knowledge of their content. This
chapter does not address the mechanisms by which physicians become
informed or knowledgeable but does address issues of creating an
operational system to incorporate the knowledge in practice and monitor performance. Physicians should think of heart failure guidelines as

without shoes and overcoats. Deviations from the standard approach to weighing the patient should be recorded in the record. Measures of blood pressure, commonly obtained by nursing staff, should also be standardized as deviations from recommended standards of obtaining blood pressure measurements are common. These deviations may result in measurement errors, and just as problematic, they may result in intra- and intervariations in measurement. Thus, using the appropriate technique is important, but, consistency, whatever the technique, is equally important. The nurse can check the medications in the patient's possession with a medication list maintained in the medical record.

DIAGNOSTIC STUDIES

Laboratory and imaging studies of patients with heart failure are typically filed in the medical record with a host of other laboratory and imaging studies unrelated to heart failure. A review of the records to determine whether and when a given test such as an echocardiogram has been ordered requires a tedious review of multiple records. Here again, a flowchart of the pertinent tests relevant to heart failure can be incorporated in the record. This process would allow the office to determine easily when the last serum study or imaging study had been obtained.

PHARMACOLOGIC MANAGEMENT

Other chapters have focused on the choice and the appropriate dosing of medications in patients with heart failure. The choice of medication is a function of the pathophysiology underlying the congestive heart failure (CHF) systolic vs diastolic dysfunction and comorbidities and contraindications. Therefore, an effective monitoring system should incorporate the underlying pathophysiology of heart failure rather than the designation of "heart failure or CHF" in a list of diagnoses that can be easily reviewed. The medication checklist should also include room for a checkoff of the potentially critical contraindications to heart failure medications—hypotension, hyperkalemia, and renal failure—so that the physicians will not have to review a long list of progress notes to determine whether a contraindication has occurred in the past.

Nonpharmacologic Management Issues and Patient Education

CHF is a chronic disorder in which patient and family education about lifestyle changes are crucial to the successful long-term management. Diet and lifestyle are crucial aspects of the management of heart failure. In addition to avoidance of smoking and limiting the salt intake to about 2 grams of sodium per day, exercise is beneficial. Exercise training does not improve cardiac function, but it can increase peak cardiac output, leading to a reduction in symptoms such as dyspnea and fatigue. As part of the overall management, home-based interventions involving nurses and other health professionals have decreased the rate of unplanned readmissions and improved mortality. Thus, the progress notes and the checklist should indicate whether the patient was counseled about the lifestyle issues.

Heart failure patients over age 70 have a readmission rate as high as 57% within 90 days of discharge. Factors associated with readmission include inadequate follow-up, poor social situations, noncompliance with a low-salt diet, and noncompliance with medication. It is essential that these issues be addressed as soon as heart failure is diagnosed. Patients should be taught to recognize the symptoms of worsening heart failure, particularly dyspnea on exertion and weight gain, and advised to notify the practitioner if these symptoms arise. Thus, a category for patient education should be included on the checklist.

Most practices do not have a social worker on site. Therefore, the physician or nurse must decide who will inquire about the stability of the social network (persons available to assist the patient, living arrangement, ability to pay for medications), factors important because they influence adherence with medications, diet, and even visits to health practices *(4)*.

The practitioner should arrange for follow-up contact by phone or in person within one week of instituting new medications or after discharge from the hospital. During this contact, the proper use of medication and compliance with diet should be addressed. Because weight gain is a crucial objective sign of fluid overload, patients should be instructed to weigh themselves almost daily and to report a weight gain of 3–5 pounds. Here the critical element is determining who within the office practice will conduct the monitoring and education. This process must continue indefinitely as patients typically do well for 3–4 months after an acute episode then begin to decompensate because of deviations from management recommendations or the development of noncardiac clinical problems that exacerbate heart failure.

ADDITIONAL RESOURCES

Some practices will have access to advanced practice nurses and physician assistants, disease management systems and critical pathways. Physicians should understand how these resources complement the physician's care and know which patients to refer. It is not feasible or necessary for every patient with heart failure to receive such resources. However, patients who are frequently unstable as manifested by frequent emergency visits or hospitalizations and those in whom the physician is unable or uncomfortable treating should be referred. A burgeoning literature has shown that advanced practice nurses can decrease utilization and improve the quality of life of patients with heart failure by maintaining an ongoing monitoring system and providing frequent (commonly weekly) feedback to patients, families, and physicians. Thus, physicians should always take advantage of this resource when available.

DISEASE MANAGEMENT SYSTEMS

Clinical practice guidelines chosen to maximize cost-effectiveness for individual patients often do not maximize cost effectiveness for populations of patients (5). Disease management systems were established to combine evidence with population control for the purpose of maximizing use of resources in a widespread manner. Disease management is not new; for centuries, clinicians have been identifying and treating patients using information gleaned from their training, the medical literature, and personal experience. What is new about the current model of disease management is that it does much more than evaluate known practices and suggest guidelines; it systematically defines a relevant population, analyzes clinical encounters, introduces interventions according to a proscribed manner, and evaluates outcomes. Thus, disease management is a systematic information-driven population approach. Interventions are conducted sometimes from a distance through telephone or telecommunications, and results are compared against outcomes. The information that drives this process involves a shift from consensus-based medicine to evidence-based medicine (6), the emerging science of integrating information from credible clinical trials to make decisions.

Variations in the performance of disease management systems may occur for several reasons: whether the individual practitioner determines when to enter the patient into the system, or whether a process external to the patient uses a variety of data-driven protocols to automatically enter patients (5,6). Persons who meet certain criteria at the screening level receive additional service, such as referral to a specialist, reminders to perform certain test or referrals. Ultimately, disease-management systems are limited by the quality of the screening and outcome data they generate. The other limitation is that the data and the interventions are generally limited to medical (as opposed to social) interventions.

CRITICAL PATHWAYS

For hospitalized patients, another variation on clinical guidelines was developed. Critical pathways are management plans that display goals for patients and provide the corresponding ideal sequence and timing of staff actions to achieve those goals with optimal efficiency. Critical pathways have varying formats and are known by many names, including critical paths, clinical pathways, and care paths (7). These pathways were first developed and applied to health care in the 1980s, when prospective payment systems focused greater interest on potential methods to improve hospital efficiency. Interest in critical pathways has increased tremendously during the past several years, as early anecdotal reports of their cost-saving potential have been disseminated usually outside the peer-reviewed medical literature. Interpreted formally, a critical pathway is the sequence of events in a process that takes the greatest length of time. Like the techniques of continuous quality improvement, critical pathway techniques were first developed for use in industry as a tool to identify and manage the rate-limiting steps in production processes. However, when applied to hospital care, efforts to capture the sequence of timed events have proved to be more complex than that of inert industry processes.

A typical pathway denotes the steps that should be taken each day. They provide a sequential or algorithm approach to managing the patient with heart failure. Multiple barriers have interrupted critical pathways. Many patients with heart failure do not enter the pathway immediately upon admission for a variety of reasons: the identification and notification system is not structured adequately and uncertainty of the diagnosis. Sometimes hospitals are not adequately staffed to provide the recommended services in a timely manner. In other instances, complications as a result of other medical illnesses interrupt the sequence.

THE FUTURE OF HEART FAILURE GUIDELINES AND DISEASE MANAGEMENT

Enhanced care of patients with heart failure will require balancing the needs of individuals with the needs of populations, a hurdle for most physicians who view the two issues as synonymous. Nevertheless, innovations in technology may allow physicians and health systems to more effectively care for patients with heart failure. Monitoring devices for home use by patients are being developed that provide feedback directly to patients and to physician offices about weight and heart rate. Second, structured medical records will be designed to facilitate and encourage decisions and treatment.

Clinical practice guidelines chosen to maximize cost-effectiveness for individual patients often do not maximize cost-effectiveness for populations of patients and disease management systems can lead to fragmentation of care. To allocate resources as efficiently as possible, newer guidelines will likely include other sources of outcomes that simultaneously address both individual and societal health benefit. Heart failure guidelines of the future are likely to be based on data-driven modifications of earlier guidelines. These modifications will have occurred through a process of steps: formulating quality and utilization data, analyzing specific guideline recommendations, converting recommendations into review criteria for assessing care and operationalizing the review criteria. Moreover, outreach and dissemination programs will incorporate local opinion leaders. Finally, advances in technology will influence the use of guidelines and other tools. Computer and hand-held digital technology may make such guidelines more user-friendly to physicians, guidelines that can both mimic the sequence of decisions in clinical practice and allow physicians to enter the sequence at any point to obtain information.

REFERENCES

1. Woolf S. Practice guidelines: a new reality in medicine: impact on patient care. Arch Intern Med 1993;153:2646–2655.
2. ACC/AHA Tack Force Report. Guidelines for the evaluation and management of heart failure. J Am Coll Cardiol 1995;26:1376.
3. Cabana MD, Rand S, Powe N, et al. Why don't physicians follow clinical practice guidelines? JAMA 1999;282:1458–1465.
4. Stewart S, Vandenbroek AJ, Pearson S, Horowitz J. Prolonged beneficial effects of a home-based intervention on unplanned readmissions and mortality among patients with congestive heart failure. Arch Intern Med 1999;159:257–261.
5. Harris JM, Jr. Disease management: new wine in new bottles? Ann Intern Med 1996;124:9:838–842.
6. Epstein RS, Sherwood LM. From outcomes research to disease management: a guide for the perplexed. Ann Intern Med 1996124:832–837.
7. Pearson SD, Goulart-Fisher D, Lee TH. Critical pathways as a strategy for improving care: problems and potential. Ann Intern Med 1995;123:941–948.

INDEX